"If we know that pain and suffering

can be alleviated, and we do nothing

about it, then we ourselves

become the tormentors."

Primo Levi

Palliative Care Consultant

"Guidelines for Effective Management of Symptoms, GEMS" © 2008 HospiScript LLC

Contents

Foreword. 5

Acknowledgments 6

Editors and Authors. 7

National Consensus Project for Quality Palliative Care 9

Palliative Care World Health Organization Model. 12

Vision of Palliative Care Continuum 12

Disease Trajectory 13

Drug Administration Abbreviations 14

Medical Abbreviations 15

Medication Therapy Management Services (MTMS) in Hospice and Palliative Care 17

Interdisciplinary Team. 18

Legal Considerations 19

Recommended Preferred Drug List 20

Compounded Medications in Palliative Care 26

Polypharmacy and Drug Interactions in Palliative Care 28

CMS Guidelines for Medication Use in Long Term Care Facilities 29

Guide to Effective Management of Symptoms (GEMS) Section 32

Anorexia and Cachexia GEMS   *Margaret Thrower, Bernie Olin, Linda Tyler, Peter Teichman* 32

Anxiety GEMS   *John Shuster, Phyllis Grauer* 40

Ascites and Edema GEMS   *Bridget McCrate Protus, Phyllis Grauer* 48

Bowel Obstruction GEMS   *Kenneth Jackson II, Rodney Tucker* 56

Constipation GEMS   *Kenneth Jackson II, John Shuster* 62

Cough GEMS   *Margaret Thrower, Peter Teichman* 68

Delirium GEMS   *John Shuster, Margaret Thrower, John Redden* 78

Depression GEMS   *John Shuster, Phyllis Grauer* 86

Diarrhea GEMS   *Phyllis Grauer, John Shuster* 98

Dysphagia GEMS   *Kenneth Jackson II, Rodney Tucker* 108

Dyspnea GEMS   *Margaret Thrower, Paul Rousseau* 116

Excessive Sedation GEMS   *John Shuster, Phyllis Grauer* 124

Fever GEMS   *Phyllis Grauer, John Shuster* 134

Hiccups GEMS   *Phyllis Grauer, John Shuster* 142

Infections GEMS   *Phyllis Grauer, Bridget McCrate Protus* 150

Insomnia GEMS   *Elizabeth Kvale, John Shuster* 158

Muscle Spasms GEMS   *Rodney Tucker, Kenneth Jackson II* 166

Nausea and Vomiting GEMS   *Phyllis Grauer, John Shuster* 172

Pain Section. 180

    Pain Assessment 181

        Pain Scales. 184

        Pain Assessment in Advanced Dementia 185

    Somatic Pain GEMS   *Phyllis Grauer, John Shuster* 188

    Methadone GEMS   *Phyllis Grauer, John Shuster* 200

    Bone Pain GEMS   *John Redden, Arthur Lipman, Kenneth Jackson II* 204

    Visceral Pain GEMS   *Phyllis Grauer, John Shuster* 210

    Neuropathic Pain GEMS   *Arthur Lipman, Phyllis Grauer* 216

Pruritus GEMS   *John Shuster, Phyllis Grauer* 226

Seizures GEMS   *John Shuster, Phyllis Grauer* 234

Contents (cont'd)

Terminal Secretions or *"Death Rattle"* GEMS   *Margaret Thrower, Bernie Olin,*
   Linda Tyler, Arthur Lipman, Kenneth Jackson II 242
Thick Secretions GEMS   *Margaret Thrower* 248
Xerostomia GEMS   *Phyllis Grauer, John Shuster* 258
Wound Care 264
Heart Failure 266
Chronic Obstructive Pulmonary Disease (COPD) 269
Palliative Chemotherapy 270
Palliative Radiation 277
Centers for Medicare and Medicaid Service—Hospice Care Regulations 281
Guidelines for Determination of Hospice Eligibility Section **282**
Adult Failure to Thrive 282
Amyotrophic Lateral Sclerosis (ALS) 283
Cancer 284
Cardiovascular Disease 285
New York Heart Association (NYHA) Functional Classification (Class and Description) 285
Chronic Degenerative Neurologic Disease 286
Dementia 287
Functional Assessment Staging 288
HIV/AIDS 289
Huntington's Disease 290
Liver Disease 291
Non-Specific Terminal Illness (Debility Unspecified/End Stage Senescence) 292

Parkinson's Disease 293
Pulmonary Disease 294
Renal Failure 295
Stroke or Coma 296
Appendices **297**
Palliative Performance Scale 297
Geriatric Depression Scale (GDS) 298
The Mini-Mental State Examination (MMSE) 300
Extrapyramidal Symptoms (EPS) from Medications 301
Medications Associated with Anticholinergic Side Effects 302
Drugs That Prolong the QT Interval or Induce Torsades de Pointes 303
Medications That May Increase Risk of Falls 304
Look-Alike and Sound-Alike Drug Names 306
Method of Dosage Adjustment in Renal Failure 309
Drugs Affected by Cytochrome P450 Enzyme Metabolism 324
Glucocorticoid Equivalency Table 327
Benzodiazepine Equivalency Table 328
Insulin Comparison Chart 330
Recommended Starting Doses in Children and Adults Less than 50 kg Body Weight 332
Pediatric Recommended Maximum Dosing 335
Subcutaneous Administration of Medications Butterfly Procedure 336
Drug Information Table 341

You've just picked up the 3rd Edition of the *Palliative Care Consultant (PCC)*. Whether you are a specialist in palliative care or a novice, the *PCC* provides ready access to well researched information that will help you provide comfort and care for your seriously ill patients.

Balancing the benefits and burdens of medical care in the midst of advancing disease is becoming increasingly complex. Through listening, examining and treating our patients' concerns, we can enrich their living and dying. The provision of palliative care can be among the most fulfilling aspects of an interdisciplinary team's responsibilities and as care providers, we are blessed to be invited into the lives and homes of these patients as they strive to find comfort, understanding and contentment.

After reading this 3rd Edition of the *Palliative Care Consultant,* I'm confident you will find this a useful resource in your mission to comfort seriously ill patients. The *PCC* is among the few resources that addresses both the pharmacologic and non-pharmacologic approaches to a broad array of disease and symptom management issues. The text's guide for effective management of symptoms is generously sprinkled with clinical pearls from experts in the field and is well referenced. For those less familiar with palliative care, the algorithms for symptom management provide a step-by-step pathway for targeting treatments to meet the individual needs of patients. The *PCC* contains other valuable tools such as hospice eligibility guidelines, drug information tables and a suggested formulary.

The *Palliative Care Consultant* is a sought-after reference on the hospice and palliative care unit where I work. I highly recommend this resource for physicians, nurses, pharmacists, residents and others charged with delivering quality palliative care.

Scott T. Shreve, D.O.
National Director, Hospice and Palliative Care, Department of Veterans Affairs
Associate Professor of Clinical Medicine in the College of Medicine at
The Pennsylvania State University
1700 S. Lincoln Avenue
Lebanon, PA 17042

Disclaimer: The comments above do not reflect the opinion or constitute the endorsement of the Department of Veterans Affairs or the United States of America.

Acknowledgments

The 3rd Edition of the *Palliative Care Consultant (PCC)* was produced through a collaborative relationship with the Ohio Hospice & Palliative Care Organization (OHPCO), the Ohio Home Care Organization (OHCO) and HospiScript Services, LLC. This edition combines the work of previous *PCC* editions with an industry leader known for implementing and managing symptoms in an economical, efficient manner using effective care pathways. OHPCO/OHCO wants to extend our gratitude to HospiScript Services, LLC for their expertise, flexibility and desire to help meet an industry need. OHPCO/OHCO also wants to extend our gratitude to Kendall/Hunt Publishing for their support and persistence in keeping us on track to produce and finish the Third Edition.

To order additional copies of the PCC, contact:

Kendall/Hunt Publishing
www.kendallhunt.com

Ohio Hospice & Palliative Care Organization/Ohio Home Care Organization
www.ohpco.org

To learn more about the GEMS (Guide for Effective Management of Symptoms), contact:

HospiScript Services, LLC.
1-800-227-0848
www.hospiscript.com

For Kendall/Hunt Publishing, 1-800-228-0810.

Editors and Authors

Editor

Phyllis A. Grauer, RPh, PharmD, CGP
Assistant Clinical Professor
The Ohio State University College of Pharmacy
Columbus, Ohio
Palliative Care Consulting Group
A Division of HospiScript Services
Dublin, Ohio

Associate Editors

Bridget McCrate Protus, RPh, PharmD, CGP
Palliative Care Consulting Group
A Division of HospiScript Services
Dublin, Ohio

John Shuster, MD
Clinical Professor of Psychiatry and Psychology
The University of Alabama
Tuscaloosa, Alabama

Authors/Reviewers

Beth Delaney, APRN, OCN, BC-PC
Program Manager, Palliative Care
Miami Valley Hospital
Dayton, Ohio

Kenneth C. Jackson II, PharmD
Associate Professor
Pacific University School of Pharmacy
Hillsboro, Oregon

Elizabeth Kvale, MD
Assistant Professor of Medicine
University of Alabama at Birmingham, Division of
Gerontology, Geriatrics, and Palliative Care
Birmingham, Alabama

Arthur G. Lipman, PharmD, FASHP
Professor of Pharmacotherapy, College of Pharmacy
University of Utah Health Sciences Center
Salt Lake City, Utah

Mary Murphy RN, MS, AOCN, ACHPN
Director of Clinical Systems & CNS Oncology
Hospice of Dayton Inc.
Dayton, Ohio

Bernie R. Olin, PhD
Harrison School of Pharmacy
University Drug Information Center
Auburn University, Alabama

Rebecca J. Paessun, MD
Radiation Oncology
Clinical Assistant Professor
Department of Medicine
Boonschoft School of Medicine
Wright State University

John Redden, RPh, CGP
VP Clinical Practice Development
HospiScript Services, LLC
Montgomery, Alabama

Paul Rousseau, MD
VA Medical Center
17 W. Vernon Avenue Suite 101
Phoenix, Arizona

Sharon Starling, RPh, PharmD
Department of Pharmacy
Riverside Methodist Hospital
Columbus, Ohio

Peter Teichman, MD
Hospice and Palliative Care Physician
New Zealand

Margaret R. Thrower, PharmD, BCPS
Regional Clinical Coordinator
McKesson Medication Management
Auburn, Alabama

Rodney Tucker, MD
Assistant Professor of Medicine
University of Alabama at Birmingham, Division of
Gerontology, Geriatrics, and Palliative Care
Birmingham, Alabama

Linda S. Tyler, PharmD
Drug Information Service
University of Utah Hospitals & Clinics
Salt Lake City, Utah

Contributors

Laura Lochtefeld, BS
Ohio Hospice & Palliative Care Organization
Ohio Home Care Organization
Dublin, Ohio

Arika Lycan, BSW
Ohio Hospice & Palliative Care Organization
Ohio Home Care Organization
Dublin, Ohio

Jeff Lycan, President/CEO
Ohio Hospice & Palliative Care Organization
Ohio Home Care Organization
Dublin, Ohio

Susan Shuster, BS
Shuster Consulting
Birmingham, Alabama

Definition of Palliative Care

The goal of palliative care is to prevent and relieve suffering and to support the best possible quality of life for patients and their families, regardless of the stage of the disease or the need for other therapies. Palliative care is both a philosophy of care and an organized, highly structured system for delivering care. Palliative care expands traditional disease-model medical treatments to include the goals of enhancing quality of life for patient and family, optimizing function, helping with decision-making and providing opportunities for personal growth. As such, it can be delivered concurrently with life-prolonging care or as the main focus of care.

Palliative care is operationalized through effective management of pain and other distressing symptoms, while incorporating psychosocial and spiritual care according to patient/family needs, values, beliefs and culture(s). Evaluation and treatment should be comprehensive and patient-centered, with a focus on the central role of the family unit in decision-making. Palliative care affirms life by supporting the patient and family's goals for the future, including their hopes for cure or life-prolongation, as well as their hopes for peace and dignity throughout the course of illness, the dying process and death. Palliative care aims to guide and assist the patient and family in making decisions that enable them to work toward their goals during whatever time they have remaining. Comprehensive palliative care services often require the expertise of various providers in order to adequately assess and treat the complex needs of seriously ill patients and their families. Members of a palliative care team may include professionals from medicine, nursing, social work, chaplaincy, nutrition, rehabilitation, pharmacy and other professional disciplines. Leadership, collaboration, coordination and communication are key elements for effective integration of these disciplines and services.

Clinical Practice Guidelines for Quality Palliative Care

Excellence in specialist-level palliative care requires expertise in the clinical management of problems in multiple domains, supported by programmatic infrastructure that furthers the goals of care and supports practitioners. Eight domains were identified as the framework for these guidelines: Structure and Processes of Care; Physical Aspects of Care; Psychological and Psychiatric Aspects of Care; Social Aspects of Care; Spiritual, Religious and Existential Aspects of Care; Cultural Aspects of Care; Care of the Imminently Dying Patient; and Ethical and Legal Aspects of Care. These domains were drawn from the work of previously established Australian, New Zealand, Canadian, Children's Hospice International, and the National Hospice & Palliative Care Organization standards efforts.

These guidelines rest on fundamental processes that cross all domains and encompass assessment, information sharing, decision-making, care planning and care delivery. Each domain is followed by specific clinical practice guidelines regarding professional behavior and service delivery. These are followed by justifications, supporting and clarifying statements, and suggested criteria for assessing whether or not the identified expectation has been met. References to the literature supporting these recommendations are included in the guidelines.

Domains of Quality Palliative Care

1. Structure and Processes of Care
2. Physical Aspects of Care
3. Psychological and Psychiatric Aspects of Care
4. Social Aspects of Care
5. Spiritual, Religious and Existential Aspects of Care
6. Cultural Aspects of Care
7. Care of the Imminently Dying Patient
8. Ethical and Legal Aspects of Care

Clinical Practice Guidelines for Quality Palliative Care

Baseline Assumptions

The following assumptions are fundamental to the development of the Clinical Practice Guidelines for Quality Palliative Care:

- **Goal guidelines:** These palliative care guidelines represent goals that palliative care services should strive to attain, as opposed to minimal or lowest acceptable practices.
- **Health care quality standards:** These palliative care guidelines assume that palliative care services will follow established practice standards and requirements for health care quality such as safety, effective leadership, medical record keeping and error reduction.
- **Code of ethics:** These guidelines assume adherence to established professional and organizational codes of ethics.
- **Ongoing revision:** Palliative care guidelines will evolve as professional practice, the evidence base and the health care system change over time. These guidelines were written assuming an ongoing process of evidence-based evaluation and revision.
- **Peer-defined guidelines:** These clinical practice guidelines were developed through a consensus process including a broad range of palliative care professionals; they are not linked to regulatory or reimbursement criteria and are not mandatory. However, they are written with the intent that they will be used as guidelines to promote the development of highest-quality clinical palliative care services across the health care continuum.
- **Specialty care:** When this document refers to specialty-level palliative care services it assumes provision of services by palliative care professionals within an interdisciplinary team whose work reflects substantial involvement in the care of patients with life-threatening or debilitating chronic illnesses, and their families. Palliative care qualifications are determined by organizations granting professional credentials and programmatic accreditation.
- **Continuing professional education:** These guidelines assume ongoing professional education for all palliative care professionals in the knowledge, attitudes and skills required to deliver quality palliative care across domains established in this document.
- **Applicability of guidelines:** These guidelines should promote integration and application of the principles, philosophy and practices of palliative care across the continuum of care by both professional and certified caregiver in these settings.

To access the complete National Consensus Project for Quality Palliative Care document, go to http://www.nationalconsensusproject.org/guideline1.pdf Accessed 1/24/07

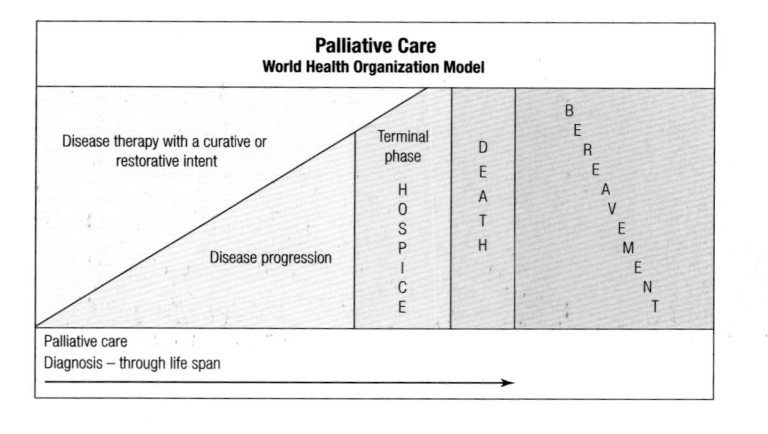

Palliative Care
World Health Organization Model

Disease therapy with a curative or restorative intent

Terminal phase

Disease progression

HOSPICE

DEATH

BEREAVEMENT

Palliative care
Diagnosis – through life span

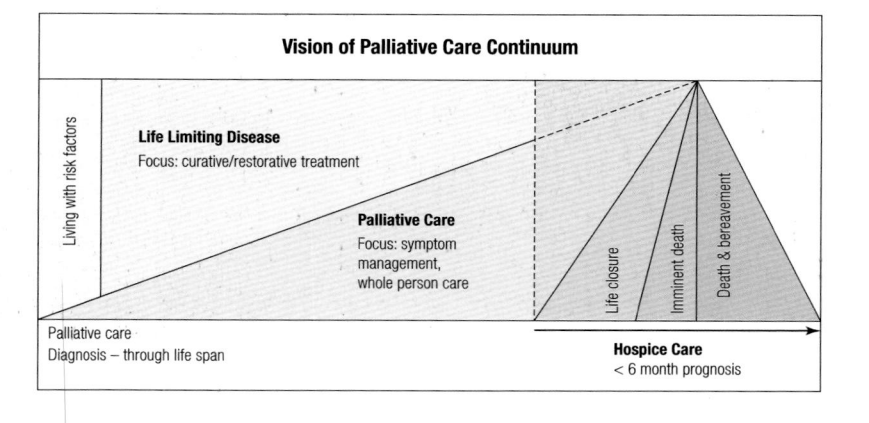

Vision of Palliative Care Continuum

Living with risk factors

Life Limiting Disease
Focus: curative/restorative treatment

Palliative Care
Focus: symptom management, whole person care

Life closure

Imminent death

Death & bereavement

Palliative care
Diagnosis – through life span

Hospice Care
< 6 month prognosis

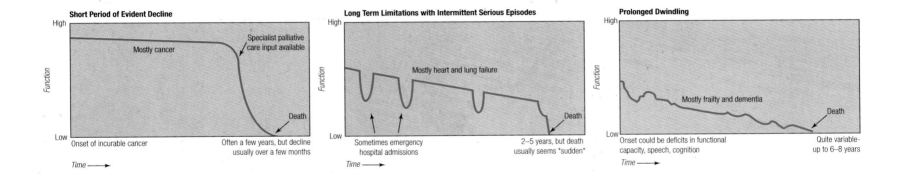

Short Period of Evident Decline

High

Mostly cancer

Specialist palliative care input available

Function

Death

Low

Onset of incurable cancer

Often a few years, but decline usually over a few months

Time ➝

Long Term Limitations with Intermittent Serious Episodes

High

Mostly heart and lung failure

Function

Death

Low

Sometimes emergency hospital admissions

2–5 years, but death usually seems *sudden*

Time ➝

Prolonged Dwindling

High

Mostly frailty and dementia

Function

Death

Low

Onset could be deficits in functional capacity, speech, cognition

Quite variable- up to 6–8 years

Time ➝

Sources: Murray, S. A et al. and Lynn J. Living Long in Fragile Health: The new demographics shape end of life care. *Improving End of Life Care: Why Has It Been So Difficult? Hastings Center Report Special Report.* 35, no. 6: S14-S18, 2005.

Drug Administration Abbreviations

Abbreviation	Definition
AC	before meals
Amp	ampule
ATC	around-the-clock
BID	twice daily
BTP	breakthrough pain
Cap	capsule
Conc	concentrate
CIVI	continuous intravenous infusion
CSCI	continuous subcutaneous infusion
D/C	discontinue
EC	enteric coated tablet
EI	elixir
GTT	drop
HS	at bedtime

Abbreviation	Definition
IM	intramuscular
inh	inhalation
inj	injection
IT	intrathecal
IV	intravenous
Liq	liquid
Loz	lozenge
MDD	maximum daily dose
NEB	nebulizer
NPO	nothing by mouth
NR	normal release
PC	after meals
PO	by mouth
PR	per rectum

Abbreviation	Definition
PRN	as needed
Q	every
Qam	every morning
QID	four times a day
Qpm	every night
q 2 h	every two hours
q 3 h	every three hours
q 4 h	every four hours
q 6 h	every six hours
q 8 h	every eight hours
q 12 h	every twelve hours
SC or SQ	subcutaneous
SL	sublingual
Sol	solution

Abbreviation	Definition
SR	sustained release
STAT	immediately
Supp	suppository
Susp	suspension
Syr	syrup
t ½	terminal half-life
Tab	tablet
TID	three times a day
Top	topical
Vag	vaginal

Medical Abbreviations

Abbreviation	Definition
APAP	acetaminophen
ASAP	as soon as possible
BM	bowel movement
BP	blood pressure
BS	blood sugar
CA	cancer
cath	catheter
CNS	central nervous system
COPD	chronic obstructive pulmonary disease
COX	cyclo-oxygenase; alternative, prostaglandin synthase
CRF	chronic renal failure
CVA	cerebrovascular accident
DM	diabetes mellitus
G tube	gastric tube
GFR	glomerular filtration rate
HA	headache
HTN	hypertension
INR	international normalized ratio
LOC	level of consciousness

Abbreviation	Definition
NG tube	nasogastric tube
NSAID(s)	nonsteroidal anti-inflammatory drug(s)
PPI(s)	proton pump inhibitor(s)
SOB	shortness of breath
SSRI(s)	selective serotonin re-uptake inhibitor(s)
TCA(s)	tricyclic antidepressants
UTI	urinary tract infection

Units of Measure

Abbreviation	Definition
°F	degrees in Farhenheit
gm	gram(s)
h	hour(s)
kg	kilogram(s)
L	liter(s)
lb	pound(s)
mcg	microgram(s)
mEq	milli-equivalent

Abbreviation	Definition
mg	milligram(s)
min	minute(s)
mL	milliliter(s)
mm	millimeter(s)
mo	month(s)
oz	ounce(s)
tbsp	tablespoon(s)
tsp	teaspoon(s)
wk	week(s)
yr	year(s)

Receptors

Abbreviation	Definition
5HT	5-hydroxytryptamine (serotonin), Type 1,2,3 and 4 alpha
AChm	acetylcholine muscarinic
δ	delta opioid
D_2	dopamine, type 2

Abbreviation	Definition
GABA	Gamma-aminobutyric acid
H	histamine, type 1 and 2
κ	kappa opioid
μ	mu opioid
NMDA	N-methyl-D-aspartate

Miscellaneous Symbols

Abbreviation	Definition
$\uparrow$	increase
$\downarrow$	decrease
$+/-$	plus or minus; approximately
$\neq$	not equal to
$>$	greater than
$<$	less than
#	number
/	divided by; fraction
:	is to; ratio
$\cong$	approximately
Δ	change to

Official "Do Not Use" List[1]

Do Not Use	Potential Problem	Use Instead
U (unit)	Mistaken for "0" (zero) the number "4" (four) or "cc"	Write "unit"
IU (International Unit)	Mistaken for IV (intravenous) or the number 10 (ten)	Write "International Unit"
Q.D., QD, q.d., qd (daily) Q.O.D., QOD, q.o.d. qod (every other day)	Mistaken for each other Period after the Q mistaken for "I" and the "O" mistaken for "I"	Write "daily" Write "every other day"
Trailing zero (X.0 mg)*	Decimal point missing	Write X mg Write 0.X mg
MS MSO$_4$ and MgSO$_4$	Can mean morphine sulfate or magnesium sulfate Confused for one another	Write "morphine sulfate" Write "magnesium sulfate"

[1]Applies to all orders and all medication-related documentation that is handwritten (including free-text computer entry) or on pre-printed forms.

*Exception: A "trailing zero" may be used only where required to demonstrate the level of precision of the value being reported, such as for laboratory results, imaging studies that report size of lesions, or catheter/tube sizes. It may not be used in medication orders or other medication-related documentation.

Additional Abbreviations, Acronyms and Symbols
(For <u>possible</u> future inclusion in the Official "Do Not Use" List)

Do Not Use	Potential Problem	Use Instead
> (greater than) < (less than)	Misinterpreted as the number "7" or the letter "L" Confused for one another	Write "greater than" Write "less than"
Abbreviations for drug names	Misinterpreted due to similar abbreviations for multiple drugs	Write drug names in full
Apothecary units	Unfamiliar to many practitioners Confused with metric units	Use metric units
@	Mistaken for the number "2" (two)	Write "at"
cc	Mistaken for U (units) when poorly written	Write "mL" or milliliters"
µg	Mistaken for mg (milligrams) resulting in one thousand-fold overdose	Write "mcg" or "micrograms"

Medication therapy is a major component of the care of patients with life-limiting illnesses. Appropriate medication therapy management results in optimal patient care outcomes, cost effective drug utilization and prevention and resolution of medication misadventures. Medication therapy management services have been defined and criteria outlined, with the support and approval of eleven pharmacy organizations. In the hospice and palliative care setting, medication therapy management can be optimized by utilizing the expertise of a palliative care pharmacist as an active member of the interdisciplinary team.

MTMS Definition and Program Criteria

Medication Therapy Management is a distinct service or group of services that optimize therapeutic outcomes for individual patients. Medication Therapy Management Services are independent of, but can occur in conjunction with, the provision of a medication product.

Medication Therapy Management encompasses a broad range of professional activities and responsibilities within the licensed pharmacist's, or other qualified health care provider's, scope of practice. These services include but are not limited to the following, according to the individual needs of the patient:

a. Performing or obtaining necessary assessments of the patient's health status;

b. Formulating a medication treatment plan;

c. Selecting, initiating, modifying, or administering medication therapy;

d. Monitoring and evaluating the patient's response to therapy, including safety and effectiveness;

e. Performing a comprehensive medication review to identify, resolve, and prevent medication-related problems, including adverse drug events;

f. Documenting the care delivered and communicating essential information to the patient's other primary care providers;

g. Providing verbal education and training designed to enhance patient understanding and appropriate use of his/her medications;

h. Providing information, support services and resources designed to enhance patient adherence with his/her therapeutic regimens;

i. Coordinating and integrating medication therapy management services within the broader health care-management services being provided to the patient.

A program that provides coverage for Medication Therapy Management services shall include:

a. Patient-specific and individualized services or sets of services provided directly by a pharmacist to the patient*. These services are distinct from formulary development and use, generalized patient education and information activities, and other population-focused quality assurance measures for medication use.

b. Face-to-face interaction between the patient* and the pharmacist as the preferred method of delivery. When patient-specific barriers to face-to-face communication exist, patients shall have equal access to appropriate alternative delivery methods. Medication Therapy Management programs shall include structures supporting the establishment and maintenance of the patient*-pharmacist relationship.

c. Opportunities for pharmacists and other qualified health care providers to identify patients who should receive medication therapy management services.

d. Payment for Medication Therapy Management Services consistent with contemporary provider payment rates that are based on the time, clinical intensity, and resources required to provide services (e.g., Medicare Part A and/or Part B for CPT & RBRVS).

e. Processes to improve continuity of care, outcomes, and outcome measures.

Definition and Program Criteria Approved: July 27, 2004 by the Academy of Managed Care Pharmacy, the American Association of Colleges of Pharmacy, the American College of Apothecaries, the American College of Clinical Pharmacy, the American Society of Consultant Pharmacists, the American Pharmacists Association, the American Society of Health-System Pharmacists, the National Association of Boards of Pharmacy, the National Association of Chain Drug Stores, the National Community Pharmacists Association, and the National Council of State Pharmacy Association Executives.

*In some situations, Medication Therapy Management Services may be provided to the caregiver or other persons involved in the patient's care.
**RBRVS = Resource-Based Relative Value Scale
CPT = Current Procedural Terminology

Interdisciplinary Team

Attending Physician
Directs medical care

Home Health Aide
Assists with personal care

Bereavement Counselor
Provides support to family

Pharmacist
Assists with symptom management

Nurse
Coordinates the care to ensure comfort

Spiritual Care
Supports patient & family spiritually

Therapists
Provide physical, occupational, speech and nutrutional services

Social Worker
Identifies community services and provides support

Patient & Family

Volunteers
Provide companionship and support

Medical Director
Consults with the team and attending physician

Legal Considerations

The principles and treatment regimens for palliative care presented in the *Palliative Care Consultant (PCC)* represent accepted standards for medical practice at the time of publication. As a result, these principles and treatment regimens should be consistent with your state's medical practice laws. Nevertheless, you should be aware of, and comply with, state laws governing medical practice, the management of chronic and acute pain and the prescribing of controlled substances. Furthermore, so long as the patient is not harmed, physicians may prescribe a drug approved by the Food and Drug Administration (FDA) for an unapproved use or in a dosage higher than that recommended by the package insert, and a pharmacist may dispense such a prescription without violating federal law or state malpractice law.

In sum, I believe the patient in need of pain and other distressing symptom management has the legal right to be treated in accordance with accepted medical practices. Every effort has been made to ensure the accuracy of this text, and that the best information available has been used. This does not diminish the requirement to exercise clinical judgment, and neither the publishers, the authors, nor the consultants can accept any responsibility for its use in practice.

David W. Grauer, JD, MSc, RPh
Partner: Squire, Sanders & Dempsey, L.L.P.
Columbus, Ohio

Recommended Preferred Drug List

DRUG (GENERIC)	BRAND NAME EXAMPLES	SYMPTON/INDICATION	DRUG CLASS
Acetaminophen	Tylenol	Fever, Pain	Non-opioid
Acyclovir	Zovirax	Viral infection	Antiviral
Albuterol	Proventil, Ventolin	Bronchospasm	Beta agonist bronchodilator
Alprazolam	Xanax	Anxiety, Dyspnea, Nausea & vomiting	Benzodiazepine
Aluminum/Magnesium Hydroxide/Simethicone	Maalox Plus	Gastritis	Antacid
Amoxicillin	Amoxil	Bacterial infection	Penicillin antibiotic
Artificial Saliva	Salivart	Xerostomia	Lubricant
Artificial Tears	Lytears	Dry eyes	Lubricant
Aspirin	Aspirin	Pain, Antiplatelet	Salicylate
Atenolol	Tenormin	Hypertension, Heart failure	Beta adrenergic blockers
Atropine	Isopto Atropine, Sal-tropine	Terminal secretions	Anticholinergic
Azithromycin	Zithromax	Bacterial infection	Macrolide antibiotic
Baclofen	Lioresal	Muscle spasm	Antispasmodic
Benzonatate	Tessalon Perles	Cough	Cough suppressant
Benztropine	Cogentin	Parkinsonism	Anticholinergic
Bethanechol	Urecholine	Urinary retention	Cholinergic
Bisacodyl	Dulcolax	Constipation	Stimulant laxative
Camphor/Menthol Lotion	Sarna	Pruritus	Topical antipruritic
Captopril	Capoten	Hypertension, Heart failure	ACE inhibitor

Carbamazepine	Tegretol	Neuropathic pain, Seizures	Anticonvulsant
Carvedilol	Coreg	Arrhythmia	Beta adrenergic blocker
Cephalexin	Keflex	Bacterial infection	Cephalosporin antibiotic
Chloral Hydrate	Noctec	Insomnia	Atypical hypnotic
Chlorpromazine	Thorazine	Anxiety, Delirium, Agitation, Hiccups, Nausea & vomiting	Phenothiazine
Ciprofloxacin	Cipro	Bacterial infection	Quinolone antibiotic
Citalopram	Celexa	Depression	Selective serotonin reuptake inhibitor
Clindamycin	Cleocin	Bacterial infection	Bacterial antibiotic
Clonazepam	Klonopin	Anxiety, Seizures	Benzodiazepine
Clonidine	Catapres	Hypertension	Alpha adrenergic agonist
Valproic Acid, Divalproex Sodium	Depakene, Depakote	Neuropathic pain, Agitation, Seizures	Anticonvulsant
Desipramine	Norpramin	Depression, Neuropathic pain	Tricyclic antidepressant
Dexamethasone	Decadron	Anorexia, Pain, Pruritus, Respiratory, Anti-inflammatory, Seizures, Nausea & vomiting	Corticosteroid
Diazepam	Valium	Anxiety, Dyspnea, Muscle spasm, Seizures	Benzodiazepine
Dicyclomine	Bentyl	Nausea & vomiting, Gastric colic	Anticholinergic
Digoxin	Lanoxin	Heart failure, Atrial fibrillation	Cardiac glycosides
Diltiazem	Cardizem	Hypertension	Calcium channel blockers
Diphenhydramine	Benadryl	Anxiety, Insomnia, Pruritus	Antihistamine
Diphenoxylate/Atropine	Lomotil	Diarrhea	Hypomotility agent
Docusate Sodium	Colace	Constipation	Stool softener
Doxazosin	Cardura	Hypertension	Alpha adrenergic blocker

Recommended Preferred Drug List (*Continued*)

DRUG (GENERIC)	BRAND NAME EXAMPLES	SYMPTON/INDICATION	DRUG CLASS
Doxepin	Sinequan	Depression, Neuropathic pain, Pruritus	Tricyclic antidepressant
Doxycycline	Vibramycin	Bacterial infection	Bacterial antibiotic
Duloxetine	Cymbalta	Depression, Neuropathic pain	Serotonin/Norepinephrine reuptake inhibitor
Erythromycin	E-Mycin, Erytab	Bacterila infection	Macrolide antibiotic
Fentanyl transdermal patch	Duragesic	Pain	Opioid
Fluconazole	Diflucan	Fungal infection	Antifungal
Fludrocortisone	Florinef	Hypotension	Mineralocorticoid
Fluoxetine	Prozac	Depression	Selective serotonin reuptake inhibitor
Fluticasone	Flovent Inhaler	Pulmonary inflammation	Corticosteroids
Furosemide	Lasix	Fluid retention	Loop diuretic
Gabapentin	Neurontin	Neuropathic pain, Agitation	Anticonvulsant
Glycopyrrolate	Robinul	Nausea & vomiting, Secretions	Anticholinergic
Guaifenesin	Robitussin, Mucinex	Cough, Pulmonary congestion	Expectorant
Guaifenesin/Dextromethorphan	Robitussin DM	Cough	Expectorant/Cough suppressant
Haloperidol	Haldol	Anxiety, Delirium, Agitation, Nausea & vomiting	Butyrophenone
Hydrochlorothiazide	Oretic	Fluid retention	Thiazide diuretics
Hydrocodone/Acetaminophen	Lortab, Vicodin	Nociceptive pain	Opioid/Non-opioid combination
Hydrocodone/Homatropine	Hycodan	Cough suppressant	Expectorant/Opioid/Anticholinergic combination
Hydrocortisone Cream	Cortaid	Topical inflammation, Rash	Corticosteroid

Hydromorphone	Dilaudid	Dyspnea, Pain	Opioid
Hydroxyzine	Atarax, Vistaril	Anxiety, Pruritus	Antihistamine
Hyoscyamine	Levsin	Bladder spasms, Nausea & vomiting	Anticholinergic
Ibuprofen	Motrin	Pain, Fever	Nonsteroidal anti-inflammatory drug
Ipratropium	Atrovent	Bronchospasm	Anticholinergics bronchodilator
Isosorbide Mononitrate	Monoket, Imdur	Angina	Nitrate vasodilator
Lactulose	Chronulac	Constipation, High ammonia	Osmotic laxative
Levodopa/Carbidopa	Sinemet	Parkinson's Disease	Antiparkinson's agents
Levofloxacin	Levaquin	Bacterial infection	Quinolone antibiotic
Lidocaine Ointment	Lidocaine Topical	Topical analgesic	Anesthetic
Lidocaine Oral	Xylocaine Viscous	Pharyngeal analgesic	Anesthetic
Lisinopril	Prinivil, Zestril	Hypertension, Heart failure	ACE inhibitor
Lorazepam	Ativan	Anxiety, Dyspnea, Nausea & vomiting, Seizures	Benzodiazepine
Losartan	Cozaar, Hyzaar	Hypertension, Heart failure	Angiotensin receptor blockers
Magnesium Hydroxide Suspension	Milk of Magnesia	Constipation	Osmotic laxative
Meclizine	Antivert	Nausea & vomiting, Vertigo	Antihistamine
Megestrol	Megace	Appetite stimulant	Progestin
Methadone	Dolophine, Methadose	Pain	Opioid
Methylphenidate	Ritalin	Depression, Fatigue	Psychostimulant
Metoclopramide	Reglan	Hiccups, Nausea & vomiting—Gastric Stasis	Prokinetic
Metolazone	Zaroxolyn	Fluid Retention	Thiazide diuretic

Recommended Preferred Drug List (*Continued*)

DRUG (GENERIC)	BRAND NAME EXAMPLES	SYMPTON/INDICATION	DRUG CLASS
Metoprolol	Lopressor, Toprol XL	Hypertension, Tachycardia	Beta adrenergic blocker
Metronidazole	Flagyl	Bacterial infection	Antibiotic
Mirtazapine	Remeron	Anorexia, Depression, Insomnia	Atypical antidepressant
Morphine	Roxanol, MS Contin	Dyspnea, Pain	Opioid
Naproxen	Naprosyn	Pain	Nonsteroidal anti-inflammatory drug
Neomycin/Polymyxin/Bacitracin	Neosporin	Topical infection	Topical antibiotic
Nitroglycerin	Nitrostat, Nitrol Ointment, Nitro Patch	Angina	Nitrate vasodilator
Nortriptyline	Pamelor	Depression, Neuropathic pain	Tricyclic antidepressant
Nystatin	Mycostatin	Fungal infection	Antifungal
Olanzapine	Zyprexa	Delirium, Agitation	Atypical antipsychotic
Omeprazole OTC	Prilosec OTC	Gastritis	Proton pump inhibitor
Oxybutynin IR	Ditropan	Bladder spasms	Anticholinergic
Oxycodone	Roxicodone Intensol, OxyContin	Dyspnea, Nociceptive pain	Opioid
Oxycodone/Acetaminophen	Percocet	Nociceptive pain	Opioid/Non-opioid combination
Pancrelipase	Pancrease	Digestive abnormalities	Pancreatic enzyme
Phenazopyridine	Pyridium	Genitourinary analgesic	Anesthetic, Antiseptic
Phenobarbital	Phenobarbital	Seizures, Delirium	Barbiturate
Phenytoin	Dilantin	Seizures	Anticonvulsant

Potassium Chloride	KlorCon	Hypokalemia	Potassium supplement
Prednisone	Deltasone	Anorexia, Pain, Pruritus, Inflammation	Corticosteroid
Prochlorperazine	Compazine	Nausea & vomiting—Chemoreceptor trigger zone	Phenothiazine
Promethazine	Phenergan	Nausea & vomiting—Chemoreceptor trigger zone	Phenothiazine
Quetiapine	Seroquel	Delirium, Agitation	Atypical antipsychotic
Ranitidine	Zantac	Gastritis	H2 antagonist
Risperidone	Risperdal	Delirium, Agitation	Atypical antipsychotic
Salmeterol	Serevent Diskus	Bronchospasm	Beta agonist bronchodilator
Scopolamine Patch	Transderm-Scop	Nausea & vomiting—Vertigo, Terminal secretions	Anticholinergic
Senna	Senokot	Constipation	Stimulant laxative
Sertraline	Zoloft	Depression	Selective serotonin reuptake inhibitor
Simethicone	Mylicon	Gas, Bloating	Anti-flatulent
Sorbitol 70% Solution	Sorbitol	Constipation, High ammonia levels	Osmotic laxative
Spironolactone	Aldactone	Fluid retention	Potassium sparing diuretic
Sulfamethoxazole/Trimethoprim	Bactrim DS	Infection—Bacterial	Sulfonamide antibiotic
Temazepam	Restoril	Insomnia	Benzodiazepine
Theophylline	Theo-Dur	Bronchospasm	Xanthines bronchodilator
Tiotropium	Spiriva	Bronchospasm	Anticholinergic bronchodilator
Trazodone	Desyrel	Insomnia, Depression	Atypical antidepressant
Venlafaxine	Effexor	Depression	Serotonin/Norepinephrine reuptake inhibitor
Warfarin	Coumadin	Thrombus	Anticoagulant

Compounded Medications in Palliative Care

Occasionally, the need arises for medications in dosage forms that are not commercially available. In those situations, pharmacists may be able to prepare or "compound" those products. However, not all compounded products are necessary, efficacious or safe and in most cases, the compounded products are costly.

The Food and Drug Administration (FDA) released guidelines in 2002 in an attempt to regulate the pharmacy practice of compounding of medications. These guidelines arose from a need to rein in some overzealous compounding pharmacies from manufacturing drug products and due to concerns for patient safety. The FDA reports that compounded drug products are at risk for contamination and often have potency less than the stated value, based on product assays. The guidelines outline 9 factors to consider:

1. Drugs may not be compounded in anticipation of prescriptions, except in very small quantities.
2. Drugs may not be compounded if they were removed from the market for safety reasons.
3. Drugs may not be compounded from bulk active ingredients that are not already components of FDA-approved drugs.
4. Drug substances used in compounding must be from an FDA-registered facility.
5. Drug substances used in compounding must meet official compendia requirements.
6. Commercial scale manufacturing or testing equipment cannot be used.
7. Compounding for third parties to resell to individual patients or offering compounded products at wholesale is prohibited.
8. Drugs products that are commercially available or that are copies of commercially available drug products may not be compounded.
9. Applicable state laws regulating the practice of pharmacy must be followed.

In addition to the 9 factors in the FDA guidance document, the health care provider must consider pharmaceutics, bioavailability, and appropriateness of compounded drug products.

- Will the medication be adequately absorbed through the non-standard route?
- Is the added expense of compounding the product justified?
- Is there bioavailability data or other research supporting efficacy of the compound?
- Are all components of the compounded product necessary to its effectiveness?
- Does the compounding pharmacy maintain and promote safe compounding practices?

Topical preparations of medications that would typically be given orally or parenterally are frequently compounded when the patient has difficulty swallowing or refuses medications. Often these medications are combinations of anxiolytics, anti-emetics, neuroleptics, and anti-histamines. Multiple drug products are combined into one topical cream or gel to be applied for symptom management. Unfortunately, there is very limited published literature on systemic bioavailability of these topical-transdermal products. Very high doses are compounded into concentrated topicals in an attempt to ensure some level of bioavailability – resulting in potential skin irritation and considerable expense to the patient. Variability in skin type and surface area of application make absorption unpredictable and inconsistent.

Compounding of rectal suppositories may be unnecessary and also adds additional expense. For example, ABHR [**A**tivan® (lorazepam), **B**enadryl® (diphenhydramine), **H**aldol®, (haloperidol), **R**eglan® (metoclopramide)] suppositories are a common drug product used for nausea and vomiting in hospice patients. Often patients who receive these multi-drug preparations are already receiving one or more of the medications, resulting in duplication of therapy and potential toxicity and adverse effects. Additionally, the individual commercially available tablet or liquid drug formulations are generally effective when administered sublingually or per rectum without the time or expense required for compounding.

Still, some compounded products are very useful for symptom management. Magic mouthwash (Maalox®, Benadryl®, Lidocaine®) is used as an oral rinse for painful stomatitis. Chlorpromazine may be compounded into an oral concentrate (100mg/ml) and used sublingually for management of agitation, hiccups, or nausea and vomiting. Medications, such as opioids, may be compounded into liquid concentrations higher than the commercially available product for sublingual use when volume is a factor.

When considering the use of compounded medications:

- Determine if all commercially available drugs, dosages, and routes have failed or are inappropriate.
- Request evidence-based, supportive literature including bioavailability data, if available.
- Always request written information on formulations including ingredients, dosages, beyond-use (expiration) dates, potential side effects, and rationale or indication for use.

*Guidline for FDA Staff and Industry. Compliance Policy Guides Manual. Sec. 460.200. Pharmacy Compounding. May 2002. Accessible at http://www.fda.gov/ora/compliance_ref/cpg/cpgdrg/cpg460-200.html

Polypharmacy and Drug Interactions in Palliative Care

Throughout disease progression, patients with life-limiting illnesses will average 12 or more symptoms at any given time. These symptoms include cachexia, pain, anorexia, xerostomia, anxiety, dyspnea, constipation, cough, depression, nausea, vomiting, and insomnia. The goal of pharmacologic therapy is to control, relieve or eliminate symptoms while minimizing polypharmacy. Polypharmacy is generally defined as the simultaneous use of 5 or more medications.

Studies have shown that polypharmacy leads to higher rates of hospitalization in older home care patients. In addition, polypharmacy tends to be associated with significant drug-related problems:

- inappropriate drug doses
- adverse drug reactions
- drug interactions
- non-compliance
- omission of drug therapy

The probability of drug interactions rises from about 13% for patients taking 2 medications to nearly 100% for patients taking 10 or more medications. Because of decreased ability to effectively metabolize and excrete medications, elderly and debilitated patients are more likely to experience medication side effects. Development of side effects of medications may in turn lead to the incorrect interpretation of the side effect as a symptom of a new medical condition with additional medications prescribed. This is a prescribing cascade that can inadvertently lead to polypharmacy.

Polypharmacy is very difficult to avoid for patients in hospice and palliative care programs. Anticipation of those common end-of-life symptoms listed above may necessitate addition of opioids for pain or dyspnea; benzodiazepines for anxiety, insomnia, and dyspnea; antipsychotic medications, such as haloperidol for nausea, vomiting, or agitation and delirium;

acetaminophen for mild pain or fever; and laxatives for prevention and management of constipation. These comfort medications are typically added to any existing therapy the patient may be prescribed related to the terminal diagnosis or other underlying conditions.

Medication regimen review should be performed upon admission to hospice and at regular intervals during the patient's hospice stay. Careful, ongoing evaluation by a pharmacist and or other qualified clinician can help:

- assist in medication selection
- avoid the addition of unnecessary medications
- prevent drug interactions
- prevent and monitor for development of potential side effects
- assist in decision-making regarding medication dosage adjustments or discontinuation

Clinician awareness of pharmacologic profiles and potential drug interactions among medications commonly used in hospice and palliative care will aid in using medications safely and effectively.

References:

Flaherty, J.H., et al, (2001). Polypharmacy and hospitalization among older home care patients. *Journals of Gerontology. Series A, Biological Sciences and Medical Sciences.* 55(10), M554–9.

Frazier, S.C. (2005). Health outcomes and polypharmacy in elderly individuals. *Journal of Gerontological Nursing*, 31(9), 4–11.

Roshon, P.A. and Gurwitz, J.H. (1997). Optimising drug treatment for elderly people: the prescribing cascade. British Medical Journal, 315(7115), 1096-9.

The Centers for Medicare & Medicaid Services (CMS) long term care facilities survey guidelines of the State Operations Manual (SOM), released on December 15, 2006, defines the criteria for use of psychopharmacologic medications, the rationale for tapering doses, the necessary documentation to explain medication use outside the guidelines and the circumstances when a gradual dose reduction (GDR) may be considered inappropriate. Although these guidelines generally emphasize the older adult resident, adverse consequences can occur in anyone at any age; therefore, these requirements apply to residents of all ages. The regulations present challenges for the palliative care team, long term care staff, and surveyors alike because medications appropriately prescribed for palliation of symptoms at the end of life may appear to violate the intent of the guidelines. The ultimate goal of the regulations and the accompanying interpretive guidelines are to assure that medication use maintains or improves the function or wellbeing of the patient. It is important to note that the guidelines DO NOT absolutely prohibit the use of any medication or class of medications. Prior to using medications and throughout the course of therapy however, the patient must be thoroughly assessed to ensure that medications are clinically indicated to treat a documented symptom or condition (this includes the use of "as needed" or "PRN" medications) and monitored for medication effectiveness and safety. The rule of primary interest in palliative / end of life care is Tag F329 §483.25(l) Unnecessary Drugs.

The Rule

F329. §483.25(l) Unnecessary Drugs *Rev. 9-20-06*

1. General. Each resident's drug regimen must be free from unnecessary drugs. An unnecessary drug is any drug when used:

   a. In excessive dose (including duplicate therapy); or
   b. For excessive duration; or
   c. Without adequate monitoring; or
   d. Without adequate indications for its use; or
   e. In the presence of adverse consequences which indicate the dose should be reduced or discontinued; or
   f. Any combinations of the reasons above.

2. Antipsychotic Drugs. Based on a comprehensive assessment of a resident, the facility must ensure that:

    (i)   Residents who have not used antipsychotic drugs are not given these drugs unless antipsychotic drug therapy is necessary to treat a specific condition as diagnosed and documented in the clinical record; and

    (ii) Residents who use antipsychotic drugs receive gradual dose reductions, and behavioral interventions, unless clinically contraindicated, in an effort to discontinue these drugs.

An additional 78 pages of "Interpretive Guidelines" for this one rule are intended to provide guidance to surveyors in determining whether medication use is in compliance with the regulations.

Medication Management is a key concept in the new regulations and has the following subsets.

• Indications for use of medication (including initiation or continued use of antipsychotic medication). *Under this section, the need for end of life or palliative care is recognized.*
• Monitoring for efficacy and adverse consequences;

• Dose (including duplicate therapy);
• Duration;
• Tapering of a medication dose/gradual dose reduction for antipsychotic medications; and
• Prevention, identification, and response to adverse consequences.

Another significant change in the regulations is the expanded role of the consultant pharmacist.

Indications for Use of Medication (including Initiation or Continued Use of an Antipsychotic Medication)

An evaluation of the resident helps to identify his/her needs, comorbid conditions, and prognosis to determine factors (including medications and new or worsening medical conditions) that are affecting signs, symptoms, and test results. The content and extent of the evaluation may vary with the situation and may employ various assessment instruments and diagnostic tools. Examples of information to be considered and evaluated may include, but are not limited to, the following:

- *An appropriately detailed evaluation of mental, physical, and functional status;*
- *Each resident's goals and preferences;*
- *Allergies to medications and foods and potential for medication interactions;*
- *A history of prior and current medication;*
- *Recognition of the need for end-of-life or palliative care; and*
- *The refusal of care and treatment.*

There are specific rules regarding antipsychotic medications and this is especially problematic in end-of-life care because these medications are often used for symptoms not related to the medication's primary indications (e.g. haloperidol for nausea and vomiting or agitation not related to a psychiatric diagnosis).

- The regulation addressing the use of antipsychotic medications identifies the process of tapering as a "gradual dose reduction (GDR)" and requires a GDR, *unless clinically contraindicated. This means,*
  - Within the first year in which a resident is admitted on an antipsychotic medication or after the facility has initiated an antipsychotic medication, the facility must attempt a GDR in two separate quarters (with at least one month between the attempts), *unless clinically contraindicated.*
  - After the first year, a GDR must be attempted annually, *unless clinically contraindicated.*

Of Particular Note in End-of-Life Care

- *For any individual who is receiving an antipsychotic medication to treat a psychiatric disorder <u>other than behavioral symptoms related to dementia</u> (for example, schizophrenia, bipolar mania, or depression with psychotic features), the GDR may be considered contraindicated, if:*
  - The resident's target symptoms returned or worsened after the most recent attempt at a GDR within the facility; and
  - The physician has documented the clinical rationale for why any additional attempted dose reduction at that time would be likely to impair the resident's function or cause psychiatric instability by exacerbating an underlying medical psychiatric disorder.

It is clear that the interpretive guidelines recognize the need to consider end-of-life care but it is advisable for palliative care teams to be prepared to provide documentation of established protocols and standards of medication use if concerns arise. Proper assessment, documentation, monitoring and follow up that establish that medications are used in the patient's best interest will clear the way for quality pharmaceutical care at the end of life.

Guidelines for Effective Management of Symptoms (*GEMS*)

Anorexia and Cachexia

Introduction and Background

- Anorexia (loss of appetite) and cachexia (severe muscle wasting and weight loss) are two of the most common and devastating signs and symptoms at the end of life. They can lead to weakness, debilitation, compromised immune function, and decreased morale.
- Unlike other symptoms that present in terminally ill patients, these symptoms are silent and sometimes receive less attention by health care professionals.
- Weight loss and lack of appetite can be very distressing to family members who often link weight and a healthy appetite with well-being.
- The goal of this guideline is to improve the patient's quality of life by improving family and patient understanding of the symptoms and treatment limitations, relieving nausea and other identifiable causes, and addressing treatments for anorexia.

Prevalence

- Anorexia (64%) and cachexia (80%) in patients with terminal illness

Causes

A thorough history and physical should be taken and possible reversible causes of anorexia/cachexia should be identified and treated, if present.

Some of the possible causes are:

- Nausea and vomiting
- Oral candidiasis
- Gastritis
- Dry mouth
- Iatrogenic (e.g. chemotherapy, radiation, drugs)
- Constipation
- Dehydration
- Weakness
- Bowel obstruction
- Hepatic metastases
- Organ failure
- Depression
- Pain

Clinical Characteristics

- Anorexia and cachexia are experienced by most terminally ill patients and are a part of the dying process.
- Malnutrition in cancer patients is not the only factor responsible for weight loss-nutritional correction may not reverse this condition.
- In cancer-associated anorexia the two most important mediating factors are:
  - Reduced intake/hypophagia due to alterations in the perception of food, nausea and vomiting, pain, and dysphagia
  - Physiologic and metabolic alteration induced by tumor

- Cancer-associated cachexia induced by profound metabolic alterations results in accelerated weight loss. Basal metabolism is increased by 50% in patients with malignant diseases leading to increased energy expenditure, resulting in fatigue, apathy, and depression.
- Cachexia due to weight loss is primarily manifested by loss of skeletal muscle and adipose tissue while visceral protein distribution remains unchanged.

Non-Pharmacologic Therapy

Reassure the family that patients:

- Generally lose their appetite and reduce food intake long before they reach the last hours of their lives.
- Can live comfortably for a long time on very little food.
- Are not starving to death and that forced feeding usually does not prolong life and may shorten it.
- May experience euphoria from the release of endogenous endorphins as a result of the natural process of dying and wasting.

Regarding foods and meal planning, consider the following:

- Involve the patient in meal planning.
- Offer small portions of the patient's favorite foods.
- Avoid foods with a strong odor, unless the patient requests them.
- Offer easy-to-swallow foods, such as pudding, gelatin, etc.
- Keep the patient company while he or she eats.
- Serve meals in a room other than where the patient sleeps.
- Serve an alcoholic drink prior to mealtime.
- Help the family redirect and find alternatives to sharing time together other than eating, (e.g. listening to music, looking at pictures, reading aloud, etc.)
- Consult a dietician experienced in end-of-life care to assist with family acceptance or for a second opinion if symptoms do not align well with disease progression, or if considering enteral or parenteral nutrition.
- Suggest alternatives for family members as they may feel a strong obligation to feed the patient. For example: Caregivers can alleviate symptoms and nurture their instinct to "do something" by moistening the patient's lips and oral cavity with a sponge.
- Assess cultural/religious issues that may interfere with understanding and acceptance. Consider enlisting pastoral care from hospice or patient's own belief system.

Pharmacotherapy

Several pharmacologic agents have been recommended and used in end-of-life care to improve the patient's appetite, improve their sense of well being, and, at times, promote weight gain.

Pharmacologic Management of Anorexia

Generic Name (Brand Name)	Usual Adult Starting Dose/Range	Common Strengths and Formulations	Comments
First Line Therapy			
Prednisone (Deltasone)	**Range:** 10–20 mg PO daily or BID	**Tablets:** 1 mg, 2.5 mg, 5 mg,10 mg, 20 mg, 50 mg **Oral Solution:** 5 mg/5 mL **Prednisone Intensol Concentrate (Oral Solution):** 5 mg/mL	• Indicated when short term therapy may be beneficial (< 6weeks) • Also useful in the conditions of bone pain, asthenia, or bronchospasm • Less expensive than dexamethasone • Start with a low dose (10 mg po daily) and monitor for efficacy weekly, can increase dose and reassess weekly
Dexamethasone (Decadron)	**Range:** 2–4 mg PO daily or BID	**Tablets:** 0.25 mg, 0.5 mg, 0.75 mg, 1 mg, 1.5 mg, 2 mg, 4 mg, 6 mg **Oral Solution:** 0.5 mg/5 mL **Dexamethasone Intensol Concentrate (Oral Solution):** 1 mg/mL	• The most comprehensively studied of the corticosteroids in palliative care • Indicated when short term therapy may be beneficial • Also useful in the conditions of bone pain or bronchospasm • Start with a low dose (4 mg po daily) and monitor for efficacy weekly, can increase dose and reassess weekly
Second Line Therapy			
Megestrol (Megace)	**Initial:** 160 mg PO daily **Maximum effective dose in anorexia/cachexia:** 800 mg PO daily	**Tablets:** 20 mg, 40 mg **Suspension:** 40 mg/mL, 125mg/mL	• Avoid in patients with limited mobility • Avoid use in patients with a history of DVT • Risk of thromboembolism and hyperglycemia-monitor patients • Start at lowest dose and monitor for efficacy every 2 weeks. If no response, increase dose by 160 mg po per 24 hours • In higher doses, liquid is preferred due to decreased pill burden and is more cost-effective. (Expensive) • Clinical trials have shown that there is no benefit at doses above 800 mg/day

Generic Name (Brand Name)	Usual Adult Starting Dose/Range	Common Strengths and Formulations	Comments
Second Line Therapy			
Mirtazapine (Remeron)	**Initial:** 7.5 mg PO daily **Range:** 7.5–45 mg PO daily **MDD:** 45 mg PO daily	**Tablets:** 15 mg, 30 mg, 45 mg	• Consider in patients with insomnia or depression combined with appetite/weight loss • Lower doses are more sedating (7.5 mg–15 mg) and more likely to stimulate appetite while higher doses are often required for depression
Third Line Therapy			
Dronabinol (Marinol)	**Initial:** 2.5 mg PO daily **Range:** 2.5–10 mg PO BID **MDD:** 20 mg PO daily	**Capsules:** 2.5 mg, 5 mg, 10 mg	• Expensive • Sometimes causes intolerable CNS side effects such as dysphoria or euphoria
Cyproheptadine (Periactin)	**Initial:** 4–8 mg PO TID **Range:** 4–20 mg PO daily **MDD:** 0.5 mg/kg/day	**Tablets:** 4 mg **Syrup:** 2 mg/5 mL	• Mechanism suggests that it would have benefit due to serotonergic activity, however very limited data regarding efficacy • Some patients may not tolerate due to dizziness and sedation

Clinical Pearls

- If patient has feeling of fullness or "squashed stomach syndrome", metoclopramide may be beneficial to increase gastric motility and reduce stomach emptying time.
- Practitioners should be prepared to discuss tube feeding as an option bearing in mind what evidence (or lack thereof) exists that tube feeding will help reach goals of treatment.
- Thalidomide 100–200 mg daily has been shown to increase weight in patients with cachexia but does not demonstrate improvement of anorexia over placebo. Thalidomide is extremely expensive and is highly teratogenic.
- Studies show anabolic agents such as oxandrolone increase muscle mass in patients with cirrhosis, COPD, AIDS and neuromuscular disorders. These medications are schedule III controlled substances due to abuse potential and are expensive.

Key References

Bruera E, Fainsinger R. Clinical management of cachexia and anorexia. In: Doyle D, Hankds GWC, MacDonald N, editors. Oxford textbook of palliative medicine. 3rd edition. Oxford: Oxford University Press; 2003:552–560.

Walsh D, Donnelly S, Rybicki L. The symptoms of advanced cancer: relationship to age, gender, and performance status in 1,000 patients. Support Care Cancer 2000;8(3):175–9.

Vainio A, Auvinen A. Prevalence of symptoms among patients with advanced cancer: an international collaborative study. Symptom Prevalence Group. J Pain Symptom Manage 1996;12(1):3–10.

Strasser F, Bruera ED. Update on anorexia and cachexia. Hematol Oncol Clin N Am 2002;16:589–617.

Tyler LS, Lipman AG. Anorexia and Cachexia in Palliative Care Patients. In: Evidence Based Symptom Control in Palliative Care. Systematic Review and Validated Clinical Practice Guidelines for 15 Common Problems in Patients with Life Limiting Disease. 1st ed. New York, NY: Pharmaceutical Products Press; 2000: 11–35.

Storey P, Knight CF. UNIPAC Four: Management of Selected Non-pain Symptoms in the Terminally Ill. 2nd edition. New York, NY: Mary Ann Liebert, Inc.; 2003: 22–28.

Ross DD, Alexander CS. Management of Common Symptoms in Terminally Ill Patients: Part I. Fatigue, Anorexia, Cachexia, Nausea and Vomiting. American Family Physician. 2001;64:807–814.

Killion K, ed. Drug Facts and Comparisons. Electronic edition. St. Louis; Facts and Comparisons, 2005, [Dexamethasone, Prednisone, Megestrol, Mirtazapine, Dronabinol, Cyproheptadine.]

Salacz M. Fast Facts and Concepts #100 Megestrol acetate for cancer anorexia/cachexia. October 2003. End-of-Life Physician Education Resource Center Available at: www.eperc.mcw.edu. Accessed on February 20, 2005.

Weissman, D. Fast Fact and Concepts #10: Tube Feed or Not Tube Feed? June, 2000. End-of-Life Physician Education Resource Center, www.eperc.mcw.edu.

Fabbro ED, Dalal S, Bruera E Symptom Control in Palliative Care—Part II: Cachexia/Anorexia and Fatigue. Journal of Palliative Medicine Apr 2006, Vol. 9, No. 2: 409–421.

G Mantovani, C Madeddu, A Maccio, G Gramignano, MR Cancer-Related Anorexia/Cachexia Syndrome and Oxidative Stress: An Innovative Approach beyond Current Treatment. Cancer Epidemiology Biomarkers & Prevention 13(10) 2004: 1651–1659.

Camps C, Iranzo V, Bremnes R, Sirera, R Anorexia–Cachexia syndrome in cancer: implications of the ubiquitin–proteasome pathway. Supportive Care in Cancer, Volume 14, Number 12 / December, 2006: 1173–1183.

Boddner D, Spencer T, Riggs AT et al. A retrospective study of the association between megestrol acetate administration and mortality among nursing home residents and clinically significant weight loss. The American Journal of Geriatric Pharmacotherapy 2007; 5 (2): 137–146.

Anorexia and Cachexia

Start

Thorough history and physical exam

Reversible causes detected

Yes → Treat

No

Anorexia still present?

No → Continue treatment and monitor

Yes → Education and appropriate reassurances*

General non-pharmacologic measures*

Prognosis >3 months + weight gain desired

Yes

No

Anorexia and Cachexia (*continued*)

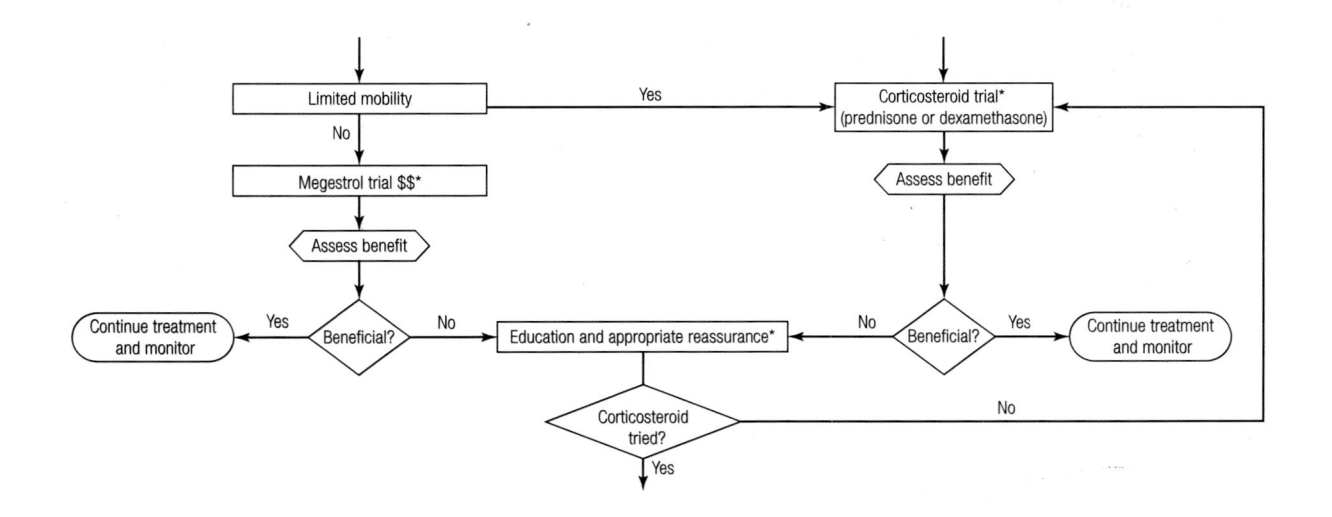

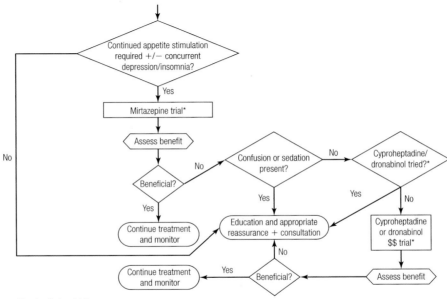

*See details in guideline
$$ expensive

Anxiety

Introduction and Background

- Anxiety is "a state of fearfulness, apprehension, worry, emotional discomfort, or uneasiness that either results from an unknown internal stimulus, is excessive, or is otherwise inappropriate to a given situation." [The Fourth Edition of the Diagnostic and Statistical Manual of Mental Disorders (DSM–IV)]
- Transient feelings of anxiety guide us to avoid situations that might lead to risk or harm and are adaptive and healthy (so-called "street smarts").
- Much like pain, when anxiety loses this adaptive or "signal" function (persists despite the absence of an anxiety-provoking stimulus or becomes excessive), it causes significant distress and suffering.
- Anxiety is closely related to fear, but fear has an identified cause or source of worry (e.g., fear of death). Fear may be more responsive to counseling than an anxiety state that the patient cannot attribute to a particular fearful stimulus.

Prevalence

- The prevalence of clinically significant anxiety in the hospice setting is not well studied, but has been reported to be as high as 72% on single-item screening.
- Surprisingly low rates of formal anxiety disorders have been found in the few studies of relevant populations, but this may reflect problems with measurement strategy.
- Anxiety disorders are the most prevalent class of mental disorders overall, so it is not surprising that anxiety is a common cause of distress at life's end.

Causes

- Patients with formal Anxiety Disorders (e.g., Panic Disorder, Generalized Anxiety Disorder, Obsessive Compulsive Disorder, Post-traumatic Stress Disorder, Phobias) usually have a history of significant anxiety that predates their terminal illness.
- Post Traumatic Stress Disorder may re-emerge as death approaches, even after decades of latency, with anxiety, avoidance behaviors, increased arousal, and vivid re-experiencing of traumatic events (as intrusive thoughts, daydreams, or nightmares).
- In addition to Anxiety Disorders, a variety of conditions can cause, mimic, or exacerbate anxiety:
  - Delirium, particularly in its early stages, can easily be confused with anxiety.
  - Physical complications of illness, especially dyspnea and undertreated pain, are common precipitants.
  - Significant anxiety is present in the majority of patients with advanced lung disease and is closely related to periods of oxygen desaturation.
  - Medication side effects, especially akathisia from older antipsychotics and antiemetics (including and especially metoclopramide) can present as anxiety.
  - Drug withdrawal states (e.g., alcohol and sedative-hypnotic drugs)
  - Interpersonal, spiritual, or existential concerns can mimic anxiety.
  - Patients with an anxious or dependent coping style are at high risk of anxiety as a complication of advanced illness.

Clinical Characteristics

- Short of making a diagnosis of a formal Anxiety Disorder, differentiating normal worry and apprehension from pathologic anxiety requires clinical judgment.
- Pathological anxiety has the following characteristics: takes on a "life of its own"; may be of an intensity that exceeds the patient's capacity to bear; lasts longer than one would expect in a given situation; and/or produces anxiety behaviors.
- Behaviors indicative of pathological anxiety include:
  - Intense worry or dread
  - Physical distress (e.g., tension, jitteriness, or restlessness)
  - Maladaptive behaviors (e.g., treatment non-adherence, social withdrawal, or avoidance)
  - Diminished coping, and inability to relax
- Pathologic anxiety may be complicated by insomnia, depression, fatigue, gastrointestinal upset, dyspnea, or dysphagia. Anxiety can also worsen these conditions if they are already present.
- Untreated anxiety may lead to numerous complications, including withdrawal from social support, poor coping, limited participation in palliative care treatment goals, and family distress.
- Reassess the patient for anxiety with any change in behavior or any change in the underlying medical condition. The following steps in assessment should be followed:
  - Search for causes of anxiety or fear—ask the patient
  - Assess for formal anxiety disorders.

Non-Pharmacologic Treatment

- Assess for other problems that might lead to the emergence of anxiety.
- Ask about anxiety that predated the hospice diagnosis and any history of effective treatments.
- Begin with clinical vigilance. Monitor for anxiety routinely and maintain a high index of suspicion for anxiety in terminal illness.
- Regardless of what treatment approach is chosen, the following principles apply:
  - Offer emotional support and reassurance when appropriate.
  - Err on the side of treatment-be willing to palliate anxiety.
  - Assess treatment response and side effects frequently.
  - Aim to provide maximum resolution of anxiety.
  - Educate patients and families about anxiety and its treatments.
- Psychotherapies can help in the management of anxiety, though the availability of trained therapists willing to make home visits and the limited stamina and attention span of seriously ill patients typically make such therapies impractical in the hospice setting.
- Cognitive and behavioral therapies can be beneficial, including simple relaxation exercises or distraction strategies (i.e., focusing on something pleasurable or at least emotionally neutral).
- Encourage chaplaincy visits especially if spiritual and existential concerns predominate.
- When an underlying cause of anxiety can be identified, treatment is initially aimed at the precipitating problem, with monitoring to see if anxiety improves or resolves as the underlying cause is addressed.

Pharmacotherapy:

- In most cases, management of pathological anxiety in the hospice setting involves pharmacologic therapies.

Pharmacologic Management of Anxiety

Generic Name (Brand Name)	Usual Adult Starting Dose/Range	Routes	Common Strengths and Formulations	Comments
First Line Therapy				
Benzodiazepines				
Lorazepam (Ativan)	0.5 mg BID–TID (scheduled or PRN) (MDD: 10 mg/day)	PO, SL, PR, IV, SQ, IM	**Tablets:** 0.5 mg, 1 mg, 2 mg **Concentrated Oral Solution:** 2 mg/mL **Injection:** 2 mg & 4 mg/mL	• (ALL DRUGS IN CLASS) May produce paradoxical agitation in elderly, demented, or brain-injured patients–start with a test dose • Short-acting • No active metabolites • Most reliably absorbed drug in class when administered parenterally • Generally the benzodiazepine of choice in hospice • Oral concentrate is expensive
Alprazolam (Xanax)	0.25 mg TID (scheduled or PRN) (MDD: 8 mg/day)	PO, SL, PR	**Tablets:** 0.25 mg, 0.5 mg, 1 mg, 2 mg **Concentrated Oral Solution:** 1 mg/mL	• Short-acting; may produce "rebound" anxiety between doses as tolerance develops • Highest risk for withdrawal if tolerant patient abruptly stops medication • Oral concentrate is expensive
Clonazepam (Klonopin)	0.5 mg BID (scheduled or PRN) (MDD: 6 mg/day)	PO, PR, SL	**Tablets:** 0.5 mg, 1 mg, 2 mg	• Long-acting; active metabolites may accumulate and contribute to sedation • Most potent of these four drugs • Can split 0.5 mg tablet in half for 0.25 mg dose
Diazepam (Valium)	2 mg BID (scheduled or PRN) (MDD: 40 mg/day)	PO, SL, IM, IV, PR	**Tablets:** 2 mg, 5 mg, 10 mg **Concentrated Oral Solution:** 5 mg/mL **Injection:** 5 mg/mL	• Most rapid onset of action with single dose • Long-acting; active metabolites may accumulate and contribute to sedation • Least potent of these four drugs • Oral concentrate is expensive

Second Line Therapy-Antipsychotics

Typical Antipsychotics

Haloperidol (Haldol)	0.5–1 mg BID–TID (scheduled or PRN)	PO, SQ, SL, IV, IM, PR	**Tablets:** 0.5 mg, 1 mg, 2 mg, 5 mg, 10 mg, 20 mg **Oral Concentrate:** 2 mg/mL **Injection:** 5 mg/mL	• (ALL DRUGS IN CLASS) Useful if anxious patient unable to tolerate benzodiazepines • (ALL DRUGS IN CLASS) May produce extrapyramidal symptoms, including akathisia (which can mimic anxiety) • (ALL DRUGS IN CLASS) May produce movement disorders • Injection is expensive
Chlorpromazine (Thorazine)	10–50 mg q4–8h (scheduled or PRN)	PO, PR, SL, IM	**Tablets:** 10 mg, 25 mg, 50 mg, 100 mg, 200 mg **Injection:** 25 mg/mL	• Especially useful if more sedation is desired • Oral concentrate and suppositories must be compounded • Can cause orthostatic hypotension

Atypical Antipsychotics

Olanzapine (Zyprexa)	2.5–5 mg daily	PO	**Tablets:** 2.5 mg, 5 mg, 7.5 mg, 10 mg, 15 mg, 20 mg **Orally Disintegrating Tablets:** 5 mg, 10 mg, 15 mg, 20 mg	• (ALL DRUGS IN CLASS) Useful if anxious patient unable to tolerate benzodiazepines AND "typical" antipsychotics • (ALL DRUGS IN CLASS) Much more expensive than "typical" antipsychotics • (ALL DRUGS IN CLASS) May produce extrapyramidal symptoms, including akathisia • Expensive
Quetiapine (Seroquel)	25 mg BID	PO	**Tablets:** 25 mg, 100 mg, 200 mg, 300 mg	• Especially useful if more sedating agent is desired • Preferred agent in patients with Parkinson's Disease due to low incidence of extrapyramidal symptoms • Expensive

Pharmacologic Management of Anxiety

Generic Name (Brand Name)	Usual Adult Starting Dose/Range	Routes	Common Strengths and Formulations	Comments
Atypical Antipsychotics				
Risperidone (Risperdal)	0.5–1 mg BID	PO	**Tablets:** 0.25 mg, 0.5 mg, 1 mg, 2 mg, 3 mg, 4 mg **Orally Disintegrating Tablets:** 0.5 mg, 1 mg, 2 mg **Oral Solution:** 1 mg/mL	• Orally disintegrating tablets are more expensive than conventional tablets • Expensive
Second Line Therapy-Antidepressants				
Selective Serotonin Reuptake Inhibitors (SSRIs)				
Citalopram (Celexa)	20 mg daily Usual therapeutic dose range: 40–60 mg	PO	**Tablets:** 10 mg, 20 mg, 40 mg **Solution:** 10 mg/5 mL	• (ALL DRUGS IN CLASS) May be especially useful if expected survival is more than a few weeks • (ALL DRUGS IN CLASS) Slow onset of action (like time course for antidepressant effects) • (ALL DRUGS IN CLASS) May worsen anxiety in the first few days to a week of therapy–consider co-administration of a benzodiazepine in the short term • Liquid not available as a generic-expensive
Escitalopram (Lexapro)	5–10 mg daily Usual therapeutic dose range: 10–20 mg	PO	**Tablets:** 5 mg, 10 mg, 20 mg **Liquid:** 5 mg/5 mL	• Reliability of reputed faster onset of action unclear
Fluoxetine (Prozac)	10–20 mg daily Usual therapeutic dose range: 20–40 mg	PO	**Tablets/Capsules:** 10 mg, 20 mg, 40 mg **Solution:** 20 mg/5 mL	• Longest half-life (by far) of the drugs in this class • Least expensive SSRI
Paroxetine (Paxil)	10 mg daily Usual therapeutic dose range: 20–40 mg	PO	**Tablets:** 10 mg, 20 mg, 30 mg, 40 mg **Suspension:** 10 mg/5 mL	• Highest incidence of anticholinergic side effects • Shortest half-life, withdrawal symptoms can occur with missed doses
Sertraline (Zoloft)	25–50 mg daily Usual therapeutic dose range: 100–200 mg	PO	**Tablets:** 25 mg, 50 mg, 100 mg **Solution:** 20 mg/mL	

Tricyclic Antidepressants (TCAs)				
Desipramine (Norpramin)	10–50 mg at bedtime **Usual therapeutic dose range:** 100–200 mg	PO	**Tablets:** 10 mg, 25 mg, 50 mg, 75 mg, 100 mg, 150 mg	• Tricyclic antidepressant • Least sedating tricyclic
Nortriptyline (Pamelor)	10–25 mg at bedtime **Usual therapeutic dose range:** 75–150 mg	PO	**Capsules:** 10 mg, 25 mg, 50 mg, 75 mg **Solution:** 10 mg/5 mL	• Tricyclic antidepressant • Least likely tricyclic to cause orthostasis

Clinical Pearls

- The primary goal of therapy for anxiety in hospice is patient comfort. Aim to prevent anxiety, not just treat it with PRN meds when it flares. Think of pain management as an analogy.
- Relief from anxiety should not require sedation.
- Start at the lower end of the dose range of a given anxiolytic agent, but recognize that standard or higher doses may be required.
- Avoid use of bupropion and psychostimulants for anxiety. While effective for depression they are ineffective for anxiety and may make anxiety worse.
- Relative potencies of benzodiazepines: (see Benzodiazepine Equivalency Chart, p. 328)

Key References

American Psychiatric Association. *Diagnostic and Statistical Manual of Mental Disorders, Fourth Edition*. Washington, DC: American Psychiatric Press, 1994.

Portenoy RK, Thaler HT, Kornblith AB, et al: The Memorial Symptom Assessment Scale: an instrument for the evaluation of symptom prevalence, characteristics and distress. *European J Cancer*. 30A:1326–1336, 1994.

Cassileth BR, Lusk EJ, Walsh WP: Anxiety levels in patients with malignant disease. *Hospice Journal*. 2: 57–69, 1986.

Hocking LB, Koenig HG: Anxiety in medically ill older patients: a review and update. *Int J Psychiatry Med*. 25: 221–238, 1995.

Stoudemire A: Epidemiology and psychopharmacology of anxiety in medical patients. *J Clin Psychiatry*. 57 Suppl 7: 64–72; 73–75, 1996.

Rubey RN, Lydiard RB: Pharmacological treatment of anxiety in the medically ill patient. *Semin Clin Neuropsychiatry*. 4: 133–147, 1999.

Anxiety

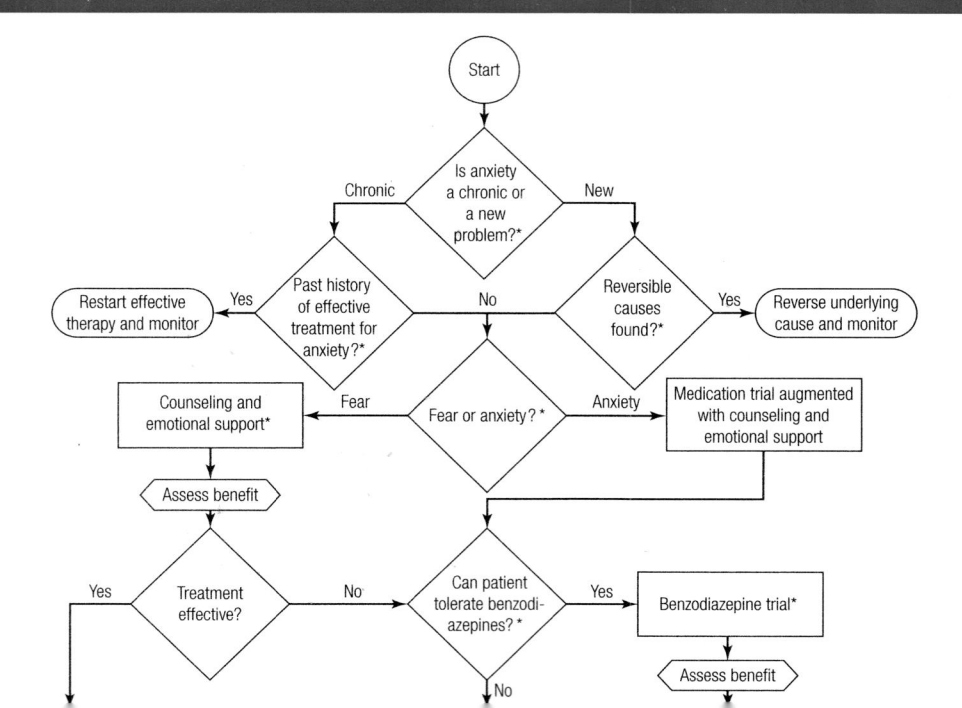

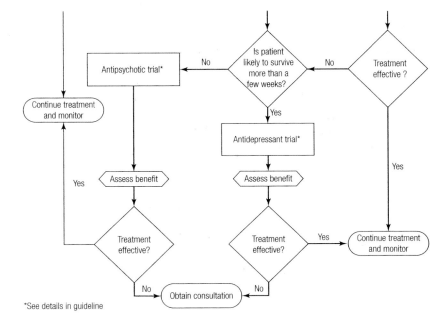

*See details in guideline

Ascites and Edema

Introduction and Background
- Edema is the accumulation of fluid in body tissues that can be generalized throughout the body or localized to one part of the body.
- Edema is common in advanced illness; underlying causes are not always identifiable or reversible.
- Edema in the palliative care setting typically results from malignancy, cardiac or liver failure, or medications.
- Ascites is excess fluid in the space between the tissues lining the abdomen and abdominal organs (the peritoneal cavity).

Prevalence
- Studies suggest frequency of edema at about 30% of patients in hospice with an advanced cancer diagnosis.
- Lymphedema is reported by 20–45% of patients following breast cancer therapy, with increasing prevalence in the years after treatment and surgery.
- Ascites can be a presenting feature in about 50% of malignancies.

Causes
- Basic causes of edema are venous obstruction, increased capillary permeability, and increased plasma volume secondary to sodium and water retention.
- Dependent edema is caused by intravascular pressure alterations resulting in uneven fluid distribution, usually affecting the legs due to reduced mobility.
- Medications:
  - Calcium channel blockers (amlodipine, verapamil), NSAIDs, steroids (prednisone, megestrol, estrogens), beta-blockers, gabapentin, pregabalin
- Heart failure results in cardiogenic pulmonary edema and often peripheral edema due to inability of the heart to pump efficiently (left ventricular dysfunction) and poor circulation.
- Hypoalbuminemia: leads to reduced oncotic pressure, decreased intravascular volume, and increased fluids in interstitial spaces. Decreased intravascular volume leads to secretion of anti-diuretic hormone and increased water retention and decreased urine output.
- Malignancy: ascites is common with ovarian, liver, and gastrointestinal cancers.

Clinical Characteristics
- Peripheral edema is the accumulation of fluid in the extremities (usually the feet, ankles, and legs), often the result of heart, kidney or liver failure.
- Ascites is the accumulation of fluid in the peritoneal cavity usually due to liver failure-either malignant or cirrhotic.
- Lymphedema is tissue swelling resulting from lymph drainage failure, typically affecting a limb with or without adjacent trunk involvement. Lymphedema is associated with chronic inflammation and fibrosis.
- Pulmonary edema is diffuse extravascular accumulation of fluid in pulmonary tissues and air spaces.
- Cerebral edema is excess accumulation of water in the extra or intracellular spaces of the brain which may result from tumors, ischemia, SIADH, or malignant hypertension.

- There are various numerical scales for grading peripheral edema. Ranging from 0 = absent or 1 = mild to 4 = severe. The precise definitions vary with each scale. Following is an example of a scale, but documentation and description of edema location, severity, and depth is better than merely documenting a number.
  1+ = Mild edema that is barely detectable.
  2+ = Slight indentation is visible when the skin is depressed.
  3+ = Deeper fingerprint returns to normal in 5 to 30 seconds.
  4+ = Severe, extremity may be 1.5 to 2 times normal size.
- Patients on diuretic therapy may monitor weight loss from ascites fluid to maintain at 0.5–1 kg-loss/day, more daily weight loss may be expected if significant peripheral edema is present along with ascites.

Non-Pharmacologic Treatment
- Elevate affected extremities using pillows, wedges, footstools, or a recliner.
- Fluid and salt restricted (<2000 mg/day) diets should only be followed if the restriction is not overly burdensome to the patient.

- Paracentesis for symptomatic ascites:
  - Fluid removal from paracentesis is only temporary and will not reverse the underlying cause.
  - Percutaneous catheters and drainage shunts may be used in patients with moderate long-term survival prognosis to aid in symptomatic drainage.
  - Large volume paracentesis (3–5 liters) may lead to hypotension, intravascular volume depletion and dehydration. More frequent (e.g., weekly), smaller volume (1–2 liters) fluid removal is usually more easily tolerated.
- Lymphatic massage
  - Involve interdisciplinary team's massage therapist or physical therapist for range of motion and massage training for patient and caregivers.
  - Elevate limb being massaged. Direction of the massage should be toward the body (from feet towards knees, or fingertips towards elbows).
- Wraps
  - Compression wrapping, bandaging, or stockings may help to reduce or relieve swelling in limbs.

Pharmacologic Management of Edema

Generic Name (Brand Name)	Usual Adult Starting Dose/Range	Maximum Daily Dose	Common Strengths and Formulations	Comments
Loop Diuretics (Potassium-wasting)				
First Line Therapy				
Furosemide (Lasix)	20–80 mg daily	600 mg/day	**Tablets:** 20 mg, 40 mg, 80 mg **Injection:** 10 mg/mL **Solution:** 10 mg/mL	• Can be given PR • Oral bioavailability about 50% • IV dose is ½ of equivalent PO dose
Second Line Therapy				
Bumetanide (Bumex)	0.5–2 mg daily	10 mg/day	**Tablets:** 0.5 mg, 1 mg, 2 mg **Injection:** 0.25 mg/mL	• Oral bioavailability about 100% • PO and IV doses are same • May work if resistant to furosemide • Can give with caution to patients allergic to furosemide
Torsemide (Demadex)	10–20 mg daily	200 mg/day	**Tablets:** 5 mg, 10 mg, 20 mg, 100 mg **Injection:** 10 mg/mL	• Oral bioavailability about 100% • PO and IV doses are same • May work if resistant to furosemide
Carbonic Anhydrase Inhibitor				
Acetazolamide (Diamox)	250 mg daily	500 mg BID	**Capsules ER:** 500 mg **Tablets:** 125 mg, 250 mg	• Primarily used to decrease intracranial pressure in cerebral edema
Thiazide-type Diuretics (Potassium-wasting)				
Metolazone (Zaroxolyn)	2.5 mg daily	20 mg/day	**Tablets:** 2.5 mg, 5 mg, 10 mg	• Works synergistically with loop and thiazide diuretics • May be effective even if CrCL < 20 mL/min • 5 mg of metolazone is approx equivalent to 50 mg HCTZ

Drug	Dose	Max Dose	Formulations	Notes
Hydrochlorothiazide (Oretic)	25–100 mg daily	200 mg/day	**Capsules:** 12.5 mg **Tablets:** 25 mg, 50 mg	• No efficacy if CrCL <30 mL/min • Less beneficial for edema than loop diuretics
Chlorothiazide (Diuril)	250–1000 mg daily or BID	1000 mg/day	**Tablets:** 250 mg, 500 mg **Suspension:** 250 mg/5 mL **Injection:** 500 mg	• No efficacy if CrCL <30 mL/min • Less beneficial for edema than loop diuretics
Chlorthalidone (Thalitone)	50–100 mg daily	200 mg/day	**Tablets:** 15 mg, 25 mg, 50 mg, 100 mg	• No efficacy if CrCL <30 mL/min • Less beneficial for edema than loop diuretics
Potassium-sparing Diuretics				
Spironolactone (Aldactone)	25 mg–200 mg daily or BID	400 mg/day	**Tablets:** 25 mg, 50 mg, 100 mg	• Avoid use if CrCL <10 mL/min • Gynecomastia possible especially at higher doses
Triamterene (Dyrenium)	50 mg–300 mg daily or BID	300 mg/day	**Tablets:** 50 mg, 100 mg	• Avoid use if CrCL <10 mL/min • Usually in combination with hydrochlorothiazide

Clinical Pearls

- All commercially available diuretics contain a sulfa moiety. Avoid if documented allergy to glyburide. Patients with sulfa antibiotic allergies usually do not have cross-reactivity with sulfa diuretics due to differing molecular structure of the sulfa component.
- Prednisone has significantly more mineralocorticoid effect than dexamethasone, which may lead to peripheral edema especially at higher daily doses.
- Loop diuretic approximate oral equivalency: Furosemide 40 mg = Bumetanide 1 mg = Torsemide 10–20 mg.
- First line therapy for ascites is combination of spironolactone 100 mg and furosemide 40 mg.
- Treatment of ascites with diuretics (e.g. spironolactone and furosemide) may not be very effective unless ascites is due to portal hypertension from extensive liver metastases.
- Presence of malignant ascites is a harbinger of advanced disease, associated with a 1 year survival rate of less than 10%.
- Evaluate upper body skin turgor to determine hydration status of patient. Poor upper body skin turgor indicates volume depletion and dehydration, despite the presence of ascites and/or peripheral edema.
- Unilateral, new-onset edema may indicate presence of deep vein thrombosis (DVT).

Key References

Spira, A.I., and Brahmer, J.R. (2004). Effusions, chapter 60, In, *Clinical Oncology*, Abeloff, M.D., et al, eds. Elsesvier Churchill Livingstone: Philadelphia LexiComp's Complete Reference Library, http://www.crlonline.com, accessed 2/13/2007.

O'Brien, J.G., Chennubhotla, C.A., Chennubhotla, R.V. (2005). Treatment of edema. *American Family Physician,* 71(11), 2111–18.

Petrek JA, Senie RT, Peters M, et al.(2001). Lymphedema in a cohort of breast carcinoma survivors 20 years after diagnosis. *Cancer* 92 (6): 1368–77.

Wright, A. Edema. In, *Theranotes*. (1998). Harcourt: New York.

Ascites

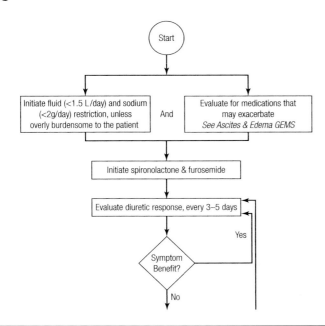

Start

↓

Initiate fluid (<1.5 L/day) and sodium (<2g/day) restriction, unless overly burdensome to the patient

And

Evaluate for medications that may exacerbate
See Ascites & Edema GEMS

↓

Initiate spironolactone & furosemide

↓

Evaluate diuretic response, every 3–5 days

↓

Symptom Benefit? — **Yes** → (back to Evaluate diuretic response)

↓ **No**

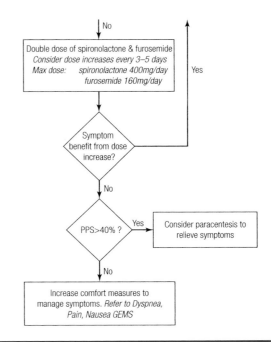

No ↓

Double dose of spironolactone & furosemide
Consider dose increases every 3–5 days
Max dose: spironolactone 400mg/day
*   furosemide 160mg/day*

↓

Symptom benefit from dose increase? — **Yes** → (back up)

↓ **No**

PPS>40% ? — **Yes** → Consider paracentesis to relieve symptoms

↓ **No**

Increase comfort measures to manage symptoms. *Refer to Dyspnea, Pain, Nausea GEMS*

Edema

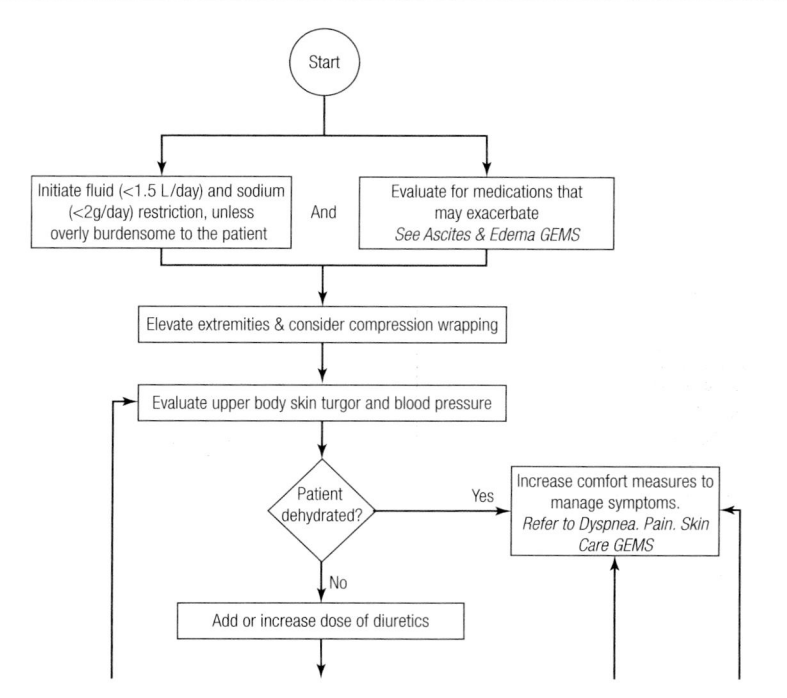

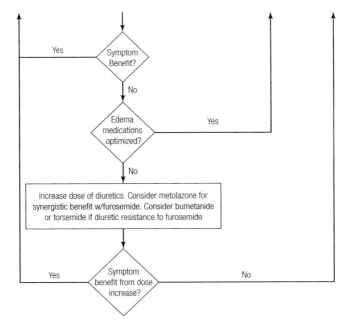

Bowel Obstruction

Introduction and Background

- The most common cancers associated with bowel obstruction are colo-rectal, stomach, and ovarian, but obstruction can occur in any advanced malignancy.
- Patients who have had abdominal surgery or abdominal radiation appear to be at higher risk of developing bowel obstruction.
- Symptoms often vary by location of the obstruction.
- Common general symptoms include abdominal pain (colicky and/or continuous), nausea and vomiting.
- Obstructions higher in the GI tract, such as the pylorus or duodenum, often produce severe emesis. This type of obstruction may be associated with less pain and distention, but often has significant volume of emesis.
- Obstruction in lower segments of the small intestine typically present with more colicky pain, moderate distention, and hyperactive bowel sounds.
- The amount of emesis may range from moderate to severe.
- Large intestine obstruction presents commonly with lower abdominal pain, and may also have a colicky component. These large intestine obstructions tend to be associated with severe abdominal distention and can have emesis which is more delayed.

Prevalence

- Eighty percent of bowel obstructions occur in the small intestine, normally secondary to adhesions and hernias.
- In the hospice setting, the rate of large intestine related bowel obstruction may be increased, especially in relation to drug-induced causes.
- Bowel obstruction is most common during the advanced stages of terminal disease.

Causes

- Understanding the cause will assist the clinician in determining the most effective method for treating this symptom.
- Mechanical causes:
  - Narrowing of the intestinal lumen (e.g., inflammation, trauma, tumor, adhesions, hernias)
  - Compression from outside the intestinal tract
- Non-mechanical causes:
  - Interference with normal intestinal muscle activity
  - Interference with normal innervation (e.g. paralytic ileus, mesenteric embolus or thrombus, and hypokalemia)

Clinical Characteristics

- The goal of medical management for patients with an intestinal obstruction is to decrease pain, nausea and distention by:
  - Decreasing the amount of secretions flowing into the bowel.
  - Reviewing the patient's medication profile to insure that no other medications are compli- cating the patient's GI motility.
- If possible, avoid the need for an NG tube and parenteral hydration.
  - If an NG tube becomes necessary, it is reasonable to discontinue when NG output is less than 100cc/day.
- Caution patients that emesis may occur if they drink or eat.
- A venting gastrostomy tube is an alternative when resumption of oral intake is desired.

Non-Pharmacologic Treatment

- Surgical approaches are considered the primary treatment for mechanical obstructions in patients without a malignancy causing their obstruction.
- For patients with a malignant bowel obstruction, there is no evidence of an improved out- come or survival following surgical correction.
- Conservative management of bowel obstruction is focused on decompression with NG tubes, supplemented with pharmacotherapy.
- The short-term use of NG tubes is often useful, but long-term use is difficult. Use of percuta- neous gastrostomy and jejunostomy tubes may prove to be useful.

Pharmacotherapy

- Pharmacotherapy is the cornerstone of treatment for bowel obstruction for patients with poor functional status and short life expectancy.
- For irreversible and complete bowel obstruction, a trial of an anticholinergic antispasmodic may decrease bowel contractions and provide pain relief.
- Parenteral opioids and anti-emetics should also be considered to relieve pain and nausea.
- Care should be used when using some anticholinergics, as they can lead to delirium.
- For a partial, functional bowel obstruction, a prokinetic agent may relieve nausea.
- Corticosteroids may prove useful in complete or partial bowel obstruction by reducing edema and inflammation around the obstruction.
- Often combination pharmacotherapy is necessary for symptom relief, and can decrease the need for larger doses of anticholinergic medications.
- The somatostatin analog, octeotide, has shown benefit for patients refractory to other therapies. Octreotide may be ineffective as a sole pharmacotherapy and may have improved efficacy in combination with an anticholinergic medication and/or corticosteroids.
- Other approaches may involve the use of stents to improve passage of GI contents, or use of endoscopic procedures. However, these approaches may not be appropriate for patients with a short life expectancy.

Pharmacologic Management of Bowel Obstruction

Generic Name (Brand Name)	Typical Regimen	Common Strengths and Formulations	Comments
First Line Therapy			
Hyoscyamine (Levsin)	0.25–0.5 mg IV/IM/SQ q6h prn colicky pain or 0.125–0.25 mg SL q4h PRN	**Injection:** 0.5 mg/mL **SL Tablets:** 0.125 mg **Oral Solution:** 0.125 mg/mL	• Do not exceed 12 tablets per 24 hours
Atropine	0.3–1.2 mg IV/IM/SQ/SL q4h PRN	**Injection:** 0.05 mg/mL, 0.1 mg/mL 0.4 mg/mL 0.5 mg/mL 1 mg/mL	• Can use atropine ophthalmic solution sublingually (unapproved route of administration)
Scopolamine (Transderm Scop)	Apply transdermally q72h Or 0.3–0.6 mg IV/IM/SQ q4h PRN	**Transdermal Patch:** 1.5 mg scopolamine per patch **Injection:** 0.4 mg/mL solution for injection	
Glycopyrrolate (Robinul)	0.1–0.2 mg IM/IV/SQ q6h colicky pain	**Injection:** 2 mg/mL	• Does not cross the blood-brain barrier
Metoclopramide (Reglan)	10 mg IM/IV/SQ/PR q6h N/V	**Injection:** 10 mg/mL	• Doses up to 120 mg per day have been reported to be of benefit • Discontinue if colic occurs
Haloperidol (Haldol)	0.5–2 mg IV/IM/SL/PR q6h PRN N/V	**Injection:** 5 mg/mL **Oral Solution:** 2 mg/mL	• Associated with prolongation of QT interval, especially when administered by the IV route in high doses

Dexamethasone (Decadron)	4 mg IM/IV/SQ Daily-BID N/V	Injection: 4 mg/mL	• Give over 5–10 minutes, rapid bolus associated with perianal pain
Second Line Therapy			
Octreotide (Sandostatin)	50–100 mcg IV/SQ q8h or continuous IV/SQ infusion initiated at 10–20 mcg/hr	Injection: 50 mcg/mL	• May require additional pharmacotherapy with an anticholinergic and/or steroid. Very expensive

Clinical Pearls

- Aggressively treat nausea and reduce vomiting.
- Promote effective pain relief with opioids as appropriate.
- Discontinue all stimulant laxatives.
- Consider use of a stool softener (e.g. docusate) if partial obstruction.
- Assess for delirium with anticholinergic use.
- Consider combination pharmacotherapy for complete and partial bowel obstruction. Consider adding an additional medication class if the patient has a partial response but maintains symptom problems after 2–3 doses of previous agent.

Key References

Ripamonti C, Mercadante S: How to use octreotide for malignant bowel obstruction. *J Support Oncol.* 2: 357–364, 2004.

von Gunten C and Muir, JC: Fast Facts and Concepts #45; 2nd Edition Medical Management of Bowel Obstruction August, 2005. End-of-Life Physician Education Resource Center www.eperc.mcw.edu.

Mercadante S: Assessment and management of mechanical bowel obstruction. In: Portenoy RK, Bruera E, eds.: *Topics in Palliative Care.* Volume 1. New York, NY: Oxford University Press, 1997, pp. 113–30.

Feuer DJ, Broadley KE: Systematic review and meta-analysis of corticosteroids for the resolution of malignant bowel obstruction in advanced gynaecological and gastrointestinal cancers. Systematic Review Steering Committee. *Ann Oncol.* 10: 1035–1041, 1999.

Feuer DJ, Broadley KE: Corticosteroids for the resolution of malignant bowel obstruction in advanced gynaecological and gastrointestinal cancer. *The Cochrane Database of Systematic Reviews* 1999, Issue 3.

Jatio A, Podratz KC, Gill P, Hartmann LC: Pathophysiology and Palliation of Inoperable Bowel Obstruction in Patients With Ovarian Cancer. *J Support Oncol.* 2: 323–337, 2004.

Bowel Obstruction

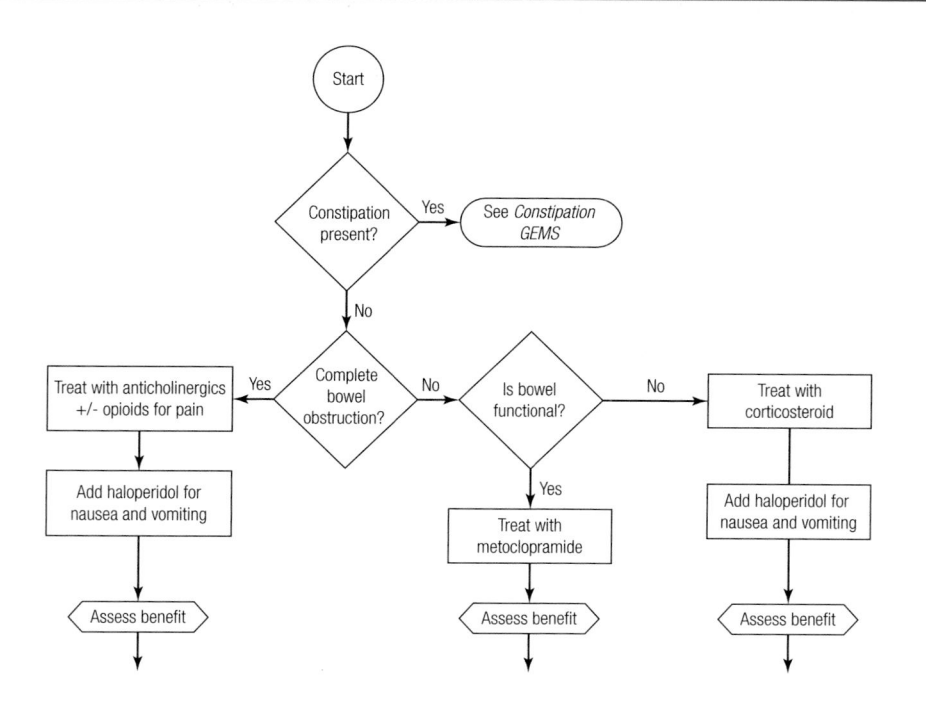

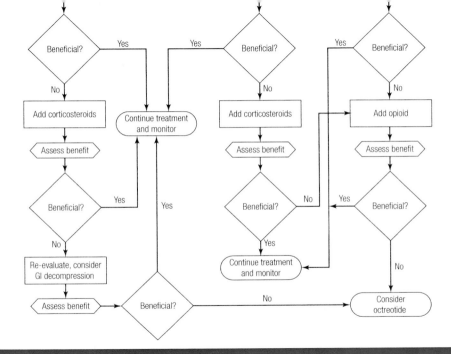

Constipation

Introduction and Background

- Constipation can be defined as the slow movement of fecal matter through the large intestine.
- This delayed elimination often results in the painful passage of dry, hard stools.
- This symptom occurs frequently in hospice and palliative care settings, especially as a result of opioid analgesic use.
- Even in the absence of opioids, constipation remains a significant issue for patients with a limited life expectancy.

Prevalence

- Constipation is a common complaint seen in healthcare settings, occurring in up to 20% of the general population.
- Rates of constipation in patients treated with maintenance opioids approach 90%.
- Recent literature suggests that approximately 50% of hospice patients without opioid pharmacotherapy have problems with constipation.

Common Causes

- Numerous factors play a role in the development and maintenance of constipation. These include:
  - Inadequate fiber intake
  - Inadequate fluid intake
  - Altered bowel habits
  - Lack of significant physical activity

- *In cancer patients*, constipation can be the result of tumor mass in the gastrointestinal tract as well as treatments related to their diagnosis.
- Additional considerations for patients at the end of life include end-organ failure, decreased mobility, and mood disturbances.
- Medication use can complicate constipation, as many drugs are associated with constipation. Consider whether reducing the dose or discontinuing medications associated with constipation is appropriate. Common offending agents include:
  - Opioid analgesics (especially codeine)
  - Nonsteroidal anti-inflammatory agents
  - Tricyclic antidepressants
  - Phenothiazines
  - Haloperidol
  - Antiparkinsonian agents
  - Diuretics
  - Calcium supplements
  - Iron supplements
  - Calcium and aluminum-containing antacids

Clinical Characteristics

- Proper assessment is essential in providing good laxative care for patients with a terminal diagnosis.
- Patients' normal bowel pattern and habits should be established, including understanding their prior and current use of laxatives.
- Care should be taken to note any changes in dietary intake (including fluids), as well as any change in physical activity.

Non-Pharmacologic Treatment

Fluid Intake

- Patients should be encouraged to increase fluid intake where appropriate and practical, assuming there are no medical contraindications.
- A goal of drinking eight 8-ounce (240 mL) glasses of fluid daily will be useful for many patients.
- Patients should be encouraged to increase their physical activity where appropriate.
- Use of warm or hot beverages 30 minutes prior to anticipated time of defecation can also be useful.

Fiber

- There are no specific fiber recommendations for patients at the end of life, but it seems reasonable to encourage consumption of foods with high fiber content.
  - Examples include fruit (apples, prunes, raisins), vegetables (broccoli, carrots, celery, squash), and whole-grain cereals, breads, and bran.
- Patients should be cautioned that increased fiber intake must be accompanied by increased fluid intake or constipation may worsen.
- High-fiber intake should be used cautiously for patients on opioid analgesics, and is contra-indicated for patients with an increased risk of bowel obstruction. This includes patients with a past history of a bowel obstruction or status-post colostomy.

Privacy

- Try to provide patients with appropriate privacy and quiet time. Bedside commodes and other appropriate assisting devices should be provided if possible.

Pharmacotherapy

The goal of pharmacotherapy should be focused on preventing constipation where possible and aggressively treating patients who have become constipated.

- Patients who require opioids to treat pain and/or dyspnea:
  - Initiate a stimulant laxative, with or without a stool softener, for all patients being initiated on an opioid regimen.
  - Alternatives could include use of osmotic laxatives such as lactulose or sorbitol.
- Patients who are not using opioids:
  - Stool softeners such as docusate (e.g. Colace) may be preferred.
  - Bulk-forming laxatives may be useful for some, but these require adequate fluid intake.
  - Bulk-forming laxatives can cause abdominal distention and early satiety.
- Patients with rectum containing hard feces:
  - Glycerin suppositories may assist with stimulating defecation. In addition to the stimulating effect, the suppositories will soften and lubricate the fecal mass allowing for easier evacuation.
  - If the patient is not using a stool softener, this should be added to their regimen.
  - If they are using a stool softener, fluid intake should be evaluated and the dose increased if appropriate.
- Patients with a full rectum containing soft feces:
  - Treat with an oral contact (stimulating) laxative (e.g. senna or bisacodyl) to stimulate bowel motility.
  - Stimulant laxatives should be added to the preventative regimen.

Pharmacologic Management of Constipation

Generic Name (Brand Name)	Typical Regimen	Routes	Common Strengths and Formulations	Comments
First Line Therapy				
Stool Softeners				
Docusate (Colace)	100–200 mg PO daily to BID	Oral	**Capsules:** 50 mg, 100 mg, 240 mg, and 250 mg	• Must be used with adequate fluid intake to maximize benefit and safety
Stimulants				
Bisacodyl (Dulcolax)	5–15 mg PO daily 10 mg daily to BID PRN	Oral Rectal	**Tablets:** 5 mg **Suppositories:** 10 mg	• May be used with stool softener • Suppositories may be poorly effective if rectum full of stool
Senna (Senokot)	2–4 tabs PO daily to BID	Oral	**Tablets:** 8.6 mg sennosides	• May be used with stool softener • Available as a combination product with docusate
Docusate Sodium + Senna (Senokot S)	1–2 PO daily to BID	Oral	**Tablets:** Docusate sodium 50 mg/senna 8.6 mg tablet	• Combination is more expensive than dosing components separately
Second Line Therapy				
Glycerin	1 PR daily to BID PRN	Rectal	**Suppository**	• For "as needed" use if hard dry stool in rectal vault
Milk of magnesia	30–60 mL PO daily to BID	Oral	**Liquid** **Tablets**	• Osmotic laxative • Associated with increased cramping and electrolyte disturbances; rapid onset (30 min to 3 hrs)
Sorbitol 70%	15–30 mL PO daily to QID	Oral	**Liquid**	• Osmotic laxative • More costly than stimulants with no improved efficacy • Associated with increased cramping and flatulence. Onset 24–48 hours

| Lactulose (Chronulac) | 30 mL PO daily to BID | Oral | **Liquid:** 10g/15 mL | • Osmotic laxative
• More costly than stimulants with no improved efficacy
• Associated with increased cramping and flatulence. Onset 24–48 hours
• More expensive than Sorbitol |
| Polyethylene glycol 3350, NF (Miralax) | 17gms in 8oz of fluid daily | Oral | **Powder** | • Osmotic laxative
• May cause nausea, bloating, cramping and flatulation
• May take 2–4 days to produce bowel movement |

Clinical Pearls

- Avoid mineral oil liquid, particularly in bedbound patients, due to high risk of aspiration.
- For high impactions, give 3–6 "Vaseline Balls" orally instead of liquid mineral oil.
  - "Vaseline Balls": Pea size frozen balls of white petrolatum rolled in powder sugar.

Key References

Fallon M, O'Neill B: ABC's of palliative care. Constipation and diarrhea. *BMJ* 315: 1293–1296, 1997 Nov 15.

Mancini I, Bruera E: Constipation in advanced cancer patients. *Support Care Cancer*. 1998;6(4):356–364.

Hallenbeck, J: Fast Facts and Concepts #15: Constipation: What makes us go. August 2005, 2nd Edition. End-of-Life Physician Education Resource Center www.eperc.mcw.edu.

Goodman mL,Wilkinson S: Laxatives for the management of constipation in palliative care patients. (Protocol) *The Cochrane Database of Systematic Reviews* 2001, Issue 4.

Sykes N: Constipation and diarrhoea. In: Doyle D, Hanks G, Cherny NI, et al, editors. *Oxford Textbook of Palliative Medicine*. 3rd edition. Oxford (UK)7 Oxford University Press; 2003. pp. 483–495.

Beckwith MC: Constipation in Palliative Care Patients. In: *Evidence Based Symptom Control in Palliative Care. Systematic Review and Validated Clinical Practice Guidelines for 15 Common Problems in Patients with Life Limiting Disease*. 1st ed. New York, NY: Pharmaceutical Products Press; 2000: pp. 47–57.

Constipation

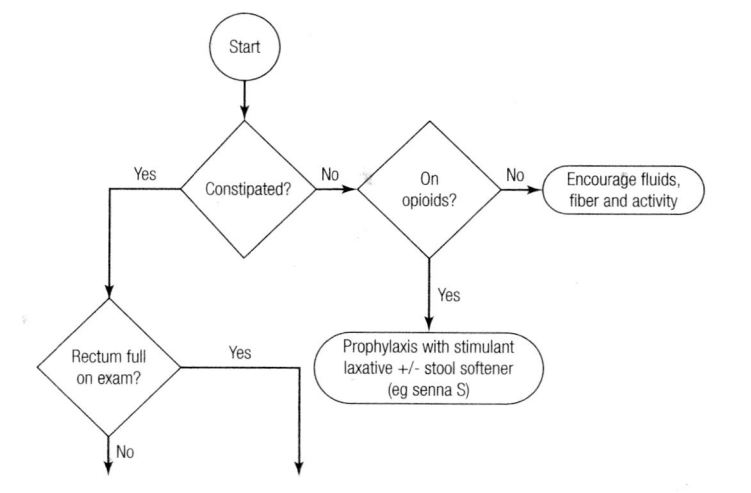

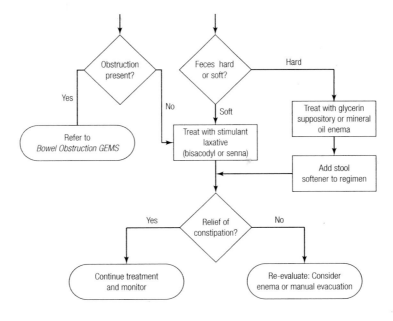

Obstruction present?
- Yes → Refer to *Bowel Obstruction GEMS*
- No →

Feces hard or soft?
- Hard → Treat with glycerin suppository or mineral oil enema → Add stool softener to regimen
- Soft → Treat with stimulant laxative (bisacodyl or senna)

Relief of constipation?
- Yes → Continue treatment and monitor
- No → Re-evaluate: Consider enema or manual evacuation

Cough

Introduction and Background

- Educate family and patient that worsening of cough is often a marker of disease progression and can be very difficult to treat.
- The goal of therapy is to improve patient comfort and decrease the cough.

Prevalence

- Cough is experienced by about 30–50% in all patients at end of life.
- In lung cancer, cough is one of the most common symptoms occurring in 47–86% of patients.

Causes

A thorough history and physical should be taken and possible reversible causes of cough should be identified and treated, if present. Some of the possible causes are:

- Heart failure
- Viral and bacterial respiratory infections
- Tuberculosis or opportunistic infections in AIDS
- Lung cancer
- Bronchospasm—albuterol (nebulizer or inhaler) or corticosteroids.
- COPD (albuterol, ipratropium, or corticosteroids)
- Pleural effusion—(confirmed by chest x-ray and treated by aspiration).
- Drugs (ACE-Inhibitors can cause cough)
- GERD (diet modifications, H2 blocker, or Proton Pump Inhibitor)

- Secretions (drying agents, such as hyoscyamine, scopolamine, or glycopyrrolate)
- Cold or post nasal drip (nasal decongestants)
- Allergies (antihistamines)
- Psychogenic cough

Clinical Characteristics

- Persistent coughing can cause anorexia, vomiting, insomnia, musculoskeletal pain, a cough fracture of a rib, exhaustion, urinary incontinence, syncope, social isolation and can lead to decreased quality of life.

Non-Pharmacologic Treatment

- Avoid smoking and second hand smoke.
- Humidified air may soothe irritated airways.
- Hard candies and lozenges can soothe throat irritation and may decrease coughing.
- Upright positioning (elevate head of bed).
- Education of family members and patient that many causes of cough are a part of disease progression such as heart failure, COPD, and lung cancer. In addition, cough is often a marker for active dying.

Pharmacotherapy

It should be determined whether the cough is productive or nonproductive.

1. Productive cough—expectorants are first line therapy (See Table 1)
2. Nonproductive "dry" cough—suppressants are first line therapy (See Table 2)

Table 1. Pharmacologic Management of Productive Cough

Generic Name (Brand Name)	Usual Adult Starting Dose/Range	Maximum Daily Dose	Common Strengths and Formulations	Comments
First Line Therapy				
Guaifenesin Immediate Release (Robitussin)	2–4 tsp PO q4h scheduled or PRN	2,400 mg/day	**Liquid:** 100 mg/5 mL	• If immediate release is effective converting to sustained release may increase adherence
Alternative				
Guaifenesin Sustained Release (Mucinex)	1–2 tablets PO q12h	2,400 mg/day	**Tablets, Extended-release (OTC):** 600 mg	• Do not crush, chew, or break tablet. Take with a full glass of water without regard to meals • Use of the extended release product, may increase adherence, if product is effective and needed around the clock
Second Line Therapy				
Nebulized Saline	Inhale 3 mL (1 vial) with nebulizer q4h scheduled or PRN	n/a	n/a	• Loosens secretions to make the cough more productive

Table 2. Pharmacologic Management of Nonproductive Cough

Generic Name (Brand Name)	Usual Adult Starting Dose/Range	Maximum Daily Dose	Common Strengths and Formulations	Comments
First Line Therapy				
Guaifenesin/Dextromethorphan Liquid (Robitussin DM)	10 mL PO q4h scheduled or PRN	60 mL/day	**Liquid:** 10 mg dextromethorphan/ 100 mg guaifenesin in 5 mL (most common strength)	• Causes fewer GI and CNS effects than opioid therapy
Hydrocodone/Homatropine Syrup or Tablets (Hycodan)	One tablet PO or 5 mL of syrup q4h scheduled or PRN	6 tablets or 30 mL in 24 hours	**Syrup or Tablets:** 5 mg hydrocodone bitartrate/1.5 mg homatropine in 5 mL	• Less constipation and less CNS effects than codeine containing preparations • If regular doses are used consider initiating a stool softener/ stimulant laxative to prevent constipation
Second Line Therapy				
Benzonatate (Tessalon Perles)	100 mg PO TID If needed, may give 100 mg PO up to q4h	600 mg/day	**Capsules:** 100 mg, 200 mg	• Swallow whole, do not crush or chew
Third Line Therapy				
Guaifenesin/Codeine Liquid (Robitussin AC)	5 to 10 mL PO q4h scheduled or PRN	60 mL per day	**Liquid:** 10 mg codeine/100 mg guaifenesin in 5 mL	• Causes more constipation and CNS side effects than hydrocodone containing preparations • If regular doses are used consider initiating a stool softener/ stimulant laxative to prevent constipation
Nebulized Lidocaine Injection	50–200 mg nebulized up to q4h PRN	200 mg/dose	**Injection:** 1%(10 mg/mL), 2% (20 mg/mL) or 4% (40 mg/mL)	• Do not eat or drink for 30 to 60 min after nebulizing lidocaine to avoid aspiration • Monitor for signs of toxicity (headache, tinnitus, facial twitches, lightheadedness, a metallic taste)

Clinical Pearls

- If the patient is being treated for pain with opioids, controlling cough may justify increasing narcotic doses, assess and reassess patient response to opioids.
- Treatment should be taken regularly (not just PRN), at appropriate intervals to maintain suppression of cough.
- Treatment should not be delayed. Patients can become 'sensitized' to prolonged coughing, making the cough more difficult to manage.

Key References

Killion K, ed. Drug Facts and Comparisons. Electronic edition. St. Louis; Facts and Comparisons, 2005, [Guaifenesin, Dextromethorphan, Benzonatate, Hycodan, Robitussin AC].

Kay P. Notes on Symptom Control in Hospice and Palliative Care. 1st edition. Machiasport, MA: Hospice Education Institute; 2004: 90–92.

Tietze KJ. Chapter 9: Disorders Related to Cold and Allergy. In: Handbook of Nonprescription Drugs. 12th edition. Washington, DC: 2000:179–190.

Leach RM. Palliative medicine and non-malignant, end-stage respiratory disease. In: Doyle D, Hankds GWC, MacDonald N, editors. Oxford Textbook of Palliative Medicine. 3rd edition. Oxford: Oxford University Press; 2003:900–901.

Irwin RS, Madison JM. The Diagnosis and Treatment of Cough. NEJM. 2000;343:1715–21.

Miller KE. Effectiveness of Guaifenesin in the Treatment of Cough. American Family Physician. 2004;July 15, 2004.

Irwin RS, Madison JM. The Persistently Troublesome Cough. Am J Respir Crit Care Med. 2002;165:1469–1474.

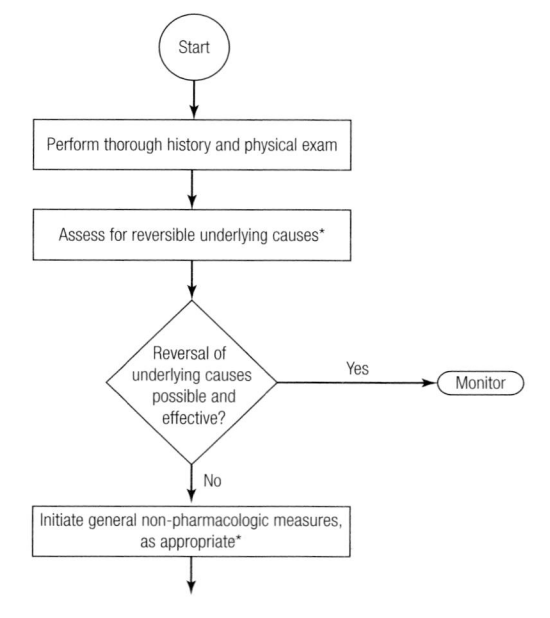

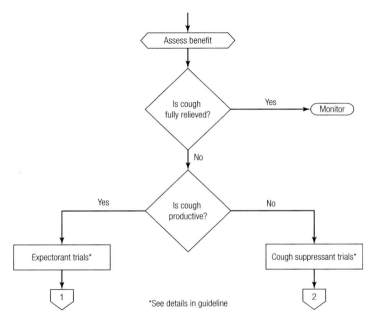

Assess benefit

Is cough fully relieved?

Yes → Monitor

No

Is cough productive?

Yes → Expectorant trials* → 1

No → Cough suppressant trials* → 2

*See details in guideline

Cough (*continued*)

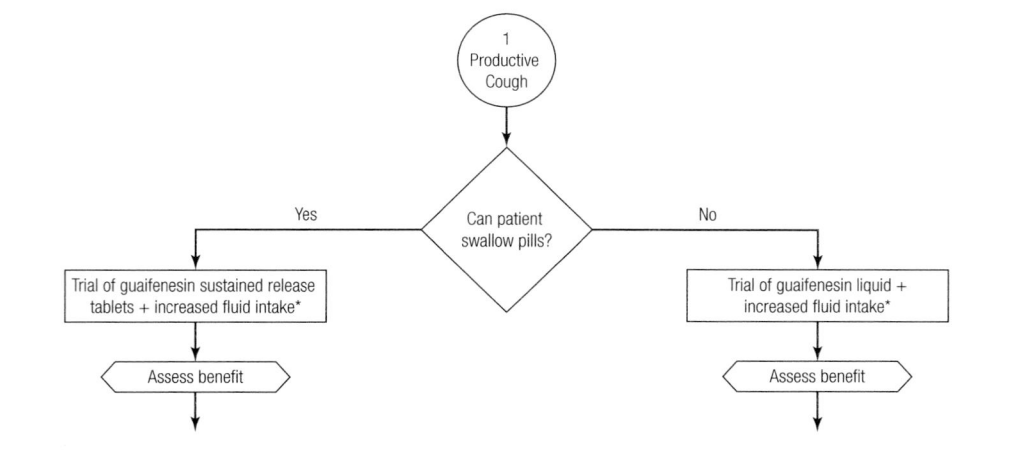

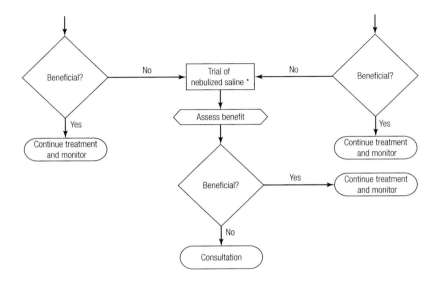

Beneficial?

No → Trial of nebulized saline *

Yes ↓
Continue treatment and monitor

Trial of nebulized saline * ← No ← Beneficial?

Beneficial? Yes ↓
Continue treatment and monitor

Assess benefit

Beneficial?

Yes → Continue treatment and monitor

No ↓
Consultation

Cough (*continued*)

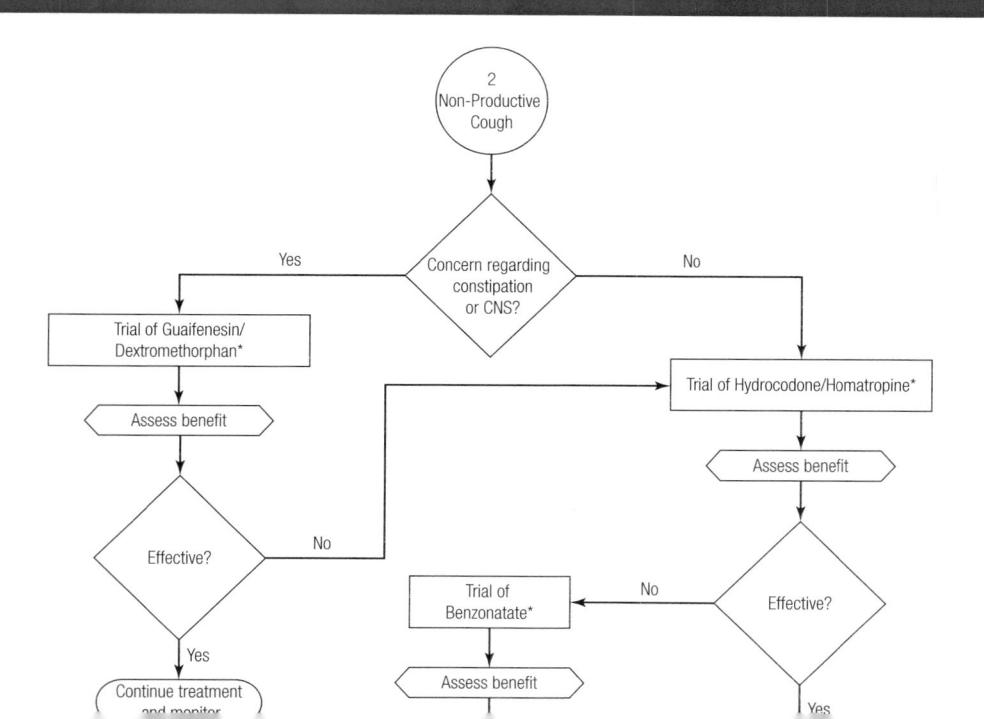

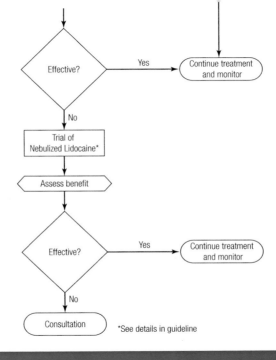

Delirium

Introduction and Background

- Delirium is a very common disorder in hospice, especially in the last few days of life.
- By definition, delirium is caused by a "general medical disorder" affecting the brain.

Prevalence

- By some estimates, more than 80% of all terminally ill patients will develop delirium prior to their death.
- The frequency with which this disorder presents and the distress it causes patients and families makes delirium a very important problem to detect and manage.

Causes

- Potential causes of delirium in the hospice setting include:
  - urinary retention
  - constipation
  - infection
  - withdrawal states
  - hypoxia
  - metabolic disturbances
  - drug side effects
- Given the advanced state of illness in this patient population, multiple causes of delirium may simultaneously coexist, adversely affecting the metabolic environment of the whole brain.

- Dopaminergic, serotonergic, and cholinergic systems are apparently involved in the pathophysiology of delirium.
- If the underlying cause or causes of the delirium can be corrected, delirium usually resolves in a matter of hours to days. Common reversible causes of delirium include:
  - urinary retention
  - constipation
  - dehydration
  - infection
  - electrolyte imbalances (e.g., hypercalcemia, hypo- or hypernatremia)
  - medication side effects (e.g., anticholinergic medications, accumulation of opiate metabolites)

Clinical Characteristics

- Classic symptoms of delirium are clouding of consciousness (including altered capacity to maintain or shift attention) and global impairment of cognitive functioning (not limited to a memory disturbance as in early dementia).
- A shift in the diurnal cycle is very common, with daytime sleepiness and nighttime agitation and restlessness ("sundowning").
- Symptoms characteristically fluctuate in severity during the course of the day (even within the course of a single hour) and from day to day.

- Delirious patients who exhibit agitation are easy to identify, but those whose cognitive disturbance leads to withdrawal and diminished responsiveness ("quiet" delirium) present a more challenging diagnosis.
- Evidence shows that both behavioral agitated and quiet subtypes of delirium respond similarly to treatment.
- If the diagnosis is in doubt and electroencephalography is available, diffuse slowing on the EEG tracing confirms the diagnosis. This procedure is seldom necessary since the diagnosis is usually apparent to careful clinical examination.

Non-Pharmacologic Treatment

- Screen for precipitants, especially reversible causes (e.g., drug side effects, pain, infection, dehydration, fecal impaction, bladder distention) and initiate measures to reverse, if possible.
- Establish a safe, soothing environment (familiar objects, photographs, and familiar music can be helpful).
- Minimize risk of injury (especially for agitated patients).
- Educate caregivers about delirium, its causes, and the plan of treatment.

Pharmacotherapy

- The most important initial step is to determine whether the goal of care is 1) to reverse the delirium and restore the patient to the best cognitive status possible or 2) to initiate palliative sedation (in the case of the actively dying patient with irreversible agitated delirium).
- If possible, reversing delirium should be pursued as this restores the patient's meaningful cognitive connection to family and others.
- Patients who are irreversibly delirious but not agitated may not require specific treatment beyond comfort measures.
- ***Treatment of delirium is an "off-label" indication for all the drugs listed in the following table.***

Pharmacologic Management of Delirium

Generic Name (Brand Name)	Usual Adult Starting Dose/Range	Routes	Common Strengths and Formulations	Comments
First Line Therapy				
Typical Neuroleptics				
Haloperidol (Haldol)	0.5–1.0 mg PO/SL/SQ/PR/IV q4–12h ATC or PRN	PO, SQ, IV, PR. SL	**Tablets:** 0.5 mg, 1 mg, 2 mg, 5 mg, 10 mg, 20 mg **Oral Concentrate:** 2 mg/mL **Injection:** 5 mg/mL	• Most commonly used and studied medication for delirium • Tablets and liquid can be used rectally and sublingually • Injection is expensive
Chlorpromazine (Thorazine)	12.5–50 mg PO/SL/PR/IM q4–8h ATC or PRN	PO, PR, SL, IM	**Tablets:** 10 mg, 25 mg, 50 mg, 100 mg, 200 mg **Injection:** 25 mg/mL **Oral Concentrate:** (100 mg/mL) must be compounded	• Especially useful if a more sedating agent is desired • Causes orthostatic hypotension
Second Line Therapy				
Atypical Neuroleptics				
Olanzapine (Zyprexa)	2.5–5 mg PO Daily	PO	**Tablets:** 2.5 mg, 5 mg, 7.5 mg, 10 mg, 15 mg, 20 mg **Orally Disintegrating Tablets:** 5 mg, 10 mg, 15 mg, 20 mg	• Expensive • Orally disintegrating tablets more expensive than conventional tablets
Quetiapine (Seroquel)	25 mg PO BID	PO	**Tablets:** 25 mg, 100 mg, 200 mg, 300 mg	• Most sedating of the atypical antipsychotics • Preferred agent in patients with Parkinson's Disease due to low incidence of extrapyramidal symptoms
Risperidone (Risperdal)	0.25–1 mg PO BID	PO	**Tablets:** 0.25 mg, 0.5 mg, 1 mg, 2 mg, 3 mg, 4 mg **Orally Disintegrating Tablets:** 0.5 mg, 1 mg, 2 mg **Oral Solution:** 1 mg/mL	• Expensive • Orally disintegrating tablets more expensive than conventional tablets

Clinical Pearls

- Start at the lower end of the dosage range of a given pharmacologic agent, but recognize that standard or higher doses may be required.
- Assess treatment response and side effects frequently.
- Clinical situations requiring antipsychotic medication doses in excess of those recommended for approved indications are unusual.
- Consider palliative or respite sedation if symptoms not controlled with optimal doses of antipsychotics.
- *In April 2005, the FDA issued a Public Health Advisory reporting an increased risk of mortality among dementia patients treated for agitation with atypical antipsychotics (listed here as Second Line treatments). It is not currently clear whether this apparent increase in mortality also applies to treatment of delirium in the setting of dementia. As of September 2006, all atypical antipsychotics carry a Black Box Warning: Patients with dementia-related behavioral disorders treated with atypical antipsychotics are at an increased risk of death compared to placebo (http://www.fda.gov/cder/drug/infopage/antipsychotics/default.htm).*

Key References

American Psychiatric Association: *Diagnostic and Statistical Manual of Mental Disorders,* 4th ed. Washington, DC: American Psychiatric Press, 1994.

Breitbart W, Cohen K: Delirium. In *Handbook of Psychiatry in Palliative Medicine.* New York: Oxford University Press, 2000, pp. 75–79.

Breitbart W, Marotta R, Platt MM, et al: A double-blind trial of haloperidol, chlorpromazine, and lorazepam in the treatment of delirium in hospitalized AIDS patients. Am J Psychiatry. 1996;153:231–237.

Fainsinger R, MacEachern T, Hanson J, et al: Symptom control during the last week of life on a palliative care unit. *J Palliat Care.* 1991;7:5–11.

Stiefel F, Fainsinger R, Bruera E: Acute confusional states in patients with advanced cancer. *J Pain Symptom Manage.* 1992; 7:94–98.

Shuster JL: Confusion, agitation, and delirium at the end of life. *Journal of Palliative Medicine.* 1998;1:177–186.

Delirium

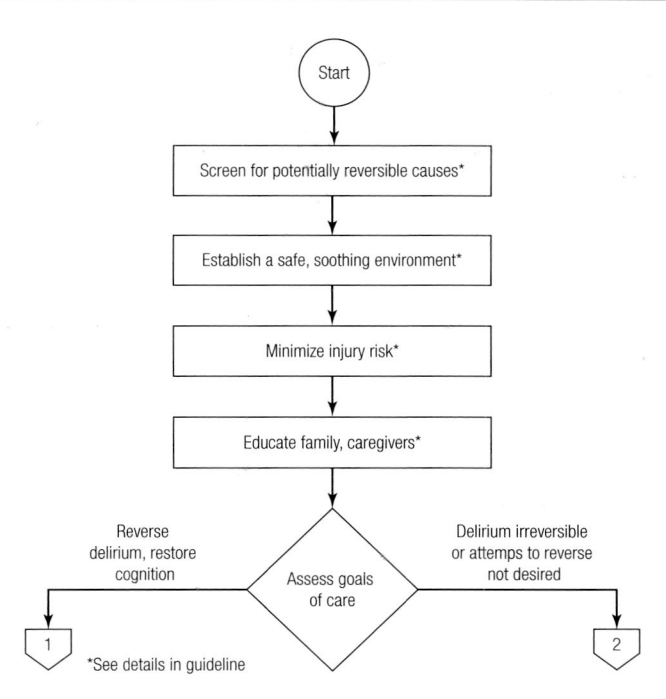

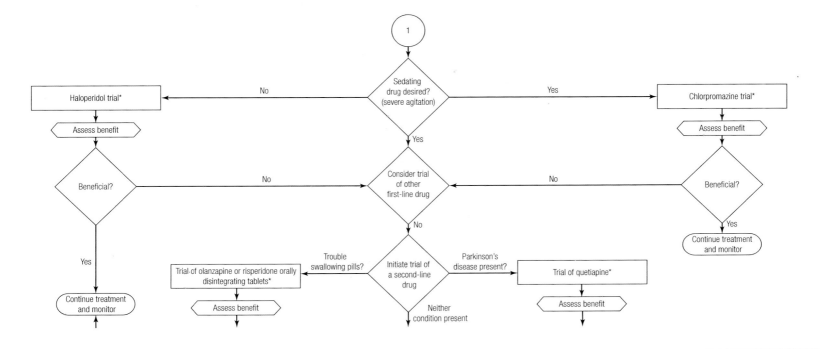

1

Sedating drug desired? (severe agitation)

No → Haloperidol trial*
Assess benefit
Beneficial?
No → Consider trial of other first-line drug
Yes → Continue treatment and monitor

Yes → Chlorpromazine trial*
Assess benefit
Beneficial?
No → Consider trial of other first-line drug
Yes → Continue treatment and monitor

Yes → Consider trial of other first-line drug

No → Initiate trial of a second-line drug

Trouble swallowing pills? → Trial of olanzapine or risperidone orally disintegrating tablets*
Assess benefit

Parkinson's disease present? → Trial of quetiapine*
Assess benefit

Neither condition present

Delirium (*continued*)

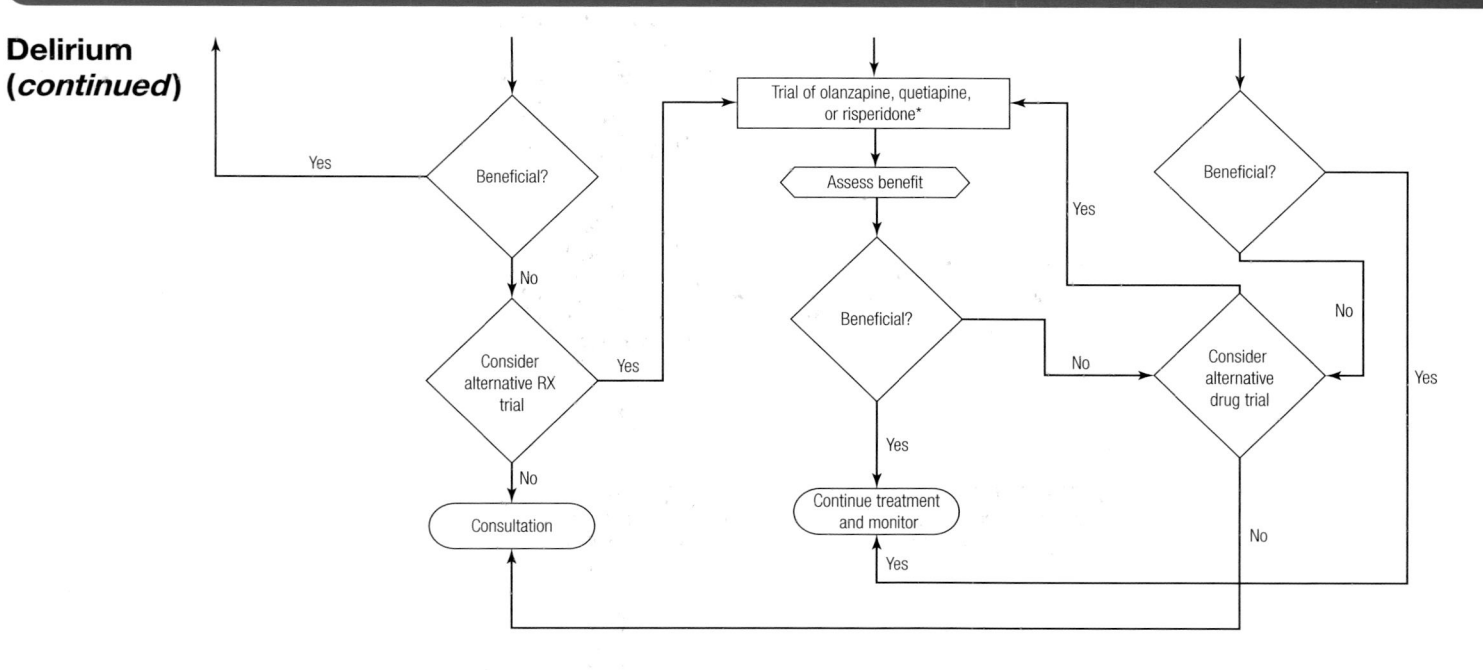

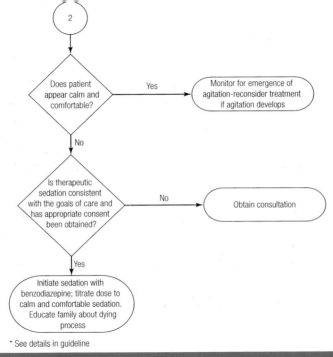

2

Does patient appear calm and comfortable?

Yes → Monitor for emergence of agitation-reconsider treatment if agitation develops

No

Is therapeutic sedation consistent with the goals of care and has appropriate consent been obtained?

No → Obtain consultation

Yes

Initiate sedation with benzodiazepine; titrate dose to calm and comfortable sedation. Educate family about dying process

* See details in guideline

Depression

Introduction and Background

- Periods of discouragement, sadness, or distress are understandable as patients adapt to a life-limiting or terminal illness. Elisabeth Kubler-Ross referred to this as the "depression" stage of grief and adaptation to loss.
- It is easy to confuse transient period of adaptation with clinical depression, characterized by a pervasive low mood, loss of interest, and despair.
- Clinical depression is properly viewed as a complication of serious illness-NEVER as a normal phase of adaptation.
- Depression is common in hospice patients and too often goes unrecognized and untreated.
- Depression is commonly associated with requests for hastened or assisted death.
- A palliative approach to treatment of depression, aimed at reducing the burden of suffering, is most reasonable.
- Effective treatment of depression will relieve suffering and enhance quality of life at the end of life.

Prevalence

- The prevalence of clinical depression in the hospice setting has been estimated at between 20% and 50%.

Causes

- Depressive disorders (e.g., Major Depressive Disorder, Dysthymia) tend to be recurrent or chronic.
- Other conditions which can cause, mimic, or exacerbate depression include anger, anxiety, delirium (of the "quiet" variety), early stages of dementia, discouragement, emotional numbing in reaction to a sudden loss or bad news, fear (particularly the fear of death), grief, interpersonal problems, a perceived loss of control over one's life situation, pain or other undertreated symptoms, or spiritual crisis.
- Some people have a pessimistic or withdrawn coping style. If this is the case, it should be characteristic of the person over the course of their lifetime and not a new pattern of behavior.

Clinical Characteristics

- The clinical features of a depressive episode include:
  - Depressed or sad mood most of the time
  - Sleep disturbance (typically early morning awakening)
  - Pervasive loss of interest or libido
  - Feelings of guilt, hopelessness, worthlessness
  - Lack of energy
  - Concentration problems
  - Appetite disturbance (typically appetite reduction with weight loss)
  - Psychomotor retardation or agitation
  - Pervasive thoughts of death or suicide

- A major depressive episode is characterized by the presence of five or more of these nine criteria (including either depressed mood or loss of interest) for at least two weeks.
- Some of these criteria could result from serious physical disease itself.
- Diagnostic confidence is increased by the presence of one or more of the following:
  - Marked anhedonia
  - Hopelessness
  - Helplessness
  - Worthlessness
  - Pervasive guilt
  - Feeling of being punished (particularly a feeling that disease itself is a punishment)
  - Suicidal ideation
  - Intense, morbid ruminations
  - Frequent tearfulness
  - Self-loathing
- Hopelessness is a particularly important indicator because of its strong association with suicidal ideation and suicide attempts.
- Always inquire about the presence of suicidal thoughts and suicidal intent in a patient with signs or symptoms of depression.
- Untreated depression not only causes prolonged suffering but places the patient at risk for a prolonged or chronic depressive episode.

- A clinical depressive episode in a hospice patient is unlikely to resolve spontaneously, so failure to recognize and treat a depression almost certainly means the patient will suffer with depression throughout his or her remaining days.

Non-Pharmacologic Treatment
- Overall goals of care for depression in hospice care are symptom reduction, social support, and the maintenance of morale.
- Treatment of depression preserves patient dignity, helps to maintain hope and meaning, and demonstrates a commitment to non-abandonment.
- Concurrent management of co-morbid physical symptoms and preservation or repair of important relationships can help reduce the severity of depression.
- General clinical approach to depression includes:
  - Assess for any history of previous depressive episodes, including family history of depression (and response to treatment).
  - Assess temporal correlation of depression onset or changes in severity to changes in general medical condition, treatment.
  - Assess substance abuse history.
  - Assess for presence of formal depressive disorders.
  - Search for factors which may complicate depression in the medically ill patient.
  - Don't be taken in by the myth of "appropriate depression" (remember, it's a complication).
  - Address any underlying general medical causes or complicating factors.

- Treatment for depression should be started when the patient meets criteria for a depressive episode.
- In the hospice and palliative care setting, a more pragmatic treatment threshold should be considered; when depressed or sad mood interferes with the patient's quality of life.
- Hospice clinicians should be willing to palliate suffering from depression.
- Psychotherapies, particularly cognitive psychotherapy and interpersonal psychotherapy, have been shown to be effective in the treatment of depression. However, the availability of trained therapists willing to make home visits, and the limited stamina and attention span of seriously ill patients typically make such therapies impractical in the hospice setting.
- Other non-pharmacologic therapies for depression include light therapy, electroconvulsive therapy (ECT), and combinations of therapies, though these interventions should be undertaken in consultation with and under the supervision of a psychiatrist.
- When an underlying cause of depression can be identified, treatment is initially aimed at the precipitating problem, with monitoring to see if depression improves or resolves as the underlying cause is addressed.
- Whenever possible, psychosocial and spiritual support of the patient should be provided by the appropriate team members in conjunction with pharmacotherapy for the treatment of depression.

Pharmacotherapy

- In most cases, management of depression in the hospice setting involves pharmacologic therapies.
- With antidepressants (other than stimulants), mood improves gradually with treatment. Insomnia may respond early (especially if sedating drug is selected). Low energy is often the symptom which persists longest. Full resolution of depressive symptoms may take longer than a few weeks.
- The goal of treatment is full resolution of symptoms and symptoms typically resolve gradually over several weeks with treatment. The same symptoms used for diagnosis are used to monitor response. Treat (and adjust dose or change therapy) until target symptoms have fully resolved and the patient's mood feels "back to normal."
- The standard recommendation for maintenance treatment for depression is an additional 16–20 weeks after achievement of full remission (a longer period is more conservative) prior to considering discontinuation. Given the prognosis of a patient eligible for hospice care, this is essentially a recommendation for lifetime maintenance for an effective and well-tolerated antidepressant treatment for hospice patients. If a decision is made to discontinue an antidepressant that has reached steady state concentration, a gradual taper over a several days to a few weeks minimizes the risk of depressive relapse.
- The FDA has required a boxed warning on labeling and in prescribing information for all antidepressants regarding the increased risk of suicidal thoughts and suicide among children, adolescents, and young adults prescribed antidepressant drugs. Data for same risk of antidepressant use among older adults is under review. Always monitor depressed patients for the emergence of suicidal ideation or intent.

Pharmacologic Management of Depression

Generic Name (Brand Name)	Usual Adult Starting Dose/Range	Routes	Common Strengths and Formulations	Comments
First Line Therapy				
Psychostimulants				
Dextroamphetamine (Dexedrine)	2.5–5.0 mg qAM (MDD: 20 mg qAM)	PO	**Tablets:** 10 mg, 5 mg	• (ALL DRUGS IN CLASS) Depression is an off-label indication • (ALL DRUGS IN CLASS) Drugs of choice in hospice (among patients who can tolerate stimulants) due to no lag time to effect • (ALL DRUGS IN CLASS) Counteract opiate-induced sedation • (ALL DRUGS IN CLASS) Exhibit synergistic analgesia with opiates • (ALL DRUGS IN CLASS) May worsen/precipitate delirium • (ALL DRUGS IN CLASS) Dose-related side effects include insomnia, hypertension, tachycardia, restlessness, hallucinations • (ALL DRUGS IN CLASS) May induce tolerance, withdrawal depression with prolonged use • Schedule II Controlled Substance
Methylphenidate (Ritalin)	2.5–5.0 mg BID (AM and noon) (MDD: 20 mg BID; AM and noon)	PO	**Tablets:** 5 mg, 10 mg, 20 mg **Solution:** 10 mg/5 mL, 5 mg/5 mL	• Frequently requires twice daily dosing • Schedule II Controlled Substance
First Line Therapy				
Serotonin Reuptake Inhibitors				
Citalopram (Celexa)	20 mg Usual therapeutic dose range: 40–60 mg	PO	**Tablets:** 10 mg, 20 mg, 40 mg **Solution:** 10 mg/5 mL	• (ALL DRUGS IN CLASS) May be especially useful if expected survival exceeds a few weeks. • (ALL DRUGS IN CLASS) Read prescribing information for Cytochrome P–450 system mediated drug interactions • (ALL DRUGS IN CLASS) Not constipating; low liability for precipitating delirium • (ALL DRUGS IN CLASS) Side effects (mostly dose-related) include GI upset, insomnia, headache, jitteriness, sexual dysfunction

Generic Name (Brand Name)	Usual Adult Starting Dose/Range	Routes	Common Strengths and Formulations	Comments
First Line Therapy				
Serotonin Reuptake Inhibitors (*continued*)				
Escitalopram (Lexapro)	5–10 mg Usual therapeutic dose range: 10–20 mg	PO	**Tablets:** 5 mg, 10 mg, 20 mg **Liquid:** 5 mg/5 mL	• Reliability of reputed faster onset of action unclear
Fluoxetine (Prozac)	10–20 mg Usual therapeutic dose range: 20–40 mg	PO	**Tablets/Capsules:** 10 mg, 20 mg, 40 mg **Solution:** 20 mg/5 mL	• Longest half-life (by far) of the drugs in this class • Least expensive SSRI
Sertraline (Zoloft)	25–50 mg Usual therapeutic dose range: 100–200 mg	PO	**Tablets:** 25 mg, 50 mg, 100 mg **Solution:** 20 mg/mL	• Solution is expensive
Second Line Therapy: Serotonin Reuptake Inhibitors				
Paroxetine (Paxil)	10 mg Usual therapeutic dose range: 20–40 mg	PO	**Tablets:** 10 mg, 20 mg, 30 mg, 40 mg **Suspension:** 10 mg/5 mL	• Highest incidence of anticholinergic side effects • Shortest half-life, withdrawal symptoms can occur with missed doses • Suspension and CR formulation expensive
Second Line Therapy				
Miscellaneous Antidepressants				
Mirtazapine (Remeron)	7.5–15 mg qHS Usual therapeutic dose range: 15–30 mg	PO	**Tablets:** 7.5 mg, 15 mg, 30 mg, 45 mg **Orally Disintegrating Tablets:** 15 mg, 30 mg, 45 mg	• Enhances central 5HT and NE • Histamine (H1) antagonist–sedation in doses 15 mg or less • 5HT2 antagonist-appetite stimulation • 5HT3 antagonist–antiemetic
Venlafaxine SR (Effexor SR)	37.5–75 mg daily (MDD: 225 mg daily)	PO	**Extended Release Capsule:** 37.5 mg, 75 mg, 150 mg	• Mixed serotonin and norepinephrine reuptake inhibitor • Can cause hypertension • Requires divided dosing • Some evidence that it reduces neuropathic pain at higher doses • Withdrawal symptoms can occur with missed doses

Second Line Therapy				
Tricyclic Antidepressants				
Desipramine (Norpramin)	12.5–50 mg Usual therapeutic dose range: 100–200 mg	PO	**Tablets:** 10 mg, 25 mg, 50 mg, 75 mg, 100 mg, 150 mg	• (ALL DRUGS IN CLASS) Greater side-effect burden compared to SSRIs: anticholinergic, sedation, tachycardia, arrhythmias, constipation, orthostasis • (ALL DRUGS IN CLASS) Effective for neuropathic pain • (ALL DRUGS IN CLASS) Can be used to stimulate appetite • Desipramine is the least sedating tricyclic
Nortriptyline (Pamelor)	10–25 mg Usual therapeutic dose range: 75–150 mg	PO	**Capsules:** 10 mg, 25 mg, 50 mg, 75 mg **Solution:** 10 mg/5 mL	• Nortriptyline is the least likely tricyclic to cause orthostasis

Psychostimulant Treatment Protocol (for use with Methylphenidate, Dextroamphetamine):

1. Begin with Starting Dose
2. Check response daily (1-2 hours after dose)
3. Raise dose daily by smallest increments until one of the following occurs:
   a. Resolution of depression
   b. Emergence of side effects
   c. "High" dose approached or exceeded

Clinical Pearls

- Any given antidepressant drug trial has about a 50–80% chance of being effective. Serial drug trials are often required to find effective, well-tolerated medication treatment for depression.
- The choice of initial antidepressant therapy should be guided by the following considerations:
   - Does the patient have a personal history of beneficial response to a particular drug? (This is the strongest and most reliable predictor of drug treatment response).
   - Does the patient have a family history of beneficial response to a particular drug? (This is the second strongest predictor of drug treatment response).
   - What is the side effect profile of the drug and are any of the typical side effects potentially beneficial for the patient (e.g., appetite stimulation commonly seen with mirtazapine or tricyclic antidepressants in a patient with anorexia and weight loss).

- What is the patient's anticipated prognosis?
- What is the cost of this drug compared to comparable alternatives?
- Generally, given the typically short survival from hospice admission to death (measured in days to weeks) and the rapid onset of action of psychostimulants for depression, stimulants are the drugs of choice for depression in hospice, but there are exceptions. Situations where one might choose a standard antidepressant over a psychostimulant include:
  - When the patient is unable to tolerate stimulants.
  - When the patient has a history of poor response to stimulants.
  - When the patient has a history of vigorous response to standard antidepressants.
  - When the patient has a relatively long life expectancy.
  - When there are other therapeutic benefits to be gained from standard antidepressant therapy (e.g., analgesic effects for neuropathic pain).
- The most common causes of antidepressant non-response are:
  - Inadequate dose
  - Insufficient duration of therapy
  - Nonadherence to treatment
  - Comorbid substance use
  - Misdiagnosis
- If a patient has a suboptimal treatment response, do the following (in this order):
  - If below the recommended therapeutic dose range, consider a dose increase.
  - If within the recommended therapeutic dose range, consider waiting 6–8 weeks while maintaining the current dose (if patient safety allows).
  - Consider changing antidepressants (probably to a drug in a different class).
  - Consider obtaining psychiatric consultation for combination or augmentation therapies.
- Unopposed antidepressants (i.e., antidepressants used without concurrent therapy with a mood stabilizer) risk precipitating mania in patients with a history of bipolar disorder. Always ask about a personal or family history of mania or bipolar disorder before starting a new antidepressant treatment trial.

Key References

American Psychiatric Association: Practice Guideline for the Treatment of Patients With Major Depressive Disorder. http://www.psych.org/psych_pract/treatg/pg/prac_guide.cfm.

Breitbart W, Bruera E, Chochinov H, Lynch M. Neuropsychiatric syndromes and psychological symptoms in patients with advanced cancer. *J Pain Symptom Manage*. 1995;10: 131–141.

Chochinov HM, Wilson KG, Enns M, Lander S: "Are you depressed?" Screening for depression in the terminally ill. *Am J Psychiatry*. 154: 674–6, 1997.

Chochinov HM, Breitbart W: *Handbook of Psychiatry in Palliative Medicine*. New York: Oxford University Press, 2000.

Masand PS, Tesar GE: Use of stimulants in the medically ill. *Psychiatr Clin North Am*. 19: 515–547, 1996.

Rodin, G., Craven, J., Littlefield, C: *Depression in the Medically Ill: An Integrated Approach*. New York: Mazel, 1991.

Shuster JL, Breitbart W, Chochinov HM: Psychiatric aspects of excellent end-of-life care. *Psychosomatics*, 40:1, 1–4, 1999.

Shuster JL, Chochinov HM, Greenberg DB: Psychiatric aspects and pharmacologic strategies in palliative care. In: Stoudemire A, Fogel BS, Greenberg DB: *Psychiatric Care of the Medical Patient*, 2nd Ed. New York: Oxford University Press, 2000, pp. 315–328.

Shuster JL: Can depression be a terminal illness? *Journal of Palliative Medicine*. 3: 493–495, 2000.

Depression

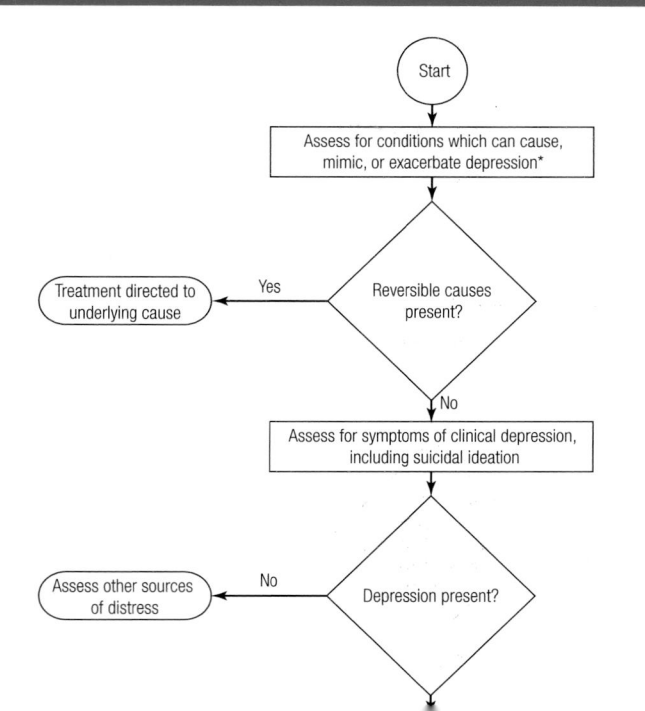

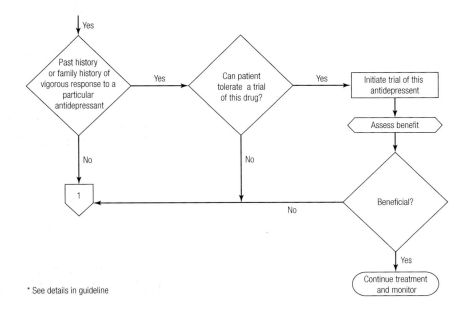

* See details in guideline

Depression (*continued*)

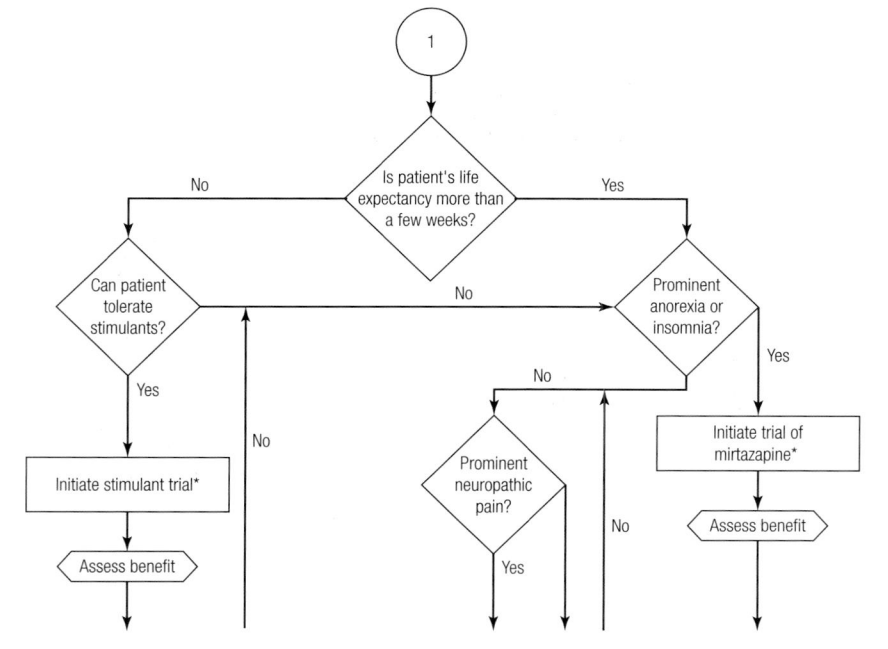

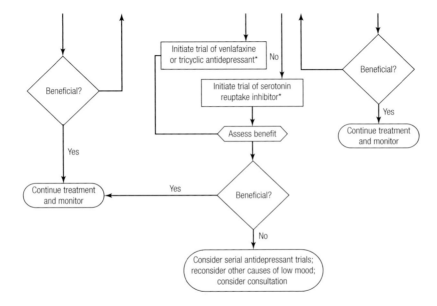

Initiate trial of venlafaxine
or tricyclic antidepressant*

No

Beneficial?

Initiate trial of serotonin
reuptake inhibitor*

Beneficial?

Yes

Continue treatment
and monitor

Assess benefit

Beneficial?

Yes

Yes

Continue treatment
and monitor

Beneficial?

Yes

Continue treatment
and monitor

No

Consider serial antidepressant trials;
reconsider other causes of low mood;
consider consultation

Diarrhea

Introduction and Background

- Diarrhea results from an imbalance of the absorption and secretion properties of the intestinal tract. The imbalance may be from decreased absorption or increased secretion.
- Diarrhea may be an acute or chronic problem.
- Investigation is warranted in order to treat the cause of the diarrhea.

Prevalence

- Diarrhea will occur in most people at some time or another. Most cases are acute and will resolve by themselves.
- Diarrhea is not common in terminally ill people, affecting less than 10%.

Causes

- Overmedication with laxatives seems to be the most common cause of diarrhea in palliative medicine.
- Cause of diarrhea directs the course of treatment:
  - Tumor-related (e.g., Carcinoid syndrome, colon cancer, lymphoma, pancreatic cancer, etc.)
  - Surgery-related or procedure-related (e.g., celiac plexus block, cholecystectomy, intestinal resection, etc.)
  - Chemotherapy-related (e.g., capecitabine, cisplatin, taxels, methotrexate, VEGFR blockers)
  - Radiation therapy–related (e.g., irradiation to the abdomen, para-aortic, lumbar, or pelvic areas)
  - Bone marrow transplantation–related (e.g., conditioning chemotherapy, total-body irradiation, graft-versus-host disease after allogeneic bone marrow or peripheral blood stem cell transplants)
  - Drug adverse effects (e.g., antibiotics-especially broad spectrum, magnesium-containing antacids, antihypertensives, fibrates, colchicine, digoxin, metoclopramide, etc.)
  - Concurrent disease (e.g., diabetes, hyperthyroidism, inflammatory bowel diseases, etc.)
  - Infection (e.g., *Clostridium species, Bacillus cereus, Giardia lamblia, Cryptosporidium, Salmonella, Shigella, Campylobacter, Rotavirus*)
  - Fecal (constipation leading to obstruction with leakage of loose stool around the obstruction)
  - Diet (e.g., Lactose intolerance, caffeine-containing products, fruit juices, high-fiber, high-fat foods, sorbitol-containing foods, spicy foods, gas-forming foods and beverages)
  - Psychological (e.g., stress, anxiety, factitious disorders, or malingering)

Clinical Characteristics

- Diarrhea can be defined as the passage of frequent loose stools with urgency. However, the definition of "frequency" is specific to the patient.
- Diarrhea may also be objectively defined as more than 200 mL of water in the stool (more than 90% water).

- It is often accompanied by gas, abdominal pain, an urgency to defecate, as well as nausea and vomiting.
- If diarrhea is accompanied by fever, occult blood, steatorrhea, appetite changes, weight loss, or tenesmus (painful, ineffective straining to defecate), these may be signs of a more serious underlying condition.
- Diarrhea may be classified into four general types, based on mechanism:
  - *Osmotic* diarrhea may be caused by a non-absorbed substance that draws fluid into the intestinal lumen. This may occur with disorders such as pancreatitis, bile duct obstruction, celiac disease, or Whipple's disease. It may also occur with ingestion of certain sweeteners or lactose intolerance.
  - *Secretory* diarrhea may be caused by bacterial toxins, viruses, and some drugs inducing intestinal secretions. 90% of acute diarrhea is caused by infection and is often accompanied by vomiting, fever and abdominal pain. Other causes include chronic alcohol ingestion, carcinoid tumor, Addison's disease, bowel resection or fistula and partial bowel obstruction or impaction.
  - *Exudative or Inflammatory* diarrhea may result from inflammation causing plasma proteins, mucus, and blood to appear in stool. It is usually accompanied by fever, pain and other manifestations of inflammation.
  - *Motility* disorders such as diabetic neuropathy, hyperthyroidism, or irritable bowel syndrome may cause decreased absorption.
- In terminal patients who are immobile and on opioid drugs, watery diarrhea may be a sign of impaction.

Non-Pharmacologic Treatment
- Temporarily stop laxative use. If diarrhea resolves, laxative may be restarted at a lower dose.
- For mild cases of diarrhea, the BRAT (bananas, rice, apples, toast) diet may reduce the frequency of stools.
- Eat small, frequent meals containing foods that are low in fiber, contain minerals, and do not stimulate or irritate the gastrointestinal tract.
- Avoid offending foods, including lactose-containing food (milk and dairy products), spicy foods, alcohol, caffeine-containing foods and beverages, certain fruit juices, gas-forming foods and beverages, high-fiber foods, and high-fat foods.
- Rehydrate the patient and replace electrolytes. Increase clear liquid intake to at least 3 liters per day (e.g., water, sports drinks, broth, weak decaffeinated teas, caffeine-free soft drinks, clear juices, and gelatin).

Pharmacologic Management of Diarrhea

Generic Name (Brand Name)	Usual Adult Starting Dose/Range	Routes	Common Strengths and Formulations	Comments
General Symptom Management: Decrease Motility				
First Line Therapy: Anti-motility Agents				
Diphenoxylate with atropine (Lomotil)	2 tablets, then 1 tablet after each loose stool (MDD: 8 per 24 hrs)	PO	**Solution:** 2.5 mg/5 mL **Tablets:** 2.5 mg	• Not recommended in patients with bacterial diarrhea
Loperamide (Immodium AD, Kaopectate II, Maalox Antidiarrheal, Pepto Diarrhea Control)	2 tablets, then 1 tablet after each loose stool (MDD: 8 per 24 hrs)	PO	**Tablets/Capsules:** 2 mg **Solution:** 1 mg/5 mL	• Not recommended in patients with bacterial diarrhea
Second Line Therapy: Anti-motility Agents				
Paregoric	5–10 mL QD-QID	PO	**Solution:** 2 mg/5 mL	• Not recommended in patients with bacterial diarrhea
Codeine	10–60 mg BID-QID	PO, IM, SQ	**Tablets:** 15, 30, 60 mg **Solution:** 15 mg/mL **Injection:** 15, 30 mg/mL	• Not recommended in patients with bacterial diarrhea • Acetaminophen with codeine may be used instead of pure codeine, for cost and ease of prescribing
First Line Therapy: Absorbents and Adsorbents				
Bismuth subsalicylate (Pepto-Bismol, Kaopectate, Maalox Total Stomach Relief)	2 tablets (or 30 mL) every 30 min to 1 hr, (MDD: 8 doses per 24 hrs)	PO	**Tablets:** Bismuth subsalicylate 262 mg **Suspension:** Bismuth subsalicylate 262 mg/15 mL	• Caution with concomitant aspirin; impaction may occur in debilitated patients • May turn stool dark or black in color • Do not use in immuno-compromised patients due to risk of bismuth encephalopathy

Bulking Loose/Watery Stool

First Line Therapy: Bulking Agents

Psyllium (Metamucil, Fiberall)	1 dose up to TID; may be followed with water	PO	**Tablets:** 4 tablets/dose **Powder:** 1 tbsp powder/ dose **Wafers:** 2 wafers/dose	• Separate drug administration times with other medication due to decreased absorption • Use with caution in dehydrated patients; must take with water
Methylcellulose (Citrucel, FiberEase)	2–4 caplets or 5–10 tsp 1 to 3 times daily	PO	**Caplets:** 500 mg **Powder**	• Use with caution in dehydrated patients; must take with water
Calcium Polycarbophil (FiberCon, Equalactin, Phillips' Fibercaps)	2 tablets (1 gm) QD-QID (MDD: 6 gm per 24 hrs)	PO	**Caplet/Tablets:** calcium polycarbophil 625 mg (equivalent to 500 mg polycarbophil)	• Epigastric pain and bloating may occur with large doses • Use with caution in dehydrated patients; must take with water

Second Line Therapy: Bulking Agents

Cholestyramine (Questran)	Use 1 packet (4 gms) QD	PO	**Powder:** 4 gm packets for reconstitution	• Effective in controlling chologenic (bile salt) or radiation-induced diarrhea

Infection

First Line Therapy: Antibiotics

Metronidazole (Flagyl)	250–500 mg TID-QID for 10 –14 days	PO, IV	**Tablets:** 250 mg, 500 mg **Suspension:** Can make extemporaneously	• Drug of choice for *C.difficile* & *Giardia* infection • May be used empirically if diarrhea follows course of antibiotics

Second Line Therapy: Antibiotics

Vancomycin (Vancocin)	125 mg QID for 10 days	PO	**Capsules:** 125 mg **Solution:** Can make extemporaneously	• PO only, IV ineffective • Very expensive–2nd line if metronidazole ineffective • Resistance occurs quickly to enterococcus • Solution: Add 20 mL sterile water to 1 g powder vial. Give 2.5 mL PO QID for 10 days

Generic Name (Brand Name)	Usual Adult Starting Dose/Range	Routes	Common Strengths and Formulations	Comments
Carcinoid Syndrome				
First Line Therapy: Carcinoid Syndrome				
Cyproheptadine (Periactin)	4 mg TID	PO	**Tablets:** 4 mg	• 12–48 mg/day in divided doses
Second Line Therapy: Carcinoid Syndrome				
Octreotide (Sandostatin)	50 mcg BID-TID titrating up as needed (mean daily dosage is 300 mcg)	IV, SQ	**Ampules:** 50, 100, 500 mcg (as acetate) **Multi-dose Vials:** 200 and 1000 mcg/mL	• For severe intractable diarrhea from carcinoid tumors • Very expensive
Steatorrhea/Pancreatic Insufficiency				
Steatorrhea				
Pancrelipase (Multiple brands)	30,000 IU pancreatic lipase with each meal	PO	**Tablets:** various strengths	• Fatty stool from pancreatic insufficiency • +/− H2 Blocker or PPI

Clinical Pearls

- Choice of agent should be individualized according to the patient's history and the primary cause of the diarrhea, if possible. Questions may be asked in order to recommend appropriate therapy:
  - When did the diarrhea begin?
  - How frequent are the episodes?
  - Are there any other symptoms that may be related to the diarrhea?
  - Have any anti-diarrheal medications been used?
  - Has the diet been altered?
  - Are there any other persons that have had diarrhea that have contact with the patient?

- What are the medications the patient is taking?
- Are there any related co-morbidities?
- Be aware of nausea associated with diarrhea or foul-smelling diarrhea, which may indicate an infectious process or toxic substance.
- Empiric treatment with metronidazole is indicated if watery, foul-smelling diarrhea is present along with any risk factors for C. difficile infection (recent hospitalization, advanced age, immunosuppression, recent or repeated use of antibiotics, especially broad-spectrum antibiotics).
- Stool studies may need to be done to determine if there are cells, mucus, fat, or blood in the stool.

Key References

Gastrointestinal Complications (PDQ®) Health Professional Version http://www.cancer.gov/cancertopics/pdq/supportivecare/gastrointestinalcomplications/healthprofessional. Accessed 3/25/06.

Sykes, N, In: *Oxford Textbook Palliative Medicine,* 3rd ed. New York: Oxford. University Press. 2005, pp. 490–496.

Ahlquist DA Camilleri M, In: Harrison's Principles of Internal Medicine, 16th Ed. New York: McGraw-Hill Medical Publishing. 2005, pp. 224–230.

Horne JS, Swanson LN: Diarrhea. *US Pharmacist.* http://www.uspharmacist.com. Accessed 3/27/06.

Jackson Gastroenterology. Diarrhea. http://www.gicare.com. Accessed 3/17/06.

Palliative care and hospice. http://www.healthinaging.org. Accessed 3/17/06.

Merck Manual Home Edition. Digestive Disorders: Diarrhea. http://www.merck.com. Accessed 3/17/06.

Diarrhea

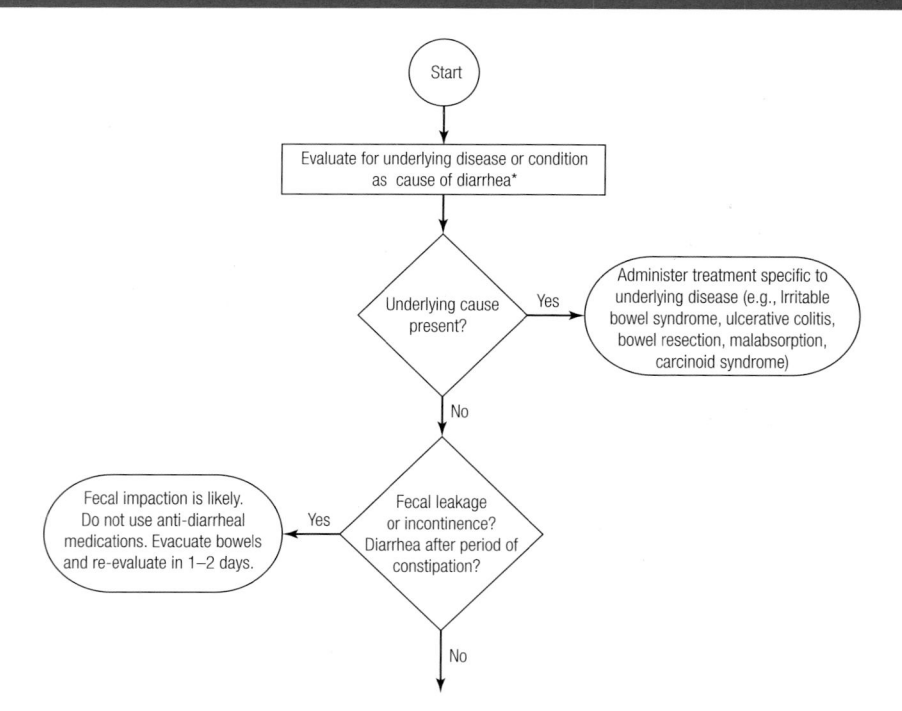

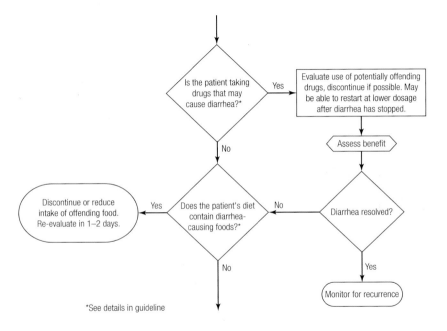

Is the patient taking drugs that may cause diarrhea?*

Yes → Evaluate use of potentially offending drugs, discontinue if possible. May be able to restart at lower dosage after diarrhea has stopped.

Assess benefit

No

Diarrhea resolved?

Yes → Monitor for recurrence

No → Does the patient's diet contain diarrhea-causing foods?*

Yes → Discontinue or reduce intake of offending food. Re-evaluate in 1–2 days.

No

*See details in guideline

Diarrhea (*continued*)

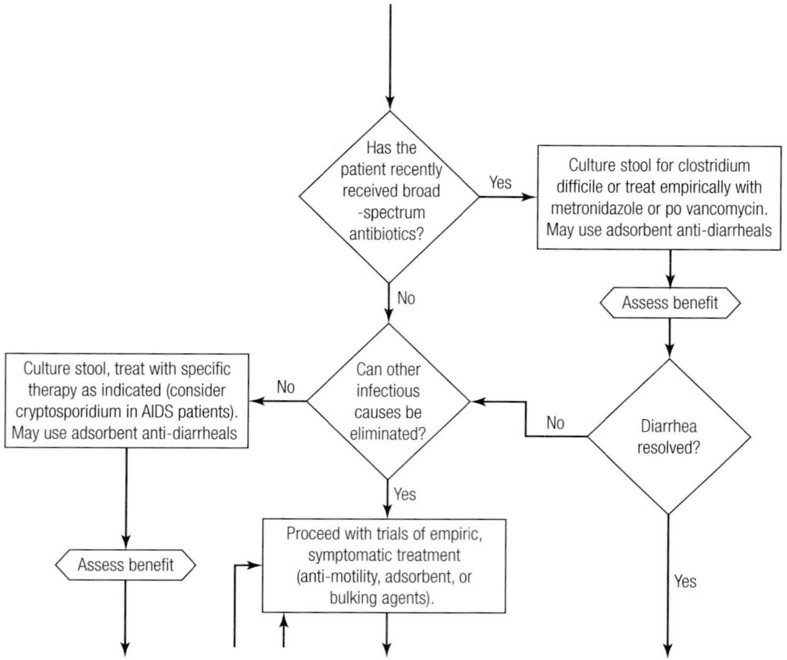

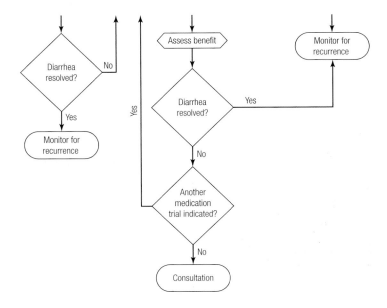

Dysphagia

Introduction and Background

- Inability to maintain a normal swallow reflex can be a very troubling symptom for patients at the end of life.
- Terminally ill patients and families should recognize that the inability to maintain nutrition through the oral route as a consequence of dysphagia is a harbinger of an overall clinical deterioration.
- Appearance of this symptom may need to stimulate a conversation on goals of care and the need for a change in focus of therapies.
- Deglutition is the act of swallowing, through which a food or liquid bolus is transported from the mouth through the pharynx and esophagus into the stomach. Normal swallowing is a smooth coordinated process that involves a complex series of voluntary and involuntary neuromuscular contractions and typically is divided into distinct phases: (1) oral, (2) pharyngeal, and (3) esophageal. If stages are impaired by pathologic condition, specific symptoms may result.

Prevalence

- Because of the multiple potential etiologies, it has been difficult to define the scope of the problem.
- Two of the more common situations associated with dysphagia include stroke (incidence ranges 22–70%) and esophageal cancer (incidence 70%).

- A major contributing factor for patients with advanced disease is *Candida*, which may be present in up to 80% of this population.

Causes

- Weakness and de-conditioning due to progression of underlying disease
- Medications (e.g., neuroleptics, anticholinergic drugs, alcohol, drugs that cause esophageal or mucosal injury)
- Radiation therapy
- Esophageal strictures
- Reflux esophagitis
- Local tumor burden (head and neck, thyroid)
- Impaired motor function (e.g. stroke)
- Neurodegenerative disease (Parkinson's disease, stroke, multiple sclerosis, Alzheimer's disease)
- Localized infection (e.g. candidiasis, HIV, herpes)
- Poor or absent dentition

Clinical Characteristics

- Dysphagia is usually associated with coughing or choking on food or fluids, but may also present as inability to swallow medications.

- Patients may describe the sensation of food being stuck in the throat, vocal changes, pain while swallowing, shortness of breath following eating or drinking, or the appearance of drooling.
- Dysphagia may also present as an increase in time to consume meals or recent decreased weight.
- Treatment of dysphagia should be guided by reversing causes where appropriate and promoting improvement in the presenting symptom such as pain.
- Prevention of aspiration is a significant goal for many patients, and should be considered. However, some patients may prefer to continue oral intake as a quality of life and comfort measure, and as such prevention of aspiration may not be reasonable.
- Simple dietary modifications (e.g. thickening agents, pureed foods) may prove beneficial.
- Postural changes (e.g. raising the head of the bed) may be useful as well as assuring proper upright positioning during meals.
- Removing environmental distractions during meal times may also be important in certain settings.
- Families may also benefit from continued reassurance that dysphagia may represent an expected part of the patient's decline.
- Signs and symptoms of dysphagia by phases:
  - Oral or pharyngeal dysphagia:
    - Coughing or choking with swallowing
    - Difficulty initiating swallowing
    - Food sticking in the throat
    - Sialorrhea
    - Unexplained weight loss
    - Change in dietary habits
    - Recurrent pneumonia
    - Change in voice or speech (wet voice)
    - Nasal regurgitation
  - Esophageal dysphagia:
    - Sensation of food sticking in the chest or throat
    - Oral or pharyngeal regurgitation
    - Change in dietary habits
    - Recurrent pneumonia

Non-Pharmacologic Treatment
- A variety of surgical and stenting procedures have been used with varying rates of success. These aggressive approaches have little value in most hospice patients.
- Palliative chemotherapy or radiation therapy may be of some benefit for patients where tumor burden is the main concern.
- There is no improved quality of life associated with use of enteral nutrition in this patient population. This approach does not prevent aspiration, and may actually complicate this problem.

- As dysphagia is often associated with patients who are approaching their death, it is more important to focus on good oral care including the use of artificial saliva and lip balms.

Pharmacotherapy

- Medication use in dysphagia follows two paths:
  - Treating underlying causes
  - Providing symptom relief
- Combine both treatment of underlying causes and symptomatic relief whenever possible.
  - Candidiasis associated dysphagia
    - Non-systemic antifungals such as nystatin suspension possibly combined with a local anesthetic such as lidocaine if localized pain is present.
    - If ineffective or undesirable, use fluconazole and an opioid.

- Xerostomia or mucositis induced dysphagia
  - Topical viscous lidocaine as a single ingredient or in combination with other agents to provide for localized analgesia.
  - Use caution with local anesthetics, as some patients may have worsening of their swallowing reflex.
- Swelling with an anatomical component
  - Steroids such as dexamethasone may be useful for temporary reduction.
- Reflux/GERD or compromised lower esophageal sphincter tone
  - H_2 blockers and/or proton pump inhibitors may prove useful.
- Diffuse esophageal spasm
  - Anticholinergic medications.

Pharmacologic Management of Dysphagia

Generic Name (Brand Name)	Typical Regimen	Common Strengths and Formulations	Comments
Antifungal for Candidiasis			
Nystatin (Mycostatin)	500,000 units Swish and swallow QID $\times$ 14 days	**Suspension:** 500,000 units/5 mL	
Fluconazole (Diflucan)	200 mg PO day 1 then 100 mg PO QD $\times$ 13 days	**Tablets:** 50, 100, 150, 200 mg **Suspension:** 10 mg/mL, 40 mg/mL	• Can be crushed • Considerably more expensive than nystatin
H2 Antagonist for GERD/reflux			
Famotidine (Pepcid)	10–20 mg PO BID	**Tablets:** 10, 20, 40 mg **Suspension:** 40 mg/mL	• Reduce dose in geriatric patients or with renal failure • May cause confusion
Ranitidine (Zantac)	75–150 mg PO BID	**Tablets:** 75, 150, 300 mg **Suspension:** 15 mg/mL	• Reduce dose in geriatric patients or with renal failure • May cause confusion
Proton Pump Inhibitor for GERD/reflux			
Omeprazole (Prilosec)	20 mg PO QD	**Tablets:** 20 mg (OTC) **Capsules:** 10, 20, 40 mg	• OTC least expensive • Do not crush
Lansoprazole (Prevacid)	30 mg PO QD	**Capsules:** 15, 30 mg **Granules:** 15, 30 mg **SoluTabs:** 15, 30 mg	• Capsule contents and granules may be sprinkled in liquids or applesauce • Solutabs dissolve in mouth or may be dissolved in water for administration
Pantoprazole (Protonix)	40 mg PO QD	**Delayed Release Tablets:** 20, 40 mg	• Do not crush

Generic Name (Brand Name)	Typical Regimen	Common Strengths and Formulations	Comments
Corticosteroid for Swelling			
Dexamethasone (Decadron)	4 mg IV/IM/PO/SQ q6h	**Tablets:** 0.75, 2, 4 mg **Injection:** 4 mg/mL	• Give IV over 5–10 minutes, rapid bolus associated with perianal pain
Anticholinergic Agents for Esophageal Spasms			
Hyoscyamine (Levsin)	0.125–0.25 PO/SL q4h PRN	**Tablets:** 0.125 mg oral and SL **Solution:** 0.125 mg/mL	• Do not exceed 12 tablets per 24 hours
Scopolamine (Transderm Scop)	Apply transdermally q72h or 0.3–0.6 mg IV/IM/SQ q4h PRN	Scopolamine per patch contains 1.5 mg **Injection:** 0.4 mg/mL	• Onset of action approximately 4 hours
Glycopyrrolate (Robinul)	0.1–0.2 mg IV/IM/SQ q6h PRN	**Injection:** 0.2 mg/mL	• Does not cross blood-brain barrier–less side effects • Tablet not available generically-expensive

Clinical Pearls

The National Dysphagia Diet (NDD), published in 2002 by the American Dietetic Association, established standard terminology for dietary texture modification in dysphagia management

- Dysphagia solid diets are classified as follows:
  - NDD Level 1: Dysphagia-Pureed (homogenous, very cohesive, pudding-like, requiring very little chewing ability).
  - NDD Level 2: Dysphagia-Mechanical Altered (cohesive, moist, semisolid foods, requiring some chewing).
  - NDD Level 3: Dysphagia-Advanced (soft foods that require more chewing ability).
  - Regular (all foods allowed).

- NDD levels of liquid viscosity (i.e., thickness or resistance-to-flow)
  - Thin (water, orange juice)
  - Nectar-like (tomato juice; fluid-type yogurt)
  - Honey-like (curd-type yogurt, cream soup, orange juice and thin soup with thickener)
  - Spoon-thick (pudding, mashed potatoes)
- When adding thickening agents to liquids, always start slowly and add more, rather than adding too much at once.
- Some thickeners can adversely affect the taste of foods.
- Foods need to look good to stimulate the appetite. Blend the meat and vegetables separately to ensure the food remains colorful.

Key References

Sreedharan A, Wortley S, Everett SM, Harris K, Crellin A, Lilleyman J, Forman D: Interventions for dysphagia in oesophageal cancer. (Protocol) *The Cochrane Database of Systematic Reviews* 2004, Issue 4.

Terre R, Mearin F: Oropharyngeal dysphagia after the acute phase of stroke: predictors of aspiration. *Neurogastroenterol Motil.* 18: 200–205, 2006.

Weissman, DE: Fast Facts and Concepts #85. Swallow studies, tube feeding and the death spiral. February 2003. End-of-Life Physician Education Resource Center www.eperc.mcw.edu.

Dahlin C, Lynch M, Szmuilowicz E, Jackson V; Management of Symptoms Other than Pain. *Anesthesiology Clin N Am.* 24: 39–60, 2006.

Rosielle D: Fast Facts and Concepts #147. Oropharyngeal Candidiasis. December, 2005. End-of-Life Physician Education Resource Center www.eperc.mcw.edu.

Levy A, Dominguez-Gasson, Brown E, Frederick C: Technology at End of Life Questioned. *The ASHA Leader,* July 20, 2004, pp. 1–14.

Dahlin C, Goldsmith T: Dysphagia, xerostomia, and hiccups. In: Ferrell BR, Coyle N, editors. *Oxford Textbook of Palliative Nursing.* New York: Oxford University Press; 2001. p. 122–138.

Lind CD: Dysphagia: evaluation and treatment. *Gastroenterol Clin N Am.* 32: 553–575, 2003.

American Dietetics Association. National Dysphagia Diet: Standardization for Optimal Care, 2002.

Dysphagia

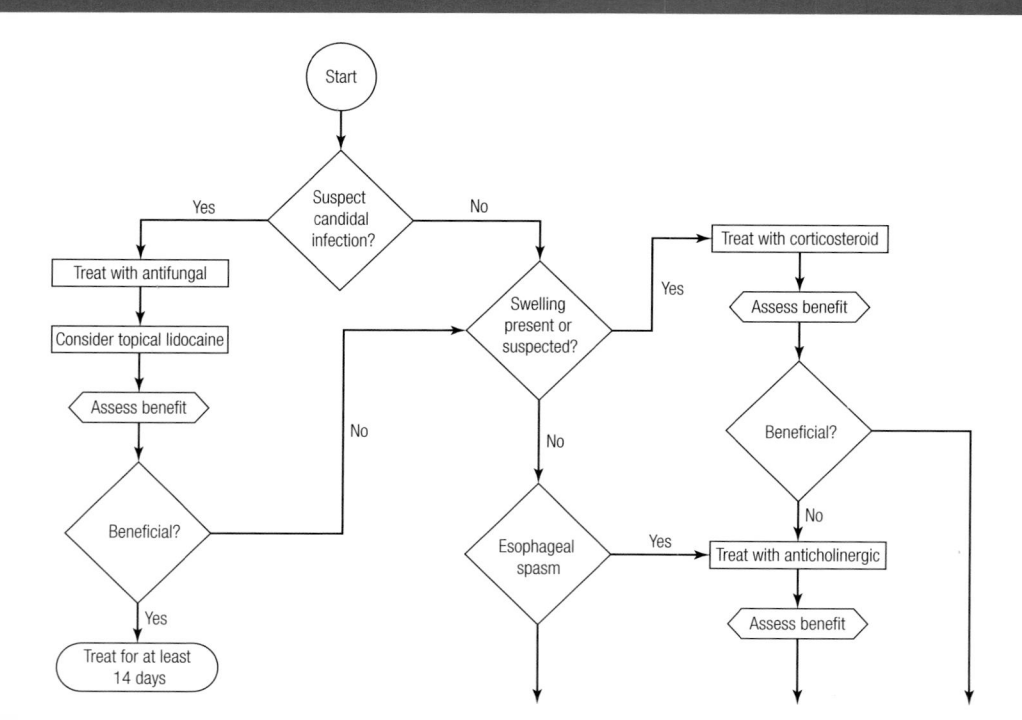

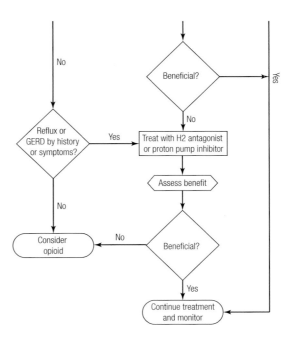

Dyspnea

Introduction and Background
- Dyspnea is one of the most distressing symptoms for patients and their loved ones.
- The goal of therapy is to decrease the patient's perception of breathlessness.

Prevalence
- The prevalence of dyspnea varies from 12–74% and tends to worsen as death approaches. Prevalence increases in the last week of life in terminally ill cancer patients to between 50–70%.

Causes
A thorough history and physical should be taken and possible reversible causes of dyspnea should be identified and treated, if present. Some of the possible causes are:

- Bronchospasm or COPD exacerbation–Albuterol, ipratropium and/or oral steroids.
- Thick secretions–If cough reflex is strong, loosen secretions with guaifenesin or nebulized saline. If the cough is weak hyoscyamine, glycopyrrolate, or scopolamine patch can effectively dry secretions.
- For anxiety associated with dyspnea–benzodiazepines (e.g. diazepam, lorazepam).
- For pleural effusions, consider therapeutic thoracentesis.

- For low hemoglobin–consider red blood cell transfusion (controversial) or erythropoietin (rarely used in hospice, but might have a larger role in palliative care patients).
- Infections–Antibiotic therapy as appropriate.
- Pulmonary emboli–Anticoagulants for prevention and treatment or vena cava filter placement, (rarely used in hospice, but might have a larger role in palliative care patients).
- Rales–Due to volume overload. Reduction of IV fluids or diuretic therapy as appropriate.

Clinical Characteristics
- Dyspnea is described as an uncomfortable awareness of breathing, it is a subjective sensation, and patient self report is the only reliable indicator. Respiratory rate or pO_2 often correlate poorly with the feeling of breathlessness.
- Respiratory effort and dyspnea are not the same. Patients may report substantial relief of dyspnea from opioids, with no change in respiratory rate.

Non-Pharmacologic Treatment
- Gather, provide information and reassure patient and family.
- Discuss meaning of symptoms with patient and family.
- Anticipate and proactively prepare the patient and family for worsening symptoms.
- Identify what triggers dyspnea attacks and minimize these triggers as much as possible.

- Discuss patient, family or staff concerns about using opioids to relieve dyspnea.
- Provide companionship since isolation and spiritual issues can worsen symptoms.
- Encourage relaxation, reduce the number of visitors in the patient's room and reduce the need for exertion.
- Reposition to comfort, usually to a more upright position or with the compromised lung down.
- Avoid strong odors, perfumes, and smoking in the patient's presence or in close proximity.
- Improve air circulation/quality:
  - Provide a draft, use fans or open windows.
  - Adjust temperature/humidity with air conditioner or humidifier.

Pharmacotherapy
- When no treatable etiology can be identified or when these treatments do not completely alleviate distressing symptoms, opioids are first line therapy for treating dyspnea because they suppress respiratory awareness, decrease response to hypoxia and hypercapnia, vasodilate and have sedative properties.
- Appropriately titrated opioids have been shown to be safe and effective in the treatment of dyspnea.
- Benzodiazepines have a role if anxiety is significant, as they can provide additional and sustained anxiolytic properties.
- Oxygen therapy may be useful to patients with dyspnea and can reverse hypoxemia.

Pharmacologic Management of Dyspnea

Generic Name (Brand Name)	Usual Adult Starting Dose/Range	Maximum Daily Dose	Common Strengths and Formulations	Comments
First Line Therapy–Opioids–Opioid Naïve Patients				
Morphine Immediate Release (MSIR, Roxanol)	Morphine sulfate immediate release 2.5–5 mg PO/SL/SC/PR/IV q4h	No ceiling dose with appropriate titration	**Immediate Release Tablets (MSIR):** 15 mg, 30 mg **Soluble Tablets:** 10 mg **Concentrated Oral Solution (Roxanol):** 20 mg/mL **Injection:** 10 mg/mL, 15 mg/mL	• For opioid tolerant patients, increase the baseline opioid dose by 25–50% and titrate • For breakthrough symptoms, 30–50% of the amount taken over 4 hours can be given q 1 hour, as needed • Consideration of inpatient hospice/palliative care setting may be helpful for patients with severe dyspnea, due to the necessity of close monitoring • Addition of benzodiazepines may also be necessary if anxiety is a significant contributor to breathlessness • Studies have been inconsistent regarding the efficacy of nebulized morphine (See below) • An interdisciplinary team should be involved in any interventions for severe dyspnea which may include palliative sedation
Oxycodone (Oxydose, Oxyfast, OxyIR, Roxicodone)	Oxycodone immediate release 5 mg PO/SL/PR q4h	No ceiling dose with appropriate titration	**Immediate Release Tablets and Capsules** (OxyIR, Roxicodone): 5 mg, 15 mg, 30 mg **Concentrated Oral Solution (Roxicodone Intensol, Oxydose, Oxyfast):** 20 mg/mL	
Hydromorphone (Dilaudid)	Hydromorphone immediate release 1 mg PO/SL/SC/PR/IV q4h	No ceiling dose with appropriate titration	**Immediate Release Tablets:** 2 mg, 4 mg, 8 mg **Oral Solution:** 1 mg/mL **Injection:** 2 mg/mL, 4 mg/mL, 10 mg/mL	

Benzodiazepines—Add If Anxiety Is Present

Lorazepam (Ativan)	0.5–1 mg PO/PR/SL/PR/SC/IV q4–6h scheduled or PRN	10 mg/day	**Tablets:** 0.5 mg, 1 mg, 2 mg **Concentrated Oral Solution (Lorazepam Intensol):** 2 mg/mL **Injection:** 2 mg/mL	• Benzodiazepines can decrease anxiety associated with breathlessness • Begin with low, non-sedating doses and titrate to effect. Breakthrough doses may be necessary to settle dyspnea • Can be used together with opioids with careful titration of each agent
Diazepam (Valium)	2–10 mg PO/SL/PR/IV q6–8h scheduled or PRN	60 mg/day	**Tablets:** 2 mg, 5 mg, 10 mg **Concentrated Oral Solution (Diazepam Intensol):** 5 mg/mL **Injection:** 5 mg/mL	• Longer acting agents are preferred for the treatment of dyspnea to avoid pronounced peak and trough effects that could lead to rebound anxiety
Alprazolam (Xanax)	0.25–0.5 mg PO/SL/PR q4–6h scheduled or PRN	10 mg/day	**Tablets:** 0.25 mg, 0.5 mg, 1 mg, 2mg **Concentrated Oral Solution (Alprazolam Intensol):** 1 mg/mL	• Intensol® solutions are expensive

Second Line Therapy—Nebulized Furosemide

Nebulized Furosemide	20 mg Nebulized QID		**Injection:** 10 mg/mL	• Mix 20 mg/2mL injection with 3 mL normal saline • Beneficial for refractory dyspnea

Third Line Therapy—Nebulized Opioids

Nebulized Fentanyl	25–50 mcg Nebulized q2–4h	100 mcg/dose	**Injection:** 50 mcg/mL	• Mix injection with normal saline • Causes less bronchospasm than nebulized morphine

Clinical Pearls

- When using opioids for patients with severe pulmonary disease, such as COPD, start at 50% of the above doses and titrate more conservatively, with increments of 25% every 24 hours, as needed.
- When an effective dose of an opioid has been established, convert to an extended-release preparation to simplify dosing.
- When using opioids, anticipate side effects and prevent constipation by initiating a stimulant laxative/stool softener combination upon initiation of opioid. Titrate to effect if dose increases.
- The use of **Nebulized Opioids** for the treatment of dyspnea is controversial. The results of studies have been inconsistent.
  - Nonrandomized studies, case reports, and chart reviews describe anecdotal improvement in dyspnea using nebulized opioids.
  - Several controlled studies using nebulized opioids have provided inconclusive or negative results.

- Disadvantages of nebulized opioids compared to oral or other dosage forms include increased costs and a more complicated method of delivery.
- Nebulized opioids may be advantageous in patients that are not able to or willing to take an oral agent or cannot tolerate adverse effects of systemic administration.
  - Fentanyl appears to be the safest nebulized opioid.
- *Nebulized furosemide* appears effective for dyspnea refractory to other conventional therapies.
  - Hypothesized mechanism of action of nebulized furosemide is its ability to enhance pulmonary stretch receptor activity, inhibition of chloride movement through the membrane of the epithelial cell and its ability to increase the synthesis of bronchodilating prostaglandins.

Key References

Brown, mL, Carrieri VK, Janson-Bjerklie S, Dodd M. Lung cancer and dyspnea: the patient's perception. Oncol Nurs Forum. 1986;13:19–24.

Tyler LS, Lipman AG. Dyspnea. In: Evidence Based Symptom Control in Palliative Care. Systematic Review and Validated Clinical Practice Guidelines for 15 Common Problems in Patients with Life Limiting Disease. 1st ed. New York, NY: Pharmaceutical Products Press; 2000:109–124.

Storey P, Knight CF. UNIPAC Four: Management of Selected Non-pain Symptoms in the Terminally Ill. 2nd edition. New York, NY: Mary Ann Liebert, Inc. 2003; 29–35.

Killion K, ed. Drug Facts and Comparisons. Electronic edition. St. Louis; Facts and Comparisons, 2005, [Various drug monographs for the classes of opioids and benzodiazepines.]

Thomas JR, vonGunten CF. Management of Dyspnea. J Support Oncol. 2003;1:23–24.

LeGrand SB, Khawam EA, Walsh D, Rivera NI. Opioids, respiratory function, and dyspnea. Am J Hosp Palliat Care. 2003;1:57–61.

Weissman DE. Fast Facts and Concepts #27: Terminal Dyspnea, November, 2000. End-of-Life Physician Education Resource Center. Available at URL: www.eperc.mcw.edu. Accessed on May 6, 2005.

Rousseau PC. Nonpain symptom management in terminal care. Clin Geriatr Med. 1996;12:313–27.

Farmcombe M, Chater S, Gillin A. The use of nebulized opioids for breathlessness: a chart review. Palliat Med. 1994;8:306–312.

Zepetella G. Nebulized morphine in the palliation of dyspnea. Palliat Med. 1997;267–275.

MacLeod R, King BJ, Potter M. Relieving breathlessness with nebulized morphine. Palliat Med. 1995;9:169.

Masood A, Thomas SH, Systemic absorption of nebulized morphine compared with oral morphine in healthy subjects. Br J Clin Pharmacol. 1996;41:250–252.

Ferraresi V. Inhaled opioids for the treatment of dyspnea. Am J Health-Syst Pharm. 2005;62:319–20.

Emanuel LL, von Gunten CF, Ferris FD, HauserJM, eds. The Education for Physicians on End-of-life Care (EPEC) Curriculum. 2003. Module 10: Common Physical Symptoms. p. 5–10.

Kohara H, Ueoka H, Aoe K, et al. Effect of Nebulized Furosemide in Terminally Ill cancer Patients with Dyspnea. J Pain Symptom Manage 2003;26:962–967.

Shimoyama N, Shimoyama M. Nebulized Furosemide as a Novel Treatment for Dyspnea in Terminal Cancer Patients. *J Pain Symptom Manage* 2002;23:73–76.

Stone P, Kurowska A. Re: Nebulized Furosemide for Dyspnea in Terminal Cancer Patients. *J Pain Symptom Manage* 2002;24:274–275.

Dyspnea

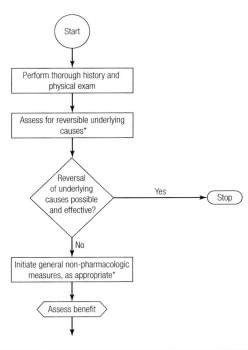

Dyspnea (*continued*)

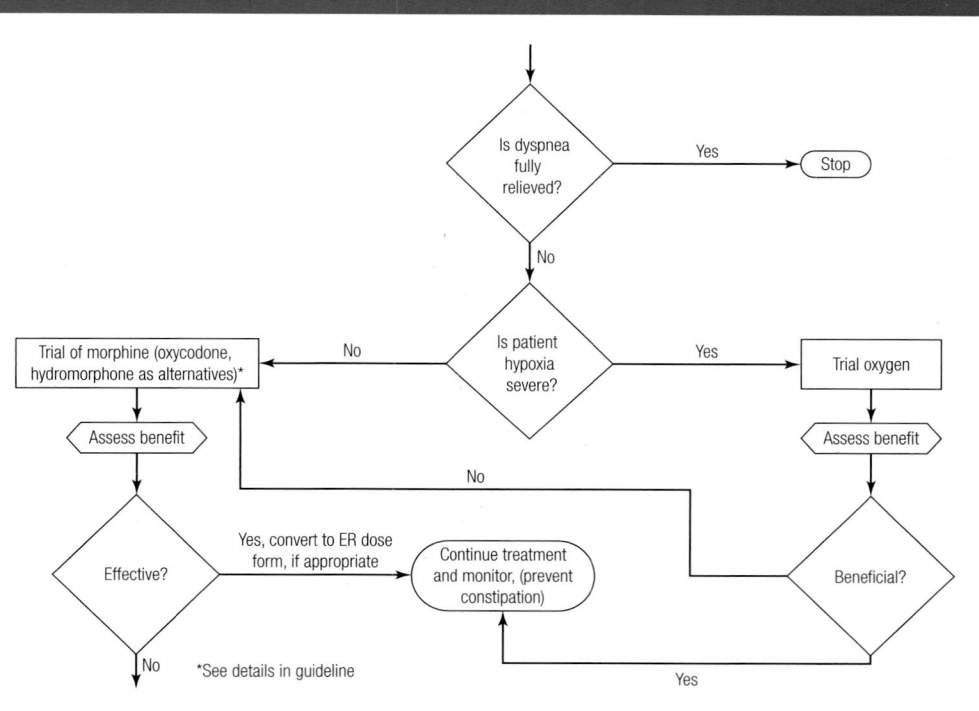

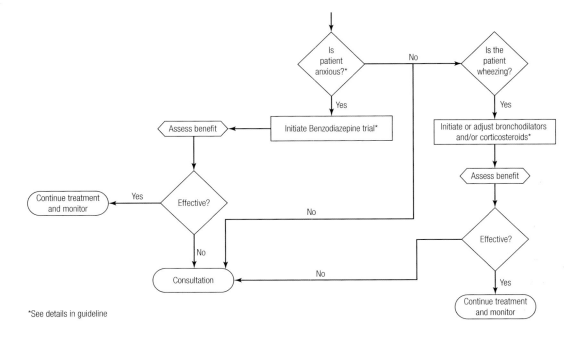

Is patient anxious?*

No → Is the patient wheezing?

Yes → Initiate Benzodiazepine trial*

No → Initiate or adjust bronchodilators and/or corticosteroids*

Assess benefit

Effective?

Yes → Continue treatment and monitor

No → Consultation

Assess benefit

Effective?

No → Consultation

Yes → Continue treatment and monitor

*See details in guideline

Excessive Sedation

Introduction and Background
- Most of the hospice and palliative care literature on "sedation" has to do with either the ethical or technical aspects of palliative sedation (a.k.a. terminal sedation, comfort sedation, or intentional sedation) or sedation which presents as a consequence of opiate therapy.
- Excess sedation treads close to the topic of fatigue, which has its own extensive and growing research literature.
- Assessment and management of common causes of excessive sedation are important to assist patients to maintain alertness and meaningful presence with family and friends.

Prevalence
- Sedation is very common in patients with advanced illness.
- Clinically significant sedation is a judgment call and collaborative evaluation of this subjective problem with the patient will determine when the threshold for clinical intervention has been exceeded.

Causes
- Common causes of daytime sedation in advanced illness include:
  - Boredom and loneliness
  - Chemotherapy or radiotherapy
  - Dehydration
  - Delirium (with reversal of the sleep/wake cycle)
  - Fatigue (consider anemia, metabolic disturbances as causes)
  - Fever
  - Infections or sepsis
  - Inflammatory processes
  - Metabolic disturbances
  - Multi-system failure (active dying process)
  - Overexertion
  - Oversleeping
  - Sedating medications:
    - Anticholinergics
    - Anticonvulsants
    - Antidepressants
    - Antihistamines
    - Antihypertensives
    - Anxiolytics
    - Muscle relaxers
    - Opioids
    - Sedative/hypnotics

- Among the medications that can cause sedation in the hospice and palliative care setting, probably the most important class (and certainly the class that has received the most attention in this regard) is the opioid analgesics. Conservative dosage reductions may be appropriate if pain is well controlled and the patient is experiencing excessive sedation.
- Sleep deprivation (from depression, delirium, pain, other symptoms) is a common cause of daytime sleepiness and apparent sedation.
- Daytime oversedation or "hangover sedation" is common when a sedative/hypnotic is given to an ill or elderly patient who has trouble sleeping at night, especially if the medication is dosed late at night.

Clinical Characteristics

- Excessive sedation is easy to recognize. The patient or family complains that the patient is unable to stay awake and alert enough to assist in care, be present with family and friends, and/or maintain an acceptable quality of life.

Non-Pharmacologic Treatment

- Patient complaints of excessive sedation should lead to a search for reversible causes, as outlined above.
- Detection of and attention to one or more of these problems can be very helpful.
  - Dehydration may be addressed by encouraging oral fluid intake or by initiating low volume parenteral fluid replacement using hypodermoclysis.
- For patients who retain the physical stamina to tolerate and benefit from these measures, physical therapy or modest exercise might reduce sedation related to fatigue.

Pharmacologic Management of Excessive Sedation

Generic Name (Brand Name)	Usual Adult Starting Dose/Range	Routes	Common Strengths and Formulations	Comments
Opioid Sparing Analgesics/Antipyretics				
Acetaminophen (Tylenol)	500–650 mg as often as q4h	PO, PR	**Tablets:** 160 mg, 325 mg, 500 mg, 650 mg **Suppositories:** 120 mg, 325 mg, 650 mg	• Opioid sparing • Maximum dose in 24 hours is 4000 mg (4 grams)
Ibuprofen (Motrin)	400–800 mg TID	PO	**Tablets:** 100 mg, 200 mg, 400 mg, 600 mg, 800 mg **Suspension:** 100 mg/5 mL	• Opioid sparing
Naproxen (Naprosyn)	250–500 mg BID	PO	**Tablets:** 220 mg, 250 mg, 275 mg, 375 mg, 500 mg **Suspension:** 125 mg/5 mL	• Opioid sparing
Corticosteroids				
Dexamethasone (Decadron)	4–8 mg daily (in divided doses)	PO, IV, PR	**Tablets:** 0.25 mg, 0.5 mg, 0.75 mg, 1 mg, 1.5 mg, 2 mg, 4 mg, 6 mg **Solution:** 0.5 mg/5 mL, 1 mg/mL **Injection:** 4 mg/mL, 10 mg/mL	• Has lesser mineralocorticoid effect than prednisone
Prednisone (Deltasone)	15–60 mg daily (in divided doses)	PO	**Tablets:** 1 mg, 2.5 mg, 5 mg, 10 mg, 20 mg, 25 mg, 50 mg **Solution:** 5 mg/5 mL, 5 mg/mL	

Psychostimulants				
Dextroamphetamine (Dexedrine)	2.5–5.0 mg qAM (MDD: 20 mg qAM)	PO	**Tablets:** 5 mg, 10 mg	• (ALL DRUGS IN CLASS) Exhibit synergistic analgesia with opiates • (ALL DRUGS IN CLASS) May worsen/precipitate delirium • (ALL DRUGS IN CLASS) Dose-related side effects include insomnia, hypertension, tachycardia, restlessness, hallucinations • (ALL DRUGS IN CLASS) May induce tolerance, withdrawal depression with prolonged use • Schedule II controlled substance
Methylphenidate (Ritalin)	2.5–5.0 mg BID (AM and noon) (MDD: 20 mg BID; AM and noon)	PO	**Tablets:** 5 mg, 10 mg, 20 mg **Solution:** 10 mg/5 mL, 5 mg/5 mL	• May require twice daily dosing • Schedule II controlled substance

Clinical Pearls

- Psychostimulant Treatment Protocol:
  - Begin with Starting Dose
  - Check response daily (1–2 hours after dose)
  - Raise dose daily by smallest increments until one of the following occurs:
    - Resolution of excessive sedation
    - Emergence of side effects
    - Maximum dose approached or exceeded
- The symptom burden of fever is often underestimated and antipyretic treatment can be very beneficial.
- Prior to initiating new pharmacologic treatment for excessive sedation, always assess whether some potentially sedating medications could be discontinued or reduced in dose.
- Sedation due to opioids must be distinguished from opioid-induced respiratory suppression and apnea due to the dying process. Respiratory suppression is characterized by impaired consciousness and a respiratory rate of less than 6–8 breaths per minute in a patient treated with opioids. Though this complication is rare in patients once tolerance has developed, a sudden increase in dose or the addition of a medication that may alter metabolism of the opioid can produce this adverse effect. Respiratory suppression is carefully reversed with administration of a diluted or low dose naloxone (0.04–0.1 mg/dose), in order to prevent precipitation of opioid withdrawal. This dose may be repeated until the opioid concentration has dropped to a safe level (return of respiratory rate to > 10 breaths per minute and increased patient alertness).
- Always let the patient be the final judge of how much sedation is clinically significant.
- Modafinil (Provigil) is a newer agent indicated for the treatment of narcolepsy, obstructive sleep apnea, and other sleep disorders. It has been used off-label for treatment of fatigue in multiple sclerosis. Though dosed only once daily, cost is prohibitive at about $8.50 per 200 mg tablet.

Key References

Brunton L, Lazo J, Parker K, eds.: Goodman & Gilman's The Pharmacological Basis of Therapeutics, 11th Edition. New York: McGraw-Hill, 2005.

National Center on Sleep Disorders Research Working Group: Recognizing problem sleepiness in your patients. *Am Fam Physician*. 59: 937–944, 1999 .

Meuser T, Pietruck C, Radbruch L, Stute P, Lehmann KA, Grond S: Symptoms during cancer pain treatment following WHO-guidelines: a longitudinal follow-up study of symptom prevalence, severity and etiology. *Pain*. 93: 247–257, 2001.

Wilwerding MB, Loprinzi CL, Mailliard JA, O'Fallon JR, Miser AW, van Haelst C, Barton DL, Foley JF, Athmann LM: A randomized, crossover evaluation of methylphenidate in cancer patients receiving strong narcotics. *Support Care Cancer*. 3: 135–138, 1995.

Bruera E, Fainsinger R, MacEachern T, Hanson J: The use of methylphenidate in patients with incident cancer pain receiving regular opiates. A preliminary report. *Pain*. 50: 75–77, 1992.

Excessive Sedation

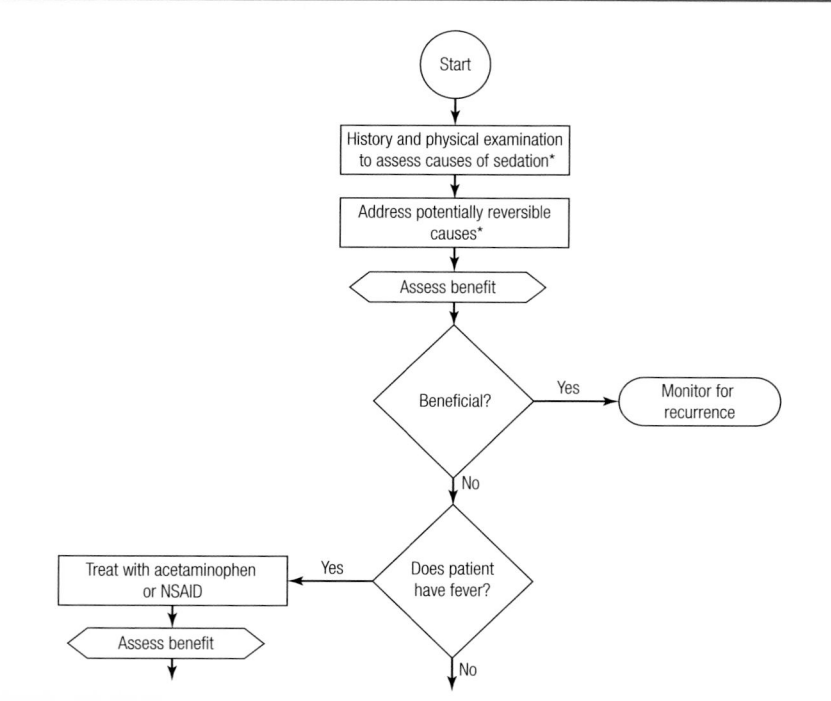

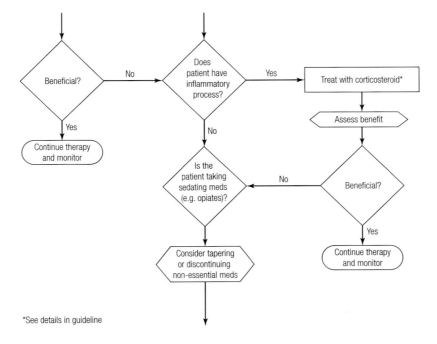

*See details in guideline

Excessive Sedation (*continued*)

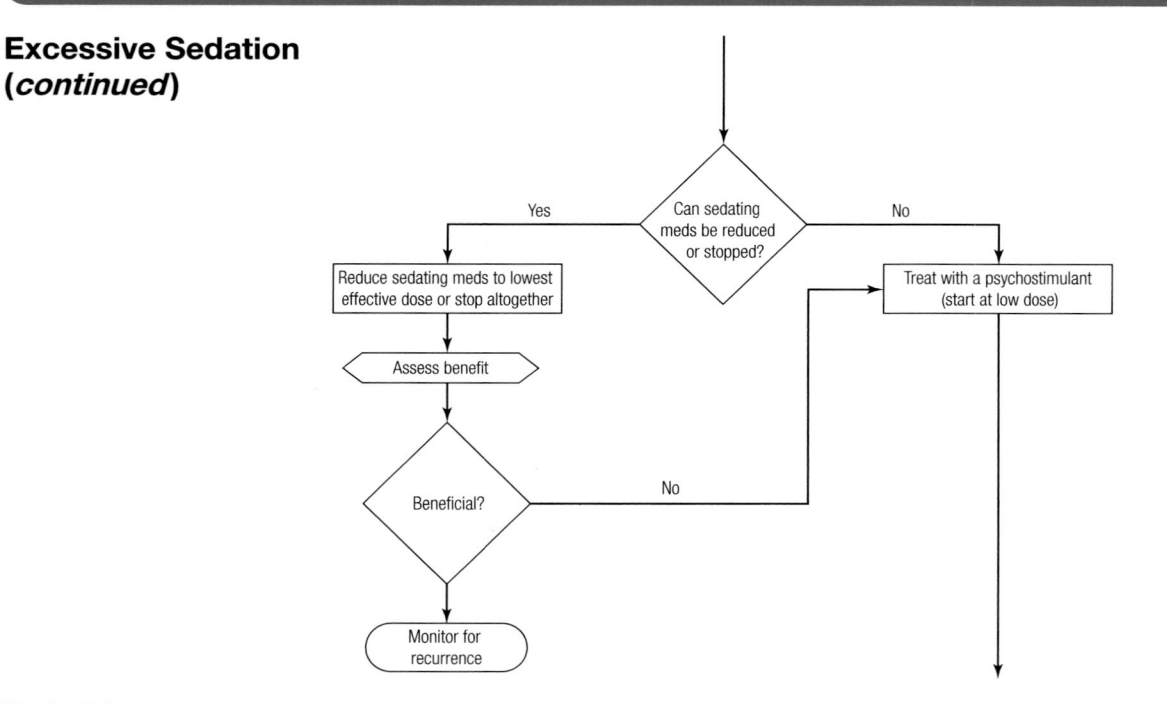

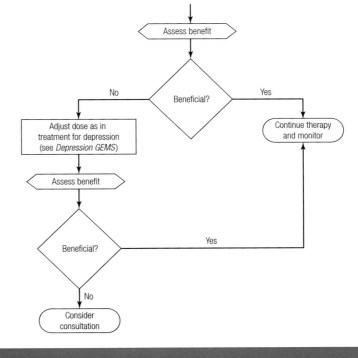

Fever

Introduction and Background

- Normal body temperature is considered to be 37°C or 98.6°F. Human body temperature normally follows a circadian rhythm.
- Body temperature is lowest—at 36.1°C (97°F) or lower in the predawn hours and rises to 37.4°C (99.3°F) or higher in the afternoon.
- A temperature greater than 38°C (100.4°F) is regarded as clinically significant.
- Fever (pyrexia) is often accompanied by other symptoms which include sweating and rigors.
- The anterior hypothalamus is the proposed neurological control center for core body temperature. This control mechanism can be reset, like a home thermostat, to a higher temperature in response to a stimulus through a process called thermogenesis.

Prevalence

- Most hospice patients will develop fever at some point in their illness.
- Though its prevalence has not been well studied in the hospice population, fever is a frequent symptom in patients when death is imminent.
- In patients with cancer, up to 70% have fever with no known infection.
- In one survey, 41% of cancer patients who underwent autopsy had documented infection as the source of their fever. In two large studies, 29% of AIDS/HIV patients experienced fever.

Causes

- Whenever possible, the cause of fever should be determined.
  - Infection is a common cause of fever in hospice patients. Identification of the organism along with antimicrobial sensitivities will expedite treatment. Infection in hospice patients may be attributed to many circumstances including alteration in physical defense mechanisms (e.g., mucositis), decreased immune response (neutropenia), presence of foreign objects (urinary or venous catheters) and aspiration.
  - Tumor fever, also known as paraneoplastic fever, can occur with several types of cancers. The most common cancers associated with fever are:
    - Hodgkin's disease
    - Lymphoma
    - Leukemia
    - Renal cell carcinoma
    - Myxoma
    - Osteogenic sarcoma
  - Drugs can cause fever particularly when patients have an allergic or hypersensitivity reaction to the medication (less than 5% of adverse events).
    - Antibiotics with the highest incidence of associated fever are *penicillins, cephalosporins, sulfonamides, nitrofurantoin and amphotericin B*.
      - Administration of a test dose to determine sensitivity, followed by premedication with acetaminophen and hydrocortisone can reduce the incidence of fever from amphotericin B therapy.

- Cytotoxic agents (bleomycin, interferon, interleukin)
- Immune therapy agents (biological response modifiers, growth factors)
- Anticonvulsants
- Allopurinol
- Hydralazine
- Central nervous system drugs
  - ❖ Neuroleptics (due to neuroleptic malignant syndrome, a rare side effect)
  - ❖ Selective serotonin reuptake inhibitors (SSRIs), tricyclic antidepressants, monoamine oxidase inhibitors(MAOI) (due to serotonin syndrome, generally a result of combining serotonergic agents. Combining a serotonergic drug with meperidine is particularly likely to precipitate serotonin syndrome)
  - ❖ Opioids and benzodiazepines (fever associated with drug withdrawal symptoms)
- Blood product transfusion
  - Premedication with acetaminophen and diphenhydramine may reduce the incidence and severity of fever
- Deep vein thrombosis or pulmonary embolus
- Gastrointestinal hemorrhage
- Graft-versus-host disease (GVHD)
- Radiation therapy
- Cardiovascular accident (CVA)

- Status epilepticus
- Rheumatoid arthritis
- Systemic lupus erythematosus

Clinical Characteristics
- Fever is almost always accompanied by headache, myalgia and malaise.
- Fever occurs in three phases:
  - When a pyrogen is introduced, initially cutaneous vasoconstriction promotes heat retention and shivering (spontaneous rapid muscle spasms), which generate additional heat.
  - When the new elevated core temperature end point is reached, heat production balances heat loss and shivering stops.
  - Finally, cutaneous vasodilatation occurs and sweating promotes heat loss to the environment.
- Sweating, along with a decrease in the quantity of pyrogen or the administration of an antipyretic agent, will reset the core temperature to a lower or normal level.
- In the elderly population, thermoregulatory mechanisms are often diminished. Consequently, hyperthermia may result in arrhythmias, ischemia, mental status changes or heart failure due to the associated increase in metabolic demands.

- The term *fever of unknown origin* (FUO) is a term that is often used incorrectly in health care settings.
  - The definition of FUO is "an illness lasting at least 3 weeks with a fever higher than 38°C on more than one occasion and which lacks a definitive diagnosis after 1 week of evaluation in a hospital".
- If possible, the cause of fever should be determined in order to appropriately treat the patient.
- In hospice patients, fever frequently occurs in the last days to hours of life, most likely due to aspiration.
- Treatment is generally limited to palliation of symptoms rather than identification and treatment of the underlying pyrogen.

Non-Pharmacologic Treatment

- Maintain patient in a dry, moderate temperature environment avoiding drafts and temperature fluctuation.
- In hot and humid environments, sponging the patient with tepid water will promote physical cooling.
- Do not use cold water or alcohol as these may lead to shivering with resulting temperature elevation and increased patient discomfort.
- Encourage fluid replacement and adequate nutrition as fever is associated with dehydration and increased metabolic demands.

Pharmacotherapy

- There are three types of agents that lower body temperature (antipyretics)—antipyretic effects of the agents in the second and third categories are side effects of these drugs, which are not typically practical for use as antipyretic agents:
  - Pure antipyretics that have no effect in the absence of a pyrogen and do not affect normal temperature, such as acetaminophen and NSAIDs.
  - Drugs that cause hypothermia in the patient who is afebrile by directly altering thermoregulatory functions, such as ethanol, phenothiazines, and sedative hypnotics. These agents cause hypothermia as a result of blunting of the shivering response.
  - Agents that are antipyretic in low doses but also cause hypothermia in high doses, such as chlorpromazine.

Pharmacologic Management of Fever

Generic Name (Brand Name)	Usual Adult Starting Dose/Range	Routes	Common Strengths and Formulations	Comments
First Line Therapy				
Acetaminophen (Tylenol)	325–650 mg q4–6h or 500–1000 mg q6–8h	PO, PR	**Tablets/Capsules:** 325 mg, 500 mg **Suppositories:** 120 mg, 325 mg, 650 mg **Syrup:** 160 mg/5 mL syrup	• Maximum daily dose = 4000 mg • Weigh risk–benefit in patients with severe liver dysfunction (e.g., cirrhosis)
NSAIDs				
Aspirin	325–650 mg q4h	PO, PR	**Tablets:** 325 mg **Suppositories:** 300 mg, 600 mg	• Associated with Reye's syndrome in children and teenagers • Use with caution in patients with decreased platelet activity
Ibuprofen (Motrin)	400–800 mg q6–8h	PO	**Tablets:** 200 mg, 400 mg, 600 mg, 800 mg **Syrup:** 100 mg/5 mL	Maximum daily dose = 3200 mg Weigh-risk benefit in patients with renal insufficiency
Naproxen (Naprosyn)	250–500 mg q8–12h	PO	**Tablets:** 250 mg, 375 mg, 500 mg **Suspension:** 125 mg/5mL	• Maximum daily dose =1250 mg/day (expressed as naproxen base, not naproxen sodium) • Aleve® (naproxen sodium) 220 mg = naproxen base 200 mg + 20 mg sodium • Weigh risk-benefit in patients with renal insufficiency • *Preferred agent for tumor fever*

Generic Name (Brand Name)	Usual Adult Starting Dose/Range	Routes	Common Strengths and Formulations	Comments
Second Line Therapy				
NSAIDs				
Indomethacin (Indocin)	25–50 mg q8h	PO	**Capsules:** 25 mg, 50 mg **Suspension:** 25 mg/5 mL	• Maximum daily dose = 200 mg/day • Causes more GI symptoms than naproxen or ibuprofen • Weigh risk-benefit in patients with renal insufficiency
Third Line Therapy				
Treatment of Malignant Hyperthermia				
Dantrolene (Dantrium)	1–2.5 mg/kg IV q6h or 4 to 8 mg/kg/day orally, in four divided doses should be administered for 1 to 3 days following a malignant hyperthermia crisis	IV, PO	**Capsules:** 25 mg, 50 mg, 100 mg **Injectable:** 20 mg/vial	• For fever > 41.5°C (106.7°F) unresponsive to NSAIDs or acetaminophen

Clinical Pearls

- Although controversial, alternating acetaminophen with a nonsteroidal anti-inflammatory drug such as ibuprofen may be beneficial when either agent alone is not producing the desired effect.
- If prognosis warrants, in neutropenic patients, determine the infectious cause of fever and treat accordingly or treat empirically if pathogen not known.
- Ethical considerations related to antibiotic treatment of the fever-causing organism may create dilemmas in patients who are approaching death. Although an antibiotic may decrease symptoms such as fever, they may also prolong the dying process. Antibiotics should be considered in patients who are near death if the patient is requesting them or if the patient is experiencing symptoms causing suffering (e.g., convulsions or pronounced mental status changes) as a result of a high fever (>40°C or 104°F). These occur most frequently in very young and very old patients.
- Aspirin should be avoided in children because of the risk of developing Reye's syndrome with resulting liver failure.

- Although not recommended as an analgesic, IV, SC or IM meperidine 12.5 to 25 mg may be used to treat fever related rigors or shivering. Do not combine with serotonergic agents due to the risk of precipitating serotonin syndrome.
- Malignant hyperthermia (characterized by fever $> 41.5°C$ or $106.7°F$) should be treated with dantrolene 1–2.5 mg/kg IV every 6 hours or 4 to 8 mg/kg/day orally, in four divided doses. Dantrolene should be administered for 1 to 3 days following a malignant hyperthermia crisis to prevent recurrence of the manifestations of malignant hyperthermia.
- Premedicating with acetaminophen, NSAIDs or steroids when administering fever producing drugs or blood products may reduce the incidence and severity of fever.
- Avoid routinely treating fever with antipyretic agents in the presence of infection which is being treated with an antimicrobial. Reducing the fever may mask antimicrobial treatment failure.

Key References

National Cancer Institute-Fever, Sweats, and Hot Flashes PDQ (2005) http://www.nci.nih.gov/cancertopics/pdq/supportivecare/fever/healthprofessional, Accessed 3/27/2006.

Cleary JF(2002) Principles & Practice of Palliative Care & Supportive Oncology 2nd Chapter 9, Lippincott Williams & Watkins, Philadelphia PA.

AidsMap Treatment and care. http://www.aidsmap.com/en/docs/3DF48BAB-BD7C-431B-ACAD-DDF2E20C4997.asp, Accessed 3/25/2006.

Dipiro JT, Talbert EL, Yee, GC, Matzke GR, Wells, BG., Posey LM. (2005) Pharmacotherapy: A Pathophysiologic Approach 6th Ed.,McGraw-Hill Medical Publishing Division.

Dinarello CA, Gelfand JA (2005) Harrison's Principles of Internal Medicine 16th Ed. Chapter 16, McGraw-Hill Medical Publishing Division.

Fever

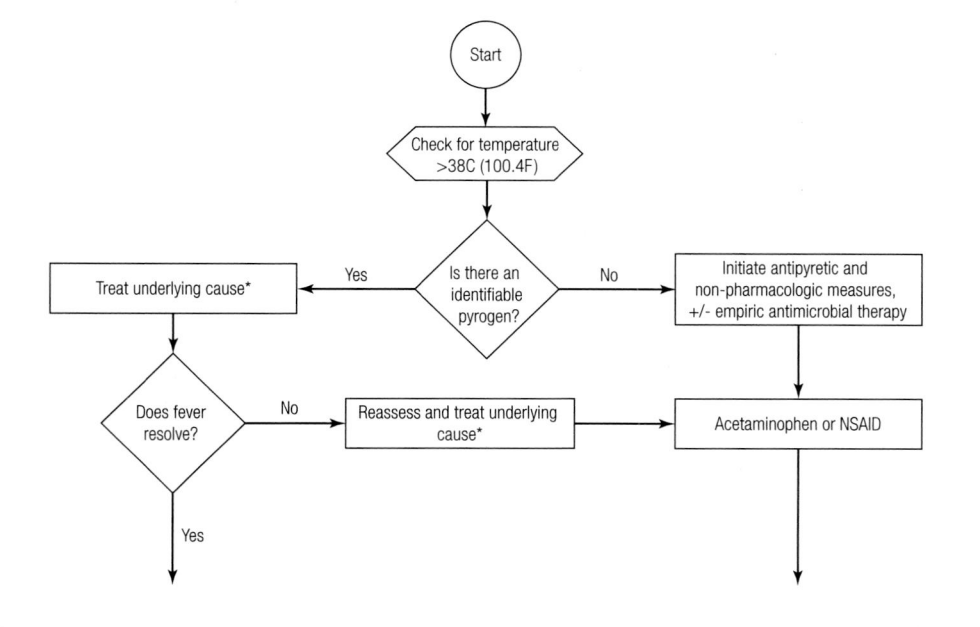

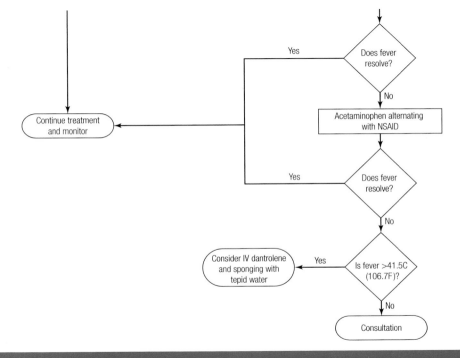

Hiccups

Introduction and Background

- Hiccups (singultus, hiccoughs) are defined as the sudden, involuntary contraction of one or both sides of the diaphragm and intercostal muscles, terminated by an abrupt closure of the glottis, producing the characteristic "hic" sound.

Prevalence

- The incidence of hiccups in advanced cancer patients or those at the end of life has not been thoroughly studied, but may occur in 1–2% (up to 9%).
- Hiccups are more frequently seen in males.

Causes

- The exact pathophysiology of hiccups is unclear. Stimulation of any members of the hiccup reflex arc, which involves the phrenic and vagal nerves, or central nervous system dysfunction may result in hiccups.
- Other causes may involve structural, metabolic, inflammatory, and infectious diseases.

- Causes of benign, self-limiting hiccups
  - Gastric distension: Excessive food or alcohol intake, aerophagia, gastric insufflation, sudden changes in gastric temperature
  - Toxins: Tobacco use, alcohol intoxication
- Causes of persistent, intractable hiccups
  - Metabolic disorders: Hyponatremia, hypocalcemia, hypocapnia, hyperuricemia, gout, fever, renal failure
  - Central nervous system: Stroke, arteriovenous malformation, cerebral contusion or hematoma, temporal arteritis, encephalitis or meningitis, neurosyphilis, multiple sclerosis, hydrocephalus, neoplasm, head trauma, anxiety
  - Peripheral nervous system: Goiter, head and neck tumors, mediastinal or lung masses
  - Surgical: Inadequate ventilation, intubation, suppression of normal inhibitory influences, hyperextension of neck (stretching phrenic nerve, manipulation of diaphragm or adjacent organs, prostatic and urinary tract surgery, laparotomy, thoracotomy, craniotomy
  - Drug-induced: Psychostimulants, sulfonamides, parenteral corticosteroids, methyldopa, benzodiazepines, short-acting barbiturates

Clinical Characteristics

- Hiccups may be one of three types:
  - Benign self-limiting
  - Persistent or chronic (more than 2 days, but less than 1 month)
  - Intractable hiccups (>1 month). They may be as frequent as 2–60 hiccups per minute.

Non-Pharmacologic Treatment

- Respiratory maneuvers (holding breath, re-breathing in a bag, valsalva manuever, compression of the diaphragm, or induction of a sneeze or cough)
- Nasal and pharyngeal stimulation (pressure on the nose, traction of the tongue, gargling, drinking water, eating sugar)
- Gastric distension relief (fasting, NG tube, lavage, induction of vomiting)
- Vagal maneuvers (digital rectal massage, ocular compression or carotid massage)

Pharmacologic Management of Hiccups

Generic Name (Brand Name)	Usual Adult Starting Dose/Range	Routes	Common Strengths and Formulations	Comments
First Line Therapy				
Chlorpromazine (Thorazine)	10–50 mg TID-QID	PO, IV, IM, PR	**Tablets:** 10, 25, 50, 100, 200 mg **CR Capsules:** 30, 75, 150 mg **Injection:** 25 mg/mL	• Centrally mediated hiccups • More sedating than haloperidol • *Only* drug with FDA indication for hiccups
Baclofen (Lioresal)	10–20 mg BID-QID	PO, IV	**Tablets:** 10, 20 mg **Injection:** 50 mcg/mL	• When muscle relaxation is needed • May cause considerable drowsiness
Metoclopramide (Reglan)	10–20 mg TID-QID	PO	**Tablets:** 5, 10 mg **Solution:** 5 g/5 mL **Injection:** 5 mg/mL	• Gastric distension mediated hiccups • Promotes gastric emptying; also has anti-emetic properties
Simethicone	40–125 mg PC & HS	PO, SL	**Softgels:** 125 mg **Chewable Tablets:** 80, 125 mg **Oral Drops:** 40 mg/0.6 mL	• Gastric distension mediated hiccups • Max = 500 mg/day
Normal Saline	Nebulize 2 mL over 5 minutes	Nebulizer	**3 mL Inhalation Dosettes**	• Suspected phrenic or vagal stimulation induced hiccups
Second Line Therapy				
Haloperidol (Haldol)	0.5–5 mg q4–8h	PO, SL, SQ, IM, IV	**Tablets:** 0.5, 1, 2, 5, 10, 20 mg **Solution:** 2 mg/mL **Injection:** 5 mg/mL	• Centrally mediated hiccups
Gabapentin (Neurontin)	300 mg TID	PO	**Capsules:** 100, 300, 400, 600, 800 mg	• Reported use as adjunct therapy
Valproate (Depakote)	15 mg/kg/day, increased by 250 mg every 2 weeks until hiccups cease or until not tolerated	PO, IV	**Delayed Release Tablets:** 125, 250, 500 mg **Sprinkles:** 125 mg **ER Tabs:** 250, 500 mg **Syrup:** 250 mg/5 mL	
Carbamazepine (Tegretol)	600–1200 mg/day	PO	**Tablets:** 100, 200 mg **ER Tablets:** 100, 200, 300, 400 mg	
Nifedipine	10–20 mg q8h	PO	**Tablets:** 10 mg **Capsules:** 10, 20 mg **ER Tablets:** 30, 60, 90 mg	• Must monitor blood pressure

Third Line Therapy				
Phenytoin (Dilantin)	15–20 mg/kg IV loading dose, 2–3 mg/kg PO BID	PO, IV	**Tablet:** 50 mg **Capsules:** 30, 100, 200, 300 mg **Suspension:** 125 mg /5 mL **Solution:** 50 mg/mL	
Midazolam (Versed)	10–15 mg IV loading dose, then 40–120 mg/ 24 hr SQ infusion	IV, IM, SQ,	**Syrup:** 2 mg/mL **Solution:** 1, 5 mg/mL	Last line therapy due to high levels of sedation

Clinical Pearls

- Identifying the underlying cause of the hiccup is vital to its treatment. Because not all underlying causes can be treated, symptomatic therapy may be warranted.
- Individual patients may respond differently to various therapies, so more than one drug trial may be necessary.
- Polypharmacy may be useful if a patient has failed several attempts with monotherapy. Combinations have been used including omeprazole and metoclopramide with baclofen, gabapentin, or both.
- Chlorpromazine is the only drug thus far with an approved indication of hiccups, but several studies have been conducted on the use of baclofen.
- Palliative sedation should remain a last resort for patients with intractable hiccups.

Key References

Berry PH: *End of Life Care: Clinical Practice Guidelines*. W.B. Saunders Company, Philadelphia, PA, 2002, Ch 26, pp. 227–331.

Dahlin C, Lynch M, Szmuilowicz E, Jackson V: Management of symptoms other than pain. *Anesthesiology Clin N Am*. 24: 39–60, 2006.

Friedman NL: Hiccups: a treatment review. *Pharmacotherapy*. 16: 986–995, 1996.

Guelaud C, Similowski T, et al: Baclofen therapy for chronic hiccup. *Eur Respir J*. 8: 235–237, 1995.

Hernandez JL, Ramos-Estebanex C, et al: Letter to the editor: Gabapentin for intractable hiccups. *Am J Med*. 177: 279–281, 2004.

Lierz P, Felleiter P: Anesthesia as therapy for persistent hiccups. *Anesth Analg*. 95: 494–495, 2002.

Sanchack KE: Hiccups: When the diaphragm attacks. *J Pall Med*. 7: 870–874, 2004.

Viera AJ, Sullivan SA: Letter to the editor: remedies for prolonged hiccups. *Am Fam Physician*. 63: 1684–1685, 2001.

Wilcock A, Twycross R: Midazolam for intractable hiccups. *J Pain Sym Manage*. 12: 59–61, 1996.

Hiccups

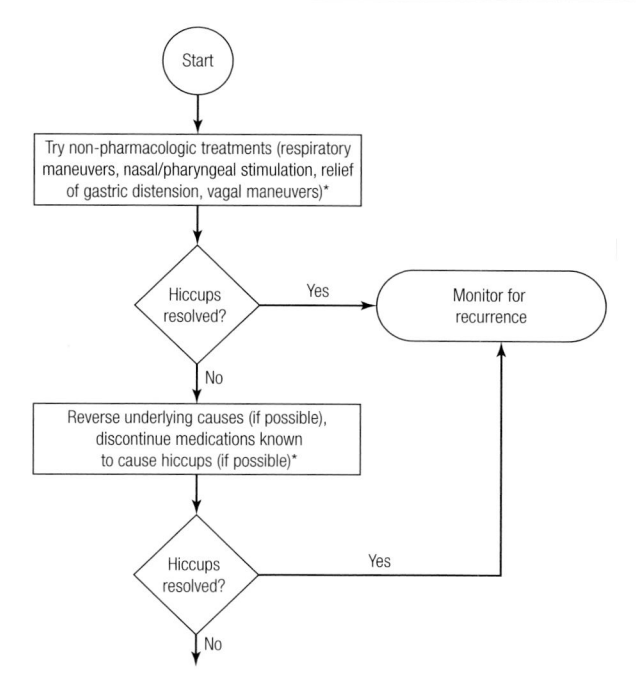

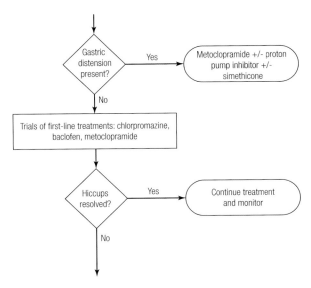

Hiccups (*continued*)

Trials of second-line treatments: haloperidol, gabapentin, valproate, nifedipine

Hiccups resolved?

Yes → Continue treatment and monitor

No → Consider trials of third-line treatments

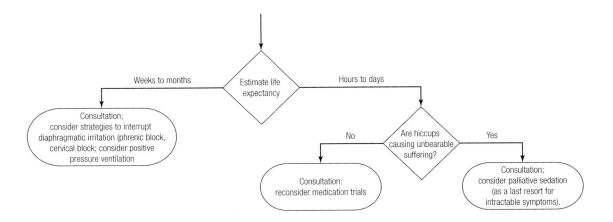

Estimate life expectancy

Weeks to months

Consultation;
consider strategies to interrupt
diaphragmatic irritation (phrenic block,
cervical block; consider positive
pressure ventilation

Hours to days

Are hiccups causing unbearable suffering?

No

Consultation;
reconsider medication trials

Yes

Consultation;
consider palliative sedation
(as a last resort for
intractable symptoms).

Infections

Introduction and Background

- Although infections in end-of-life are not uncommon, decisions about treatment are complex. In some cases, it may be appropriate to forego antimicrobial therapy for infections accompanying the dying process unless treatment is necessary to improve quality of life and reduce suffering.
- When appropriate, antibiotic therapy should be prescribed based on reasonable therapeutic goals and dosed according to the patient's clinical conditions.
- Factors such as potential adverse effects of treatment, the need for laboratory monitoring, and the patient's comfort and convenience are important to take into consideration when developing an individualized regimen.

Prevalence

- Although the exact rate of infections complicating hospice care is unknown, some studies indicate that approximately 40% (29–83%) of conscious cancer patients experience infections at the end of life. Frequently, the presence of fever is the primary factor leading to a clinical diagnosis of infection despite the fact that non-infectious causes of fever (e.g., drug-induced fever and fever secondary to underlying malignancy) may be the source.

Causes

- Infection in hospice patients may result from alteration in physical defense mechanisms (e.g., mucositis), decreased immune response (neutropenia), presence of foreign objects (urinary or venous catheters) and aspiration.
- Other contributing factors to infection include malnutrition, asthenia, decreased level of consciousness and immobility.
- The most common types of infection in terminally ill patients are:
  - Urinary tract infections
  - Upper and lower respiratory infections
  - Oral or pharyngeal candidiasis
  - Skin infections
  - Clostridium difficile colitis
  - Septicemia

Clinical Characteristics

- General signs and symptoms of an infection might include a fever higher than 100.5 degrees, chills, pain, ache, malaise, confusion, delirium and night sweats.
- Additional symptoms specific to the site of infection include:
  - Urinary tract infections; painful urination, burning, urinary frequency and urgency, flank pain
  - Upper respiratory infections; stuffiness, sore throat, headache , runny nose, cough

- Lower respiratory infection: productive cough, cough with rust-colored sputum, cough with thick yellow-green mucus, dry cough
- Oral or pharyngeal candidiasis (Thrush) ; raw red and/or white patches on throat, tongue, tonsils and mouth mucosa, painful swallowing
- Skin infections (Cellulitis): erythema, heat, swelling, pain or drainage
- *Clostridium difficile* colitis: frequent watery stools, cramping

Non-Pharmacologic Treatment

- Treat fever:
  - Maintain the patient in a dry, moderate-temperature environment avoiding drafts and extremes of temperature fluctuation.
  - In hot and humid environments, sponging the patient with tepid water will promote physical cooling.
  - Do not use cold water or alcohol as these may lead to shivering with resulting temperature elevation and increased patient discomfort.
  - Encourage fluid replacement and adequate nutrition, as tolerated.

Pharmacotherapy

- The following table contains recommendations for empiric antimicrobial therapy in hospice patients, based on known or suspected site of infection.
- When possible and consistent with the patient's goals of care, the source of the infection should be determined. Identification of the organism along with antimicrobial sensitivities will guide treatment toward antibiotic coverage most likely to be effective, but obtaining specimens for culture and sensitivity is not always consistent with the goals of care articulated by the patient and/or the family.
- Potential adverse effects of treatment, the need for laboratory monitoring, and the patient's comfort and convenience are important to take into consideration when developing an individualized treatment regimen.

Pharmacologic Management of Infections

Generic Name (Brand Name)	Usual Adult Starting Dose/Range	Routes	Common Strengths and Formulations	Comments
Respiratory Infections				
First Line Therapy				
Amoxicillin (Amoxil)	500 mg TID × 10–14 days (PO)	PO	**Capsules:** 250, 500 mg **Suspension:** 125 & 250 mg/5 mL	
Cefaclor (Ceclor)	250–500 mg q8h × 10–14 days (PO)	PO	**Capsules:** 250, 500 mg **Suspension:** 125, 250 mg/5 mL	
Doxycycline Hyclate (Vibramycin)	100 mg BID × 7–14 days (PO)	PO	**Capsules:** 50, 75, 100 mg Susp:25 mg/mL, 50 mg/mL	
Erythromycin (E-Mycin, Erytab)	250–500 mg QID × 10–14 days (PO)	PO	**Tablets:** 250, 333, 500 mg **Suspension:** 200,400 mg/5 mL	• Can cause GI upset
Sulfamethoxazole/Trimethaprim (Bactrim DS)	800/160 mg BID × 10–14 days (PO)	PO	**Tablets:** 800–160 mg **Susp:** 200–40 mg/5 mL	• Encourage fluids
Ciprofloxacin (Cipro)	250–500 mg BID × 7–10 days	PO	**Tablets:** 250, 500 mg	
Respiratory Infections				
Second Line Therapy				
Clarithromycin (Biaxin)	250–500 q12h × 7–14 days	PO	**Tablets:** 250, 500 mg: 500 mg XL **Suspension:** 125 & 250 mg/5 mL	• Extended release product (Biaxin XL) can be given once daily (500–1000 mg) • 2005 FDA warning regarding increased mortality with clarithromycin use in patients with coronary artery disease

Amoxicillin and Clavulanate (Augmentin)	875 mg q12 h or 500 mg q8h × 7–10 days	PO	**Tablets:** 250–125 mg, 500–125 mg, 875–125 mg **Chewable Tablet:** 400–57 mg **Tablets:** 1000–62.5 mg	• Adjust dose in renal failure • Take with meals to increase absorption and decrease GI intolerance
Levofloxacin (Levaquin)	250–500 mg daily × 7–10 days (PO)	PO	**Tablets:** 250, 500, 750 mg **Suspension:** 250 mg/5 mL	• Reduce dose in renal failure
Ceftriaxone (Rocephin)	1 gm daily × 5–10 days	IM, IV	**Injection:** 250, 500 mg, 1, 2 gm vials for reconstitution	• IM Injection is painful, consider mixing Lidocaine 1% with antibiotic to reduce pain

Urinary Tract Infections

First Line Therapy

Amoxicillin (Amoxil)	250–500 mg po TID × 7 days	PO	**Capsules:** 250, 500 mg **Suspension:** 125 & 250 mg/5 mL	
Cephalexin (Keflex)	250–500 mg po TID –QID × 7 days	PO	**Capsules:** 250, 500 mg **Suspension:** 125, 250 mg/5 mL susp	
Sulfamethoxazole /Trimethaprim (Bactrim DS)	1 tab BID × 7 days	PO	**DS Tablets:** 800–160 mg **Suspension:** 200–40 mg/5 mL	• Encourage fluids
Ciprofloxacin (Cipro)	100–500 mg po BID × 3–14 days	PO	**Tablets:** 250, 500, 750 mg **Solution:** 125 mg/5 mL **Injection:** 25 mg/mL	• Expensive. Adjust dose and frequency for renal insufficiency 100 mg qd × 3 days usually sufficient

Non-Odiferous Skin Infections (Cellulitis)

First Line Therapy

Cephalexin (Keflex)	250–1000 mg QID × 10–14 days	PO	**Capsules:** 250, 500 mg **Suspension:** 125, 250 mg/5 mL	
Dicloxacillin (Dynapen)	250–500 mg q6h × 10–14 days	PO	**Capsules:** 250, 500 mg	

Generic Name (Brand Name)	Usual Adult Starting Dose/Range	Routes	Common Strengths and Formulations	Comments
Non-Odiferous Skin Infections				
Second Line Therapy				
Erythromycin (E-Mycin, Erytab)	250–500 mg QID × 10–14 days	PO	**Suspension:** 250, 333, 500 mg tabs; 200, 400 mg/ 5 mL	• Can cause GI upset
Amoxicillin (Amoxil)	250–500 mg TID × 10–14 days	PO	**Capsules:** 250, 500 mg caps **Liquid:** 125 & 250 mg/5 mL	
Odiferous Skin Infections				
First Line Therapy				
Metronidazole (Flagyl)	250–500 mg TID-QID × 10–14 days	PO	**Tablets:** 250, 500 mg	• Do not take with alcohol. May use topically
Crushed Metronidazole Tablets	Sprinkle powder sparingly over affected area daily	Topical	**Tablets:** 250 mg, 500 mg	• More cost effective than gel
Second Line Therapy				
Metronidazole Gel (Metrogel 1%)	Apply a thin layer to affected area daily	Topical	**Gel:** 60 gms	• Expensive

Oral-Pharyngeal Infections (Thrush)				
First Line Therapy				
Nystatin (Mycostatin)	Swish and swallow/spit 5 mL po QID × 7–10 days	PO	**Suspension:** 100,000u/mL	

Oral-Pharyngeal Infections (Thrush)				
Second Line Therapy				
Fluconazole (Diflucan)	100–200 mg QD × 1–10 days Vaginal Infections: 1 × 150 mg dose	PO	**Tablets:** 50, 100, 150, 200 mg **Suspension:** 40 mg/mL	• Expensive. Can reduce dose and frequency in geriatric or renally compromised patients. • Also used for systemic and vaginal fungal infections

Clinical Pearls

- Although intramuscular injections are generally avoided, aminoglycosides (gentamicin, tobramycin) and ceftriaxone administered intramuscularly may be beneficial in patients who have organisms resistant to oral therapy or who are unable to take oral medication and have no intravenous access.

Key References

Nagy-Agren S, Haley H Management of Infections in Palliative Care Patients with Advanced Cancer Journal of Pain and Symptom Management. Volume 24, Issue 1, Pages 64–70 (July 2002).

Twycross R, Wilcock A (2006) HPCFUSA. Pallliativedrugs.com.

Infections

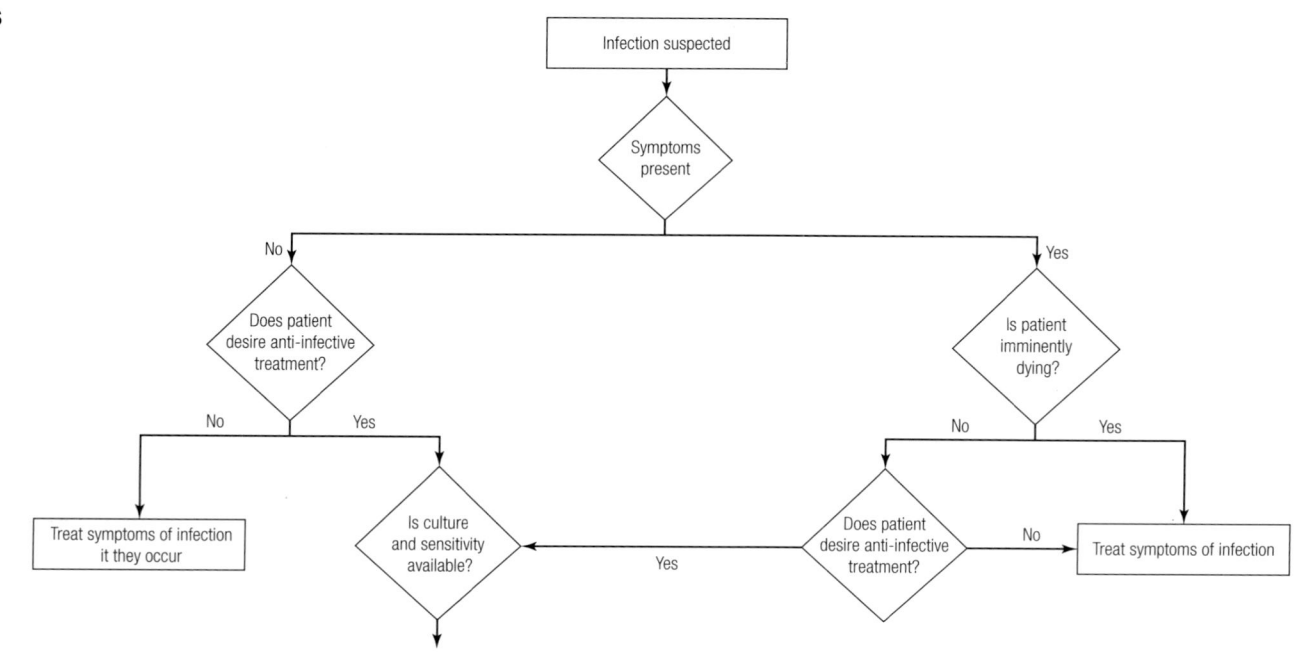

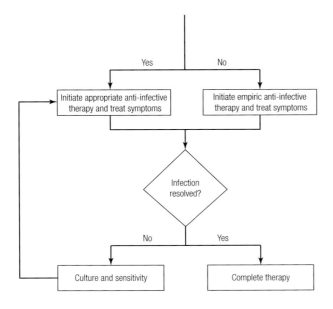

Insomnia

Introduction and Background

- Nearly half of the U.S. population reports intermittent insomnia, so it is not surprising that this pervasive symptom contributes significantly to suffering at the end of life.
- The insomnia syndrome in cancer has been defined as the occurrence of difficulty with initiating or maintaining sleep 3 or more days per week to a degree that impairs daytime function.
- Many hospice patients who do not meet formal criteria for insomnia syndrome, experience symptoms that contribute to their total suffering. Insomnia may be identified variously by individual patients as a disruption of previous sleep patterns, difficulty falling asleep, frequent waking, non-restorative sleep, or some combination of these problems.
- Insomnia diminishes quality of life for people at the end of life, and may intensify feelings of isolation and loneliness in advanced illness. It makes coping with symptoms and life stressors more difficult, and contributes to caregiver distress and fatigue.
- Effective control of this symptom requires a comprehensive assessment of contributing factors and a combination of behavioral and pharmacologic approaches to restore a restful pattern of sleep.
- The goal of treatment for insomnia is restful, restorative sleep. A target number of hours spent asleep is not as important as the results of sleep.

Prevalence

- The prevalence of insomnia symptoms in the hospice population is not well studied.
- The few studies that have been undertaken in hospice populations or populations with advanced cancer show that insomnia symptoms are common, with a prevalence of approximately 70%.

Causes

- The single most important cause of insomnia in the hospice population is poorly controlled physical symptoms.
  - Pain is known to contribute to sleep disturbance, and is common among hospice patients, particularly those with a cancer diagnosis.
  - Shortness of breath, nausea, and frequent urination are physical symptoms that are also likely to contribute to sleep disturbance if control is not optimized.
- Emotional states can impact quality of sleep, and both depression and anxiety are more common among hospice patients than they are in the general public.
- Patients with advanced disease, irrespective of the underlying pathology, are at high risk for a dysregulation of the immune system and the chemical messengers (cytokines) that play a role in maintaining the regular sleep cycle.
- Hospice patients frequently have an underlying organic disruption of circadian rhythm that contributes to sleep disturbance.

- Although the mechanism is not understood, it also appears that patients with cancer have a higher rate of restless leg syndrome than the general population.
- Hospice patients are at particularly high risk for insomnia if they experienced a significant degree of sleep disruption before the onset of illness.
- It is essential to determine whether apparent insomnia may be a prodrome of the day/night reversal of delirium.
  - Delirium is common in the hospice population, with increased prevalence for those in the final stage of their disease process.
  - This distinction is essential in determining the approach to treatment—delirium must be adequately addressed before insomnia can be treated.
  - There is evidence that treatment of delirium with benzodiazepines may be detrimental (unless the goal of care is palliative sedation).
  - Appropriate management of delirious patients with antipsychotics should address both the delirium and the associated sleep disturbance.

Clinical Characteristics
- The most common sleep disturbance reported by cancer patients is difficulty with sleep maintenance. This is also true in other medically ill populations.
- Difficulty with sleep initiation or early morning wakening is also common.
- Patients may appear to sleep an adequate number of hours at night, but report that their sleep is not restful or restorative.

- The majority of patients with insomnia report that physical discomfort or uncontrolled symptoms contribute to disturbed sleep.
- While optimization of pain and symptom management is a necessary component of the treatment plan for insomnia, treatment of insomnia as a symptom should not be delayed in this process.
- Worry and intrusive thoughts (anxiety, perseveration) are identified by patients as important contributors to the symptom of insomnia.
- Patients are often hesitant to report the symptom of insomnia, and it is important to be vigilant about screening for it through the trajectory of a patient's illness.

Non-Pharmacologic Treatment
- Addressing the behavioral component of sleep disturbance is an essential part of the overall management plan.
- Sleep may improve substantially with attention to good sleep hygiene. These common-sense recommendations include:
  - Wake up at the same time of day.
  - Minimize caffeine and nicotine use, especially late in the day or during nighttime awakenings.
  - Avoid alcohol use late at night.
  - Avoid heavy meals late at night, though a light bedtime snack may promote sleep.
  - Avoid excessive fluids before bedtime.

- ◆ Consider moderate regular exercise (if tolerated), but not close to bedtime.
- ◆ Minimize noise, light, and extremes of temperature in the bedroom.
- ◆ Try simple relaxation techniques.
- ◆ Consider a bedtime ritual (e.g., warm bath, reading) to help relax.
- Hospice patients may not have the energy or attention to adhere to all standard sleep hygiene recommendations, but even a minimal modification of behavior to reinforce a normal day/night sleep pattern can yield dramatic symptomatic improvements.
- Relaxation therapy may involve progressive muscle relaxation (avoid in persons with painful bony metastases) or imagery, and is most helpful in reducing in intrusive thoughts and promoting sleep onset.
- Sleep restriction therapy is not helpful in patients with markedly decreased functional status, but even debilitated patients can be exposed to bright light in daylight hours and spend time out of bed for portions of the day (if this does not unduly burden the patient and caregiver).
- Establishing a bedtime routine that is comforting to the patient may be helpful for the patient, and allow the caregiver to channel energy into activities such as reading, listening to music, massage, or holding hands.

Pharmacotherapy

- The goal of pharmacologic intervention is to provide the patient with a restorative night of sleep while utilizing the lowest dose possible to minimize side-effects and avoid daytime ("hangover") sedation.
- The benefit of a good night's sleep is largely measured in how rested, refreshed, and alert the patient feels the next day.

Pharmacologic Management of Insomnia

Generic Name (Brand Name)	Usual Adult Starting Dose/Range	Routes	Common Strengths and Formulations	Comments
First Line Therapy				
Benzodiazepines				
Lorazepam (Ativan)	0.5 mg HS (scheduled or PRN) (Max dose–2 mg HS)	PO, SL	**Tablets:** 0.5 mg, 1 mg, 2 mg **Concentrated Oral Solution:** 2 mg/mL	• (ALL DRUGS IN CLASS)–best for short-term or intermittent use; Tolerance to sedating effects develops with longer use • Short-acting • No active metabolites • Generally the benzodiazepine of choice in hospice • Oral concentrate expensive
Temazepam (Restoril)	7.5 mg HS (scheduled or PRN) (Max dose–30 mg HS)	PO	**Tablets:** 7.5 mg, 15 mg, 30 mg	• 7.5 mg strength is expensive
First Line Therapy				
Antidepressants				
Trazadone (Desyrel)	25 mg–200 mg HS (Usual therapeutic dose range: 50–100 mg)	PO	**Tablets:** 50 mg, 100 mg, 150 mg	• Unlikely to have significant antidepressants effect at doses used for sleep • Daytime sedation common at higher doses • Orthostasis at higher doses
First Line Therapy-Alternate				
Chloral hydrate (Somnote)	500 mg–1000 mg HS (Max dose: 2000 mg)	PO	**Capsules:** 500 mg **Syrup:** 500 mg/5 mL	• Chill syrup to mask unpleasant flavor • Do not stop abruptly if used for prolonged periods • Dangerous in overdose • Tolerance may develop to the sedating effects of chloral hydrate • Indicated for short-term or intermittent use

Second Line Therapy				
Antidepressants				
Mirtazapine (Remeron)	7.5 mg–30 mg HS	PO	**Tablets:** 15 mg, 30 mg	• May lose sedating effect at higher doses • May also stimulate appetite
Third Line Therapy				
GABA Receptor Non-benzodiazepines				
Zolpidem (Ambien)	5–10 mg HS	PO	**Tablets:** 5 mg, 10 mg	• (ALL DRUGS IN CLASS)–Little to no anxiolytic effect • (ALL DRUGS IN CLASS) – No clear advantage over benzodiazepines • (ALL DRUGS IN CLASS)– Expensive and short acting • Expensive and short acting
Zaleplon (Sonata)	5–10 mg HS	PO	**Tablets:** 5 mg, 10 mg	• Expensive and short acting
Eszopiclone (Lunesta)	1 mg HS	PO	**Tablets:** 1 mg, 2 mg, 3 mg	• Expensive and short acting
Melatonin Receptor Agonist				
Ramelteon (Rozerem)	8 mg HS	PO	**Tablets:** 8 mg	• Expensive • Not a controlled substance • Mechanism of action thought to be analogous to melatonin

Clinical Pearls

- Delirium is very common in hospice patients, and day/night reversal or sleep disturbance often occurs as a prodromal syndrome in these patients.
- Comprehensive assessment for and optimal management of contributing symptoms is essential to relieving insomnia in hospice patients. Most hospice patients have inadequately controlled symptoms that contribute to their sleep disturbance.
- Insomnia is an off-label indication for antidepressants. A sedating antidepressant is the obvious first choice treatment for insomnia when depression is the underlying cause.

Key References

Savard J, Morin CM: Insomnia in the context of cancer: a review of a neglected problem. *J Clin Oncol*. 19: 895–908, 2001.

Morin C, Colecchi C, Stone J, Sood R, Brink D: Behavioral and pharmacological therapies for late-life insomnia. *JAMA*. 281: 991–999, 1999.

Breitbart W, Marotta R, Platt MM, Weisman H, Derevenco M, Grau C, et al: A double-blind trial of haloperidol, chlorpromazine, and lorazepam in the treatment of delirium in hospitalized AIDS patients. *Am J Psychiatry*. 153: 231–237, 1996.

Hugel H, Ellershaw J, Cook L, Skinner J, Irvine C: The prevalence, key causes, and management of insomnia in palliative care patients. *J Pain Symptom Manage*. 27: 316–321, 2004.

Kvale EA, Shuster JL: Sleep disturbance in supportive care of cancer: a review. *J Palliat Med*. 9: 437–450, 2006.

Insomnia

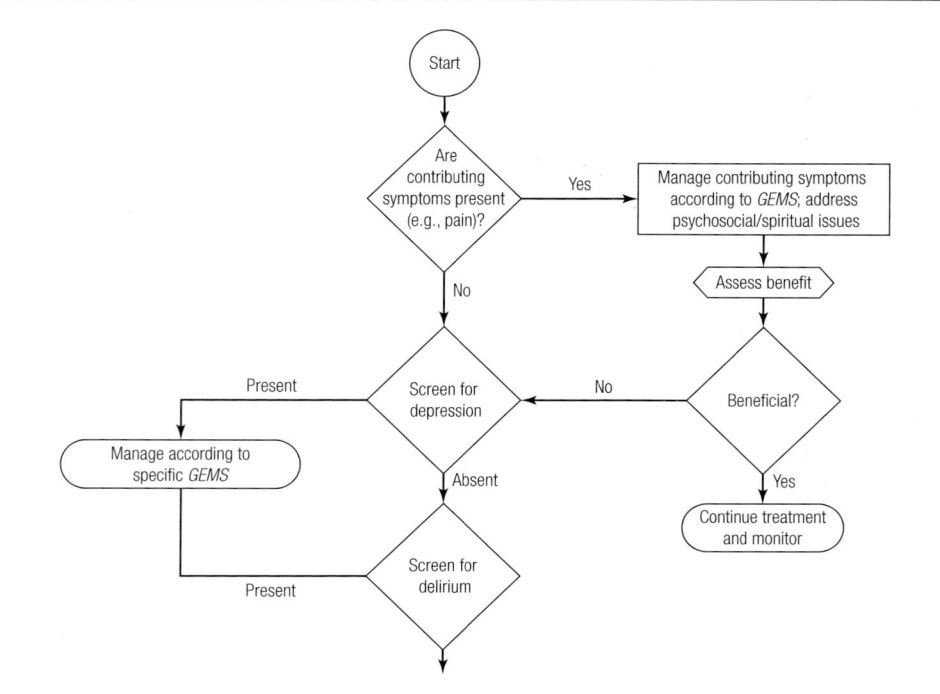

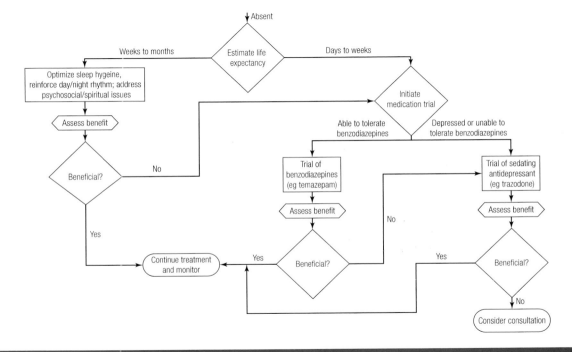

Absent

Estimate life expectancy

Weeks to months → Optimize sleep hygeine, reinforce day/night rhythm; address psychosocial/spiritual issues → Assess benefit → Beneficial?
- No → Initiate medication trial
- Yes → Continue treatment and monitor

Days to weeks → Initiate medication trial
- Able to tolerate benzodiazepines → Trial of benzodiazepines (eg temazepam) → Assess benefit → Beneficial?
  - Yes → Continue treatment and monitor
  - No → Trial of sedating antidepressant (eg trazodone)
- Depressed or unable to tolerate benzodiazepines → Trial of sedating antidepressant (eg trazodone) → Assess benefit → Beneficial?
  - Yes → Continue treatment and monitor
  - No → Consider consultation

Muscle Spasms

Introduction and Background

- Muscle spasms are a spontaneous contraction of either a single muscle or group of muscles (often used interchangeably with the terms muscle cramps and rigidity).

Prevalence

- While there has been very little study of the prevalence of muscle spasms in patients with most advanced illnesses, this condition is seen commonly as part of the overall symptom burden of patients approaching the end of life.
- Patients with malignancies, heart failure, HIV/AIDS, and advanced neuromuscular disease may be at highest risk.
- Patients with these advanced illnesses may be progressively limited in mobility, remaining in bed for prolonged periods of time.
- Inadequate levels of hydration predispose to muscle cramps or spasms and may lead to acute back muscle spasms, especially in the setting of pre-existing previous back pain or pathology.

Causes

- Multiple causes of muscle spasms are common, depending on the underlying disease state.
- Spasms have been classified by clinical feature and patient description, site of origin, or potential cause.
- Underlying causes of muscle spasm varies by disease state:
  - Patients with advanced cancer may have direct neural or muscle invasion along with biochemical abnormalities such as hypomagnesemia.
  - Patients with complex AIDS-related neuropathies may have spasms due to underlying nerve pathology or inflammation.
  - Patients with advanced heart failure may be subject to muscle spasms and cramps due to hypokalemia.
  - Patients with advanced multiple sclerosis may be at risk of spasm due to increased muscle spasticity and contractures.
- Exact causes of muscle spasms can be uncovered in most patients, particularly those with cancer.
- Muscle spasms also commonly occur in patients due to overexertion, strain, or overuse of certain muscle groups.
- Nocturnal muscle spasms or "leg cramps" are poorly understood in causation and respond to different treatments than muscle spasms in other locations.
- Restless leg syndrome (RLS) is a separate disorder that should not be confused with these types of leg cramps, although mild spasm or twitching is characteristic of RLS. RLS is considered a sleep disorder and the treatment of RLS involves medications not included in this guideline.

Clinical Characteristics

- Muscle spasms are unpredictable in occurrence.
- They range from rare to very frequent and can last for variable lengths of time, but usually not longer than several minutes.
- As with any painful condition, patient description can be wide ranging depending on the muscle group affected and the degree of muscle contraction.
- A series of contractions or a prolonged muscle spasm can lead to residual tenderness and hypersensitivity in the muscle group.

- Evaluation for potential biochemical causes should be judicious, depending on the benefit versus burden to patients with advanced illness.
- A thorough history and physical exam with particular emphasis on neurologic and musculo-skeletal systems can uncover the likely cause in most cases.
- Limited biochemical evaluation may be helpful in certain circumstances, but more extensive neurodiagnostic evaluation (e.g. CT scans, EMGs, etc.) should be reserved only for refractory cases.

Non-Pharmacologic Treatment

- Non-pharmacologic treatment of muscle spasms is very important, especially in light of the potential side effects of pharmacologic treatments for the condition.
- The following comfort measures are important in the overall management of patients with recurrent muscle spasms:
    - Comfort positioning and repositioning, particularly in bed bound patients or those with paralysis.
    - Evaluation and treatment of dehydration where possible.
    - Gentle massage and stretching of affected muscle groups.
    - Application of mild heat or topical preparations/lotions to affected muscle groups. Do not apply heat for longer than 20 minutes at a time.

Pharmacotherapy

- Pharmacologic treatment of muscle spasms is straightforward and determined partially by the frequency, severity, and potential causes of the muscle spasms.
- Review of previous usage of any pharmacologic treatments for muscle spasms and their benefit is important in selection of initial therapy.

- Patients may benefit from other classes of medications for analgesia such as acetaminophen, anti-inflammatories, or opioids if there are elements of underlying pain, tenderness, or inflammation in the affected muscle groups.
- There may be circumstances in which preparations such as supplemental magnesium or topical lidocaine are useful in the treatment of focal muscle spasms, but these are not included in the following table.
- The treatment of acute back spasm and pain may require a combination of medications including an anti-inflammatory, a muscle relaxant, and possibly a short course of opioid treatment.
- Most medications used for muscle spasms can cause primary side effects such as sedation, dry mouth, and dizziness.
- Depending on severity and frequency of spasms, the starting dose should be low and on an "as needed" basis with titration individualized to the patient's requirement.
- These agents potentiate effects of other central nervous system medications such as antidepressants, anxiolytics, and opioid pain medications and should be used with caution when prescribed in conjunction with these agents.
- Reduce doses in elderly patients.
- Most commonly used medications to treat muscle spasms are listed in the table; a diverse group of drugs that are not chemically related. These medications do not act directly on the muscle.
- Caution is indicated in their use, especially when these medications are used for longer than the two-week period customary in the setting of acute back pain or acute spasm. Tapered withdrawal may be appropriate.

Pharmacologic Management of Muscle Spasms

Generic Name (Brand Name)	Usual Adult Starting Dose/Range	Routes	Common Strengths and Formulations	Class of Agent/Comments
First Line Therapy				
Baclofen (Lioresal)	5–10 mg TID; MDD 80 mg	PO	**Tablets:** 10 mg, 20 mg	• Antispastic class • Most commonly used agent
Diazepam (Valium)	2–5 mg TID-QID; MDD 30–40 mg	PO, SL, IV	**Tablets:** 2 mg, 5 mg, 10 mg **Oral Concentrate:** 5 mg/mL	• Benzodiazepine class • Concentrate is expensive
Second Line Therapy				
Tizanidine (Zanaflex)	Usually 4 mg q6–8h; MDD 36 mg (or 12 mg/dose)	PO	**Tablets:** 2 mg, 4 mg, 6 mg	• Antispastic class • Prominent sedation a potential side effect or benefit • Significant orthostatic hypotension, structurally related to clonidine
Cyclobenzaprine (Flexeril)	5 mg TID; MDD 10 mgTID	PO	**Tablets:** 5 mg, 10 mg	• Sedative/hypnotic class • Structurally similar to tricyclic antidepressants
Third Line Therapy				
Orphenadrine (Norflex)	100 mg BID; MDD 200 mg	PO; IV available	**Tablets:** 100 mg sustained release	• Sedative/hypnotic class
Metaxalone (Skelaxin)	400–800 mg TID-QID; MDD 800 mg QID	PO	**Tablets:** 400 mg, 800 mg	• Sedative/hypnotic class
Methocarbamol (Robaxin)	750 mg– 1.5 gms QID; MDD 6 gms	PO; IV available	**Tablets:** 500 mg, 750 mg	• Sedative/hypnotic class
Carisoprodol (Soma)	350 mg QID; MDD 1400 mg	PO	**Tablets:** 350 mg	• Sedative/hypnotic class • Reports of increased abuse potential with this agent

MDD–maximum daily dose

Clinical Pearls

- The causes of muscle cramps can be uncovered in most cases; a thorough history and limited physical exam is important.
- The primary focus for patients with advanced illness is comfort and symptom control. Non-pharmacologic treatments are important along with medications.
- Medications available to treat muscle spasms can potentiate other CNS medications and should be monitored closely.
- Medication dosage, scheduling, and overall utilization should be individually titrated to meet patient's goals for symptom relief with minimization of side effects.

Key References

Berger, AM, Portenoy, RK, Weissman, DE. *Principles and Practice of Palliative Care and Supportive Oncology, Second edition.* Philadelphia, PA: Lippincott Williams & Wilkins, 2002.

Chou, R, Peterson, K, Helfand, M: Comparative Efficacy and Safety of Skeletal Muscle Relaxants for Spasticity and Musculoskeletal Conditions: A systematic Review. *Journal of Pain and Symptom Management.* 28-2: 140–175, 2004.

Smith, HS, Barton, AE: Tizanidine in the management of spasticity and musculoskeletal complaints in the palliative care population. *American Journal of Hospice and Palliative Care.* 17–1: 50–58, 2000.

Steiner, I, Siegal, T: Muscle Cramps in Cancer Patients. *Cancer.* 63: 574–577, 1989.

Lussier, D, Huskey, AG, Portenoy, RK: Adjuvant Analgesics in Cancer Pain Management. *The Oncologist.* 9: 571–591, 2004.

Agar, M, Broadbent, A, Chye, R: The Management of Malignant Psoas Syndrome: Case Reports and Literature Review. *Journal of Pain and Symptom Management.* 28: 282–293, 2004.

Muscle Spasms

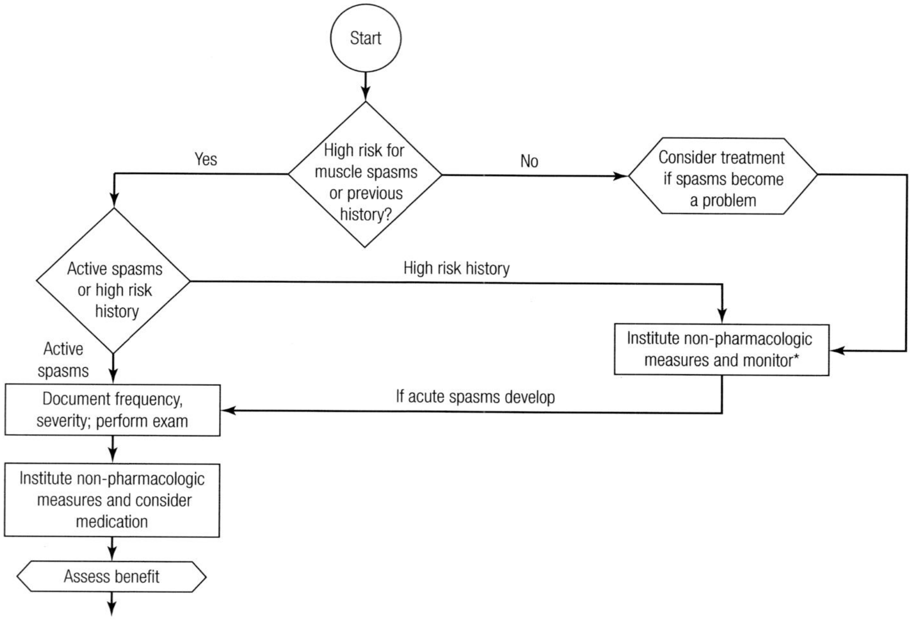

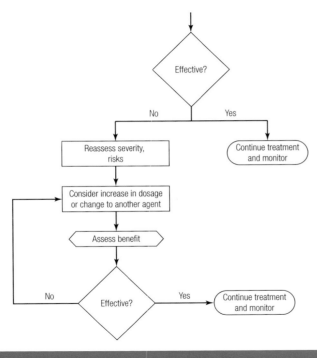

Nausea and Vomiting

Introduction and Background

- Nausea is an unpleasant feeling of needing to vomit often accompanied by autonomic symptoms of pallor, cold sweats, salivation, tachycardia and diarrhea. Nausea can range from a mild stomach upset to complete anorexia. Retching presents as spasmodic movements of the diaphragm and abdominal muscles that may progress to vomiting. Vomiting is a complex process of involuntary spasms resulting in the reflux of gastric contents through the mouth. Chronic nausea can be defined as lasting longer than a week without a well identified or self-limiting cause such as chemotherapy, radiation or infection.
- The GI tract and brain are the two organ systems involved with nausea and vomiting. In these two systems, the primary neurotransmitters that mediate these symptoms include *dopamine, histamine, acetylcholine,* and *serotonin.*
- The pathophysiology of nausea and vomiting is complex. The vomiting center located in the brain receives input from various areas within the brain as well as from the gastrointestinal tract. The figure to the right indicates the four major mechanisms for stimulation of the vomiting center.

Mechanisms Involved in Nausea & Vomiting

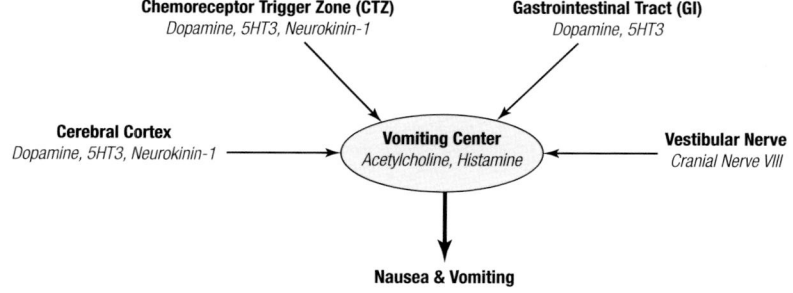

Prevalence

- Studies have demonstrated that up to 71% of palliative care patients will develop nausea and vomiting with approximately 40% experiencing these symptoms in the last six weeks of life.
- Women and younger patients tend to report higher rates then other subsets of patients.

Causes

- Major causes of chronic nausea include:
  - Autonomic dysfunction
  - Constipation
  - Antibiotics
  - Nonsteroidal anti-inflammatory drugs (NSAIDs)
  - Other drugs
  - Infection
  - Peptic ulcer disease
  - Bowel obstruction
  - Metabolic abnormalities (e.g., renal or hepatic failure, hypercalcemia)
  - Increased intracranial pressure
  - Anxiety
  - Radiation therapy
  - Chemotherapy

Clinical Characteristics

- *Chemoreceptor trigger zone* (CTZ) is located in the area postrema of the medulla. Nausea and vomiting are stimulated here by chemotherapeutic agents, bacterial toxins, metabolic products (e.g., uremia) and opioids. Dopamine (D_2), serotonin (5-HT) and neurokinin-1 are the primary neurotransmitters involved in this process. Therapy is based on blocking D2 with dopamine antagonists including butyrophenones (e.g., haloperidol), phenothiazines and metoclopramide. Serotonin (5-HT3) antagonists (e.g., ondansetron), also active here, are mainly used for chemotherapy and radiotherapy-induced nausea.

- *Cerebral Cortex* induced nausea and vomiting can be caused by anxiety, taste, and smell as well as by increased intracranial pressure. Corticosteroids are useful to decrease intracranial pressure while anxiolytics such as benzodiazepines are used to treat "anticipatory" nausea as well as gustatory and olfactory stimulation.

- *Vestibular* nausea and vomiting is triggered by motion. Opioids can sensitize the vestibular center, resulting in movement-induced nausea. Ambulatory patients are more susceptible to vestibular nausea and vomiting than bedbound patients. Since histamine and acetylcholine are the predominant neurotransmitters here, antihistamines and anticholinergics are the drugs of choice in movement-induced nausea and vomiting.

- *Gastrointestinal (GI) tract* stimulation occurs through vagal and sympathetic pathways. These pathways can be triggered by stimulation of either mechanoreceptors or chemoreceptors located in the gut. Gastric stasis, gastrointestinal obstruction, drugs, metastatic disease, bacterial toxins, chemotherapeutic agents, and irradiation can lead to nausea and vomiting. Glossopharyngeal or vagus nerve stimulation in the pharynx by sputum, mucosal lesions or infection (e.g., *Candida*) can also evoke nausea. The major neurotransmitters in the upper GI tract are dopamine, acetylcholine and serotonin (5-HT). Metoclopramide blocks 5-HT4 and increases gastric motility above the jejunum, whereas anticholinergics will decrease GI spasticity and motility in nausea induced by gut hyperactivity. In high doses, metoclopramide will also act as a 5HT3 antagonist.

- *Autonomic Failure* causes gastroparesis resulting in anorexia, nausea, early satiety and constipation. Delayed gastric emptying is frequently observed in patients with diabetes mellitus, chronic renal failure and neurological disorders. Malnutrition, cachexia, lung and pancreatic cancers, human immunodeficiency virus, radiotherapy, and drugs such as opioids, anticholinergics, antidepressants and vasodilators have been associated with autonomic failure and resulting chronic nausea, poor performance, tachycardia and malnutrition.

Non-Pharmacologic Treatment
- Relaxation techniques
- Avoid strong odors, foods, or other triggers
- Eliminate offending medications, if possible

Pharmacologic Management of Nausea and Vomiting

Generic Name (Brand Name)	Usual Adult Starting Dose/Range	Routes	Common Strengths and Formulations	Comments
Chemoreceptor Trigger Zone: First Line Therapy–Dopamine Antagonists				
Haloperidol (Haldol)	0.5–1 mg q12h or q4–6h PRN	PO, PR, SQ, IM, IV, SL	**Tablets:** 0.5, 1, 2, 5, 10, 20 mg **Oral Concentrate:** 2 mg/mL **Injection:** 5 mg/mL	• Potent D_2 antagonist • Rarely need to give over 1–2 mg BID or TID • Extrapyramidal symptoms (EPS) rare in low doses • Parenteral route may cause less EPS than oral • Causes less sedation than other anti-emetics
Prochlorperazine (Compazine)	10 mg PO q4–6h PRN 25 mg PR q6–12h PRN	PO, IM, IV, PR	**Tablets:** 5, 10 mg **Solution:** 5 mg/5 mL **Injection:** 5 mg/mL **Suppositories:** 2.5, 5, 25 mg	• May cause sedation and EPS
Chemoreceptor Trigger Zone: Second Line Therapy–Dopamine Antagonists				
Metoclopramide (Reglan)	10 mg TID-QID AC & HS	PO, PR, IV, SQ	**Tablets:** 5, 10 mg, **Solution:** 5 mg/5 mL **Injection:** 5 mg/mL	• Prokinetic: Useful if gastric stasis also present • Has 5-HT_4 agonist action in the gut • Starting dose for elderly = 5 mg TID-QID • May cause sedation, confusion and EPS
Chlorpromazine (Thorazine)	10–25 mg q4–6h PRN	PO, PR	**Tablets:** 10, 25, 50, 100, 200 mg	• Very sedating • Causes orthostatic hypotension • May cause EPS
Trimethobenzamide (Tigan)	300 mg PO TID-QID PRN	PO	**Capsule:** 300 mg **Solution:** 100 mg/mL	• Anti-emetic of choice in patients with Parkinson's disease • Trimethobenzamide suppositories have been withdrawn from the U.S. market by FDA requirement. Oral formulations are still available
Promethazine (Phenergan)	12.5–50 mg PO, PR, IV, IM q4–6h PRN	PO, IM, IV, PR	**Tablets:** 12.5, 25, 50 mg **Solution:** 6.25 mg/5 mL **Injection:** 12.5, 25, 50 mg/mL **Suppositories:** 12.5 mg, 25 mg, 50 mg	• Less effective than haloperidol, prochlorperazine or chlorpromazine • Very sedating • May cause EPS • Suppositories are expensive

Generic Name (Brand Name)	Usual Adult Starting Dose/Range	Routes	Common Strengths and Formulations	Comments
Gastric Stasis: First Line Therapy				
Metoclopramide (Reglan)	5–10 mg TID-QID AC & HS	PO, PR, IV, SQ	**Tablets:** 5, 10 mg **Solution:** 5 mg/5 mL **Injection:** 5 mg/mL	• D2 antagonist • Has 5-HT4 agonist action in the gut • Starting dose for elderly = 5 mg TID-QID • May cause sedation, confusion and EPS
Erythromycin (E-Mycin)	125–250 mg TID-QID	PO	**Tablets:** 250 mg **Suspension:** 200 mg/5 mL	• Beneficial if patient cannot tolerate metoclopramide (due to EPS)
Vestibular Nausea: First Line Therapy–Antihistamines				
Meclizine (Antivert)	12.5–25 mg q6–12h	PO	**Tablets:** 12.5, 25 mg	• Sedating
Vestibular Nausea: Second Line Therapy–Anticholinergics				
Scopolamine (Transderm Scop)	1–3 patches topically Q3 days	Topical	**Transdermal Patch:** 1.5 mg	• Sedating and constipating • May cause confusion and visual disturbances
Glycopyrrolate (Robinul)	1–2 mg PO q4–6h 0.2 mg SQ, IV q4–6h	PO, SQ, IV	**Tablets:** 1, 2 mg **Injection:** 0.2 mg/mL	• Causes less confusion and visual disturbances because it is least likely to cross the blood-brain barrier
Cerebral Cortex Nausea: First Line Therapy–Anxiolytics				
Lorazepam (Ativan)	0.5–1 mg q4–6h PRN or ATC	PO, SL, PR, SQ,IV, IM	**Tablets:** 0.5, 1, 2 mg **Oral Concentrate:** 2 mg/mL **Injection:** 2, 4 mg/mL	• Treats anxiety that causes or exacerbates nausea and vomiting • Indirect anti-emetic effect
Hydroxyzine (Atarax or Vistaril)	10–25 mg q6h PRN or ATC	PO, IM	**Tablets:** 10, 25, 50, 100 mg **Capsules:** 25, 50, 100 mg **Oral Solution:** 10 mg/5 mL (Atarax) 25 mg/5 mL (Vistaril) **Injection:** 25, 50 mg/mL	• Antihistamine • Very sedating • IM Injection is painful • Atarax (hydroxyzine HCl) and Vistaril (hydroxyzine pamoate) are different salt forms of same active ingredient
Cerebral Cortex Nausea-Increased Intracranial Pressure: First Line Therapy–Corticosteroids				
Dexamethasone (Decadron)	4 mg daily–QID	PO. IV. SQ, PR	**Tablets:** 0.5, 2, 4 mg **Solution:** 1 mg/mL **Injection:** 4 mg/mL	• May titrate to 48 mg/day

Clinical Pearls

- Potentially reversible causes of nausea and vomiting should not be overlooked (e.g., constipation, anxiety, pain, drugs).
- The clinical features of nausea and vomiting should guide the choice of antiemetics used.
- Corticosteroids may have a role in non-specific nausea and vomiting in addition to their usefulness in reducing intracranial pressure. The mechanism of this action is unknown.
- If nausea is due to gastritis, hiatal hernia, gastro-esophageal reflux disease (GERD) or peptic ulcer disease, histamine$_2$ (H$_2$) antagonists or proton pump inhibitors (PPIs) should be administered.
- Refractory cases of nausea and vomiting often require judiciously selected combinations of medications from different classes (e.g., various combinations of haloperidol, metoclopramide, diphenhydramine, lorazepam, dexamethasone).
- 5-HT3 antagonists ondansetron (Zofran), granisetron (Kytril), dolasetron (Anzemet), and palonosetron (Aloxi) have limited usefulness in nausea and vomiting due to terminal illness. They are very expensive and very neurotransmitter-selective. Their niche use is within the first 10–14 days of chemotherapy. Mirtazapine (Remeron) also has some 5-HT3 antagonist activity.
- Aprepitant (Emend) is a neurokinin-1 antagonist which is indicated for the treatment of nausea due to highly emetogenic chemotherapy and in combination with a 5-HT3 antagonist and corticosteroid, not as a sole agent.

Key References

Bruera E, Sweeney C, In: *Principles & Practices of Palliative Care & Supportive Oncology,* 2nd Ed. Philadelphia: Lippincott Williams & Wilkins. Ch 14, 2002.

Ferris FD, von Gunten CF, Emanuel LL: Ensuring competency in end-of-life care: controlling symptoms. *BMC Palliative Care.* 1:5, 2002.

Gralla RJ, Osoba D, Kris MG, et al.: Recommendations for the use of antiemetics: evidence-based, clinical practice guidelines. American Society of Clinical Oncology. *J Clin Oncol.* 17: 2971–2994, 1999.

Tyler LS: Nausea and Vomiting in Palliative Care. In: *Evidence Based Symptom Control in Palliative Care.* Binghamton, NY: The Haworth Press, Inc., 2000, pp 163–181.

Vella-Brincat J, Macleod AD: Haloperidol in palliative care. *Palliat Med.* 18: 195–201, 2004. http://www.cancer.gov/cancertopics/pdq/supportivecare/nausea/HealthProfessional/

Nausea and Vomiting

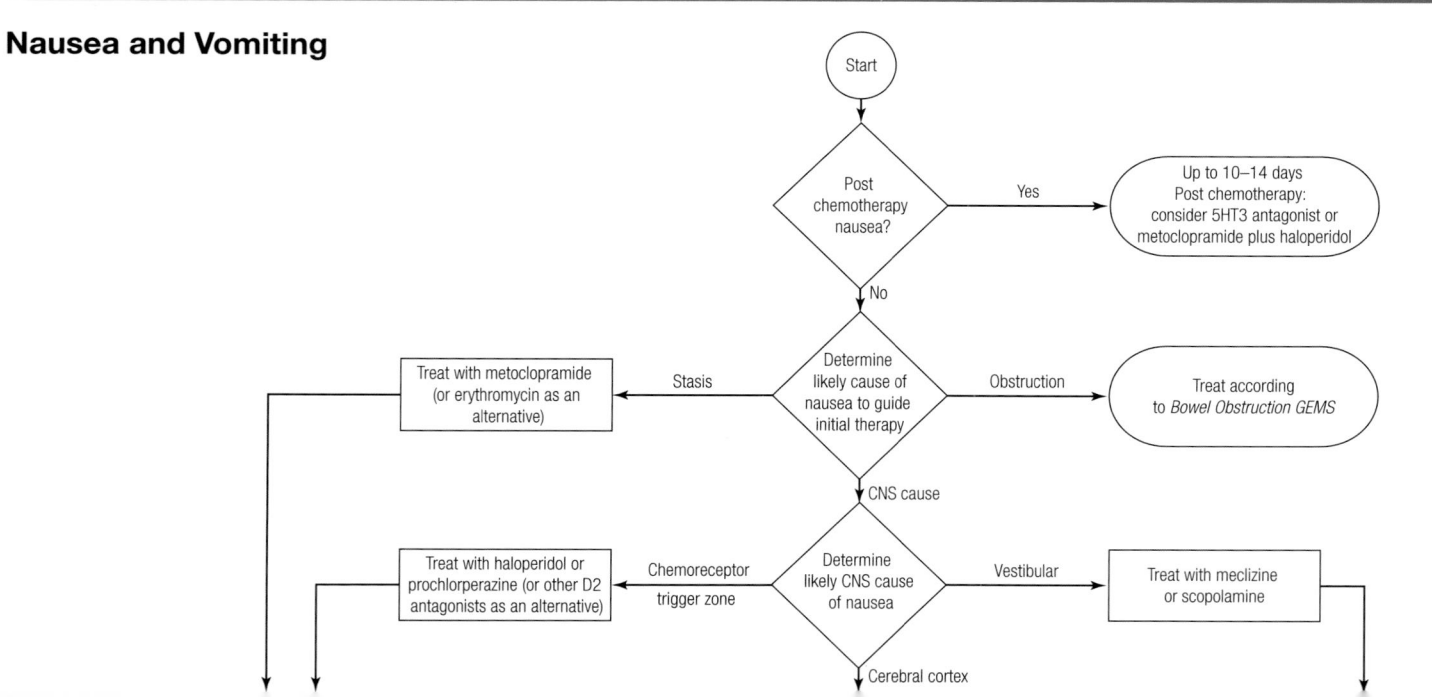

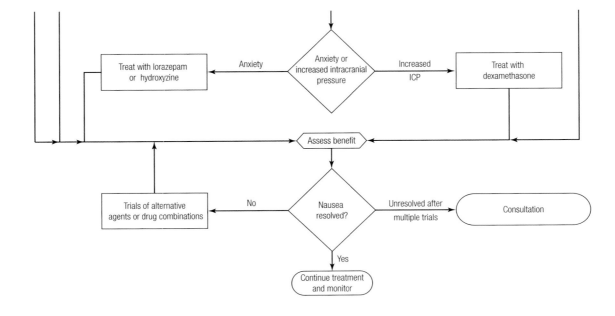

Pain

Medical Definition

- "Pain is an unpleasant sensory and emotional experience associated with actual or potential tissue damage"

  International Association for the Study of Pain, 1979

Operative Definition

- "Pain is whatever the experiencing person says it is, existing whenever he/she says it does."

  Margo McCaffery

Ideal Analgesia = Pain Control + Improved Functional Status

Pain as a Symptom

Acknowledge the presence of and contribution to pain perception of:

- Physical Pain
- Nonphysical Pain
  - Psychological or Emotional Pain
  - Behavioral Pain
  - Cognitive Pain
  - Spiritual/Existential Pain
  - Cultural or Sociological Pain

Classification of Pain

Acute pain

- Identified event, resolves days–weeks
- Usually nociceptive

Chronic pain

- Cause often not easily identified, multifactorial
- Indeterminate duration
- Nociceptive and/or neuropathic

Chemical Classes of Opioids

- *PHENANTHRENES*
  - Morphine
  - Codeine
  - Hydromorphone
  - Hydrocodone
  - Oxycodone
  - Oxymorphone
- *DIPHENYLHEPTANE DERIVATIVE*
  - Methadone
  - Propoxyphene
- *PHENYLPIPERIDINE DERIVATIVES*
  - Meperidine
  - Fentanyl

PQRST Assessment Parameters

P = Provokes
- Aggravating / Alleviating factors
- What causes pain?
- What makes it better?
- Worse?

Q = Quality
(Try to let patient describe the pain, sometimes they say what they think you would like to hear.)

- What does it feel like?
- Is it sharp?
- Dull?
- Stabbing?
- Burning?
- Crushing?

R = Radiates
- Where does the pain radiate?
- Is it in one place?
- Does it go anywhere else?
- Did it start elsewhere and now localized to one spot?

S = Severity
- How severe is the pain on a scale of 1–10?
- On average
- Worst
- Least
- Currently

T = Time
- Time / date pain started?
- How long did it last?

Opioid Adverse Effects

Common	**Uncommon**
Constipation	Bad dreams / hallucinations
Dry mouth	Dysphoria / delirium
Nausea / vomiting	Myoclonus / seizures
Sedation	Pruritus / urticaria
Sweats	Respiratory depression
	Urinary retention

Opioid-Induced Neurotoxicity

- Dependent on both the *dose* and *duration of opioid therapy*
- Other precipitating factors include:
  - Underlying delirium
  - Dehydration
  - Acute renal failure
  - Advanced age
  - Concurrent use of other psychoactive medications
  - Benzodiazepines
  - Tricyclic antidepressants
- Can occur with ALL opioids at high doses but most commonly with morphine (due to accumulation of the morphine-3 glucuronide metabolite) and hydromorphone
- Present with neuroexcitatory side effects (confusion, agitation, myoclonus) despite unrelieved pain
- Further increase of dose exacerbates excitatory behaviors
- Incidence
  - Morphine > Hydromorphone
  - Renal insufficiency > Normal renal function
  - High dose > low dose

Signs/ Symptoms of Neurotoxicity

- Myclonus–twitching of large muscle groups (intermittent, migratory)
- Delirium
- Hallucinations/Seizures
- Rapidly escalating dose requirement
- Hyperalgesia/Allodynia
- Pain "doesn't make sense"; not consistent with recent pattern or known disease

Treatment of Opioid-Induced Neurotoxicity

- Rotate to a structurally dissimilar opioid with differing receptor affinity profiles (methadone or fentanyl)
- Hydration
- Delirium—add haloperidol
- Neuromuscular excitation/myoclonus—clonazepam, lorazepam, baclofen, barbiturates
- Behavioral excitation resolves over hours to days as offending metabolites clear

Simple Descriptive Pain Intensity Scale

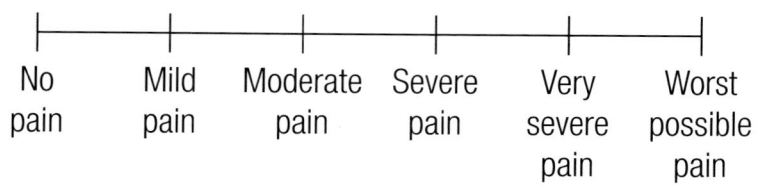

| No pain | Mild pain | Moderate pain | Severe pain | Very severe pain | Worst possible pain |

0–10 cm No Pain/Worst Pain Scale

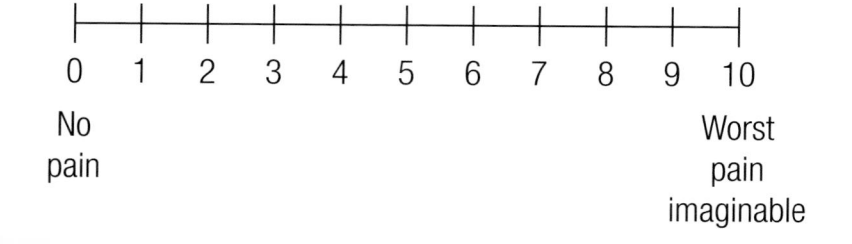

0   1   2   3   4   5   6   7   8   9   10

No pain

Worst pain imaginable

Wong-Baker FACES Pain Rating Scale

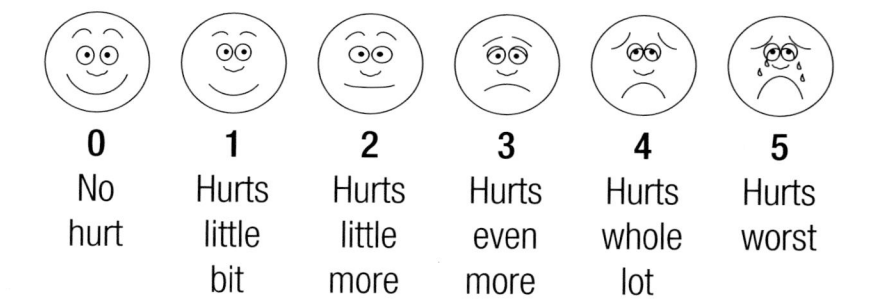

| 0 | 1 | 2 | 3 | 4 | 5 |
| No hurt | Hurts little bit | Hurts little more | Hurts even more | Hurts whole lot | Hurts worst |

Explain to the person that each face is for a person who feels happy because he has no pain (hurt) or sad because he has some or a lot of pain.

Face 0 is very happy because he doesn't hurt at all.

Face 1 hurts just a little bit.

Face 2 hurts a little more.

Face 3 hurts even more.

Face 4 hurts a whole lot.

Face 5 hurts as much as you can imagine, although you don't have to be crying to feel this bad.

Pain Assessment IN Advanced Dementia

PAINAD (Warden, Hurley, Volicer, 2003)

	0	1	2	Score
Breathing Independent of Vocalization	Normal	Occasional labored breathing. Short period of hyperventilation	Noisy labored breathing. Long period of hyperventilation. Cheyne-stokes respirations	
Negative Vocalization	None	Occasional moan or groan. Low level speech with a negative or disapproving quality	Repeated troubled calling out. Loud moaning or groaning. Crying	
Facial Expression	Smiling, or inexpressive	Sad. Frightened. Frown	Facial grimacing	
Body Language	Relaxed	Tense. Distressed pacing. Fidgeting	Rigid. Fists clenched, Knees pulled up. Pulling or pushing away. Striking out	
Consolability	No need to console	Distracted or reassured by voice or touch	Unable to console, distract or reassure	
				TOTAL

OPIOIDS: Equianalgesic Doses and Durations of Action[1]

Generic Name	Examples of Brand Names	SC,IV	Oral	Duration of Action (Hrs)
RECOMMENDED for Chronic Pain Management				
Morphine Sulfate	Roxanol	10 mg	30 mg[2]	4[3,5,6]
Hydromorphone	Dilaudid	1.5 mg	7.5 mg	4[3,6]
Oxycodone	Oxy IR or Combination of Oxycodone 5 mg with ASA or Acetaminophen[4,5] Percocet, Percodan, Tylox	—	20 mg	4
Hydrocodone	In combination with ASA or Acetaminophen[4]: Vicodin, Lortab, Lorcet	—	30 mg	4
Oxymorphone[8]	Opana, Opana ER, Numorphan	1 mg	10 mg	4–6
Fentanyl Transdermal (Recommend decreasing calculated dose by ~ 1/3 when switching from the patch to an alternative drug & route of administration)	Duragesic Transdermal System Patch	**ORAL MORPHINE EQUIV**[6]. 100 mcg/hr ≅ Morphine 200 mg/24 hrs 75 mcg/hr ≅ Morphine 150 mg/24 hrs 50 mcg/hr ≅ Morphine 100 mg/24 hrs 25 mcg/hr ≅ Morphine 50 mg/24 hrs 12.5 mcg/hr ≅ Morphine 25 mg/24 hrs		48–72 hrs

Methadone[7]	Dolophine	50% oral dose	24 hr Oral Morphine / Oral Morphine: Methadone Ratio	8–12 hours
			>30 mg — 2 : 1	
			31–99 mg — 4 : 1	
			100–299 mg — 8 : 1	
			300–499 mg — 10 : 1	
			500–999 mg — 15 : 1	
			>1000 mg — 20 : 1	

NOT RECOMMENDED for Chronic Pain Management

Codeine		130 mg	200 mg	3–4
Butorphanol	Stadol	2 mg	—	3–4
Meperidine	Demerol	100 mg	300 mg	2–4
Nalbuphine	Nubain	10 mg	—	3–4
Pentazocine	Talwin	30 mg	50 mg	3–4

Consider reducing calculated dose by 1/3–1/2 when changing from oral to parenteral route, transdermal to any other route or from one opioid to another to accommodate for incomplete cross sensitivity, absorption variability, and patient variability.

1. Adapted from American Pain Society "Principles of Analgesic Use in the Treatment of Acute Pain and Cancer Pain. 5th Ed. 2003
2. Although controlled single dose studies demonstrate an IM:PO ratio of 1:6, there is good evidence that the ratio changes to 1:2–3 with chronic dosing.
3. Oral route provides the longest duration of action.
4. Maximum dose of acetaminophen/24hrs = 4000 mg (3000 mg in geriatric patients)
5. Sustained release morphine and oxycodone should not be given any more frequently then every 8–12 hours (Exception: Avinza® or Kadian® ~ 24hrs)
6. McCaffrey, M & Pasero, C. Pain Clinical Manual, 2nd Ed., Mosby: St. Louis, 1999.
7. Storey, P. Primer of Palliative Care, 4th Ed., AAHPM 2007.
NOTE: Methadone should only be prescribed by an experienced practitioner
8. Prommer, E. Oxymorphone: A Review. Support Care Cancer. 2006; 14: 109–115.

Somatic Pain

Introduction and Background

Pain is defined by the International Association for the Study of Pain (IASP) as *"an unpleasant sensory and emotional experience associated with actual or potential tissue damage and described in terms of such damage"* (IASP, 1979). Classification of the most common types of pain by pathophysiology and duration is outlined in this figure.

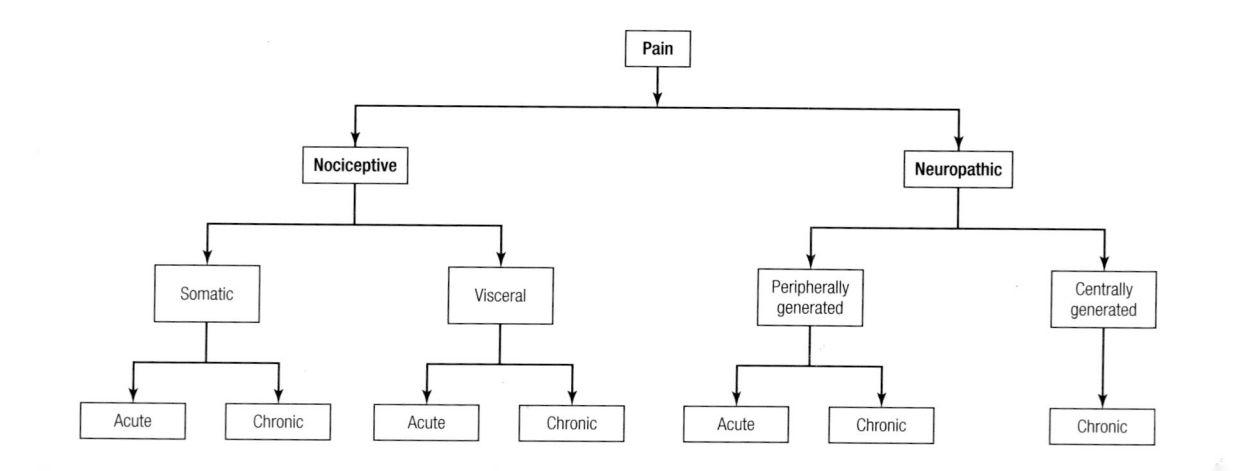

Prevalence

- The SUPPORT study (1995) demonstrated that in spite of efforts to control pain, 74 to 95% of very ill or dying hospitalized patients still experienced uncontrolled pain.
- Although the tools are available to treat over 90% of pain, some patients still suffer needlessly. This is due in part to factors related to health care professionals, including:
  - Lack of knowledge about the appropriate use of analgesics,
  - Undue concern about regulatory oversight, and
  - Undue concern about potential for abuse or addiction.

Causes

Nociceptive pain is defined as the normal processing of stimuli that either cause damage normal tissues or have the potential to do so if exposure to the stimulus is prolonged.

- Nociceptive pain involves four processes: transduction, transmission, perception and modulation.
  - *Transduction* occurs when mechanical, thermal or chemical stimuli cause tissue damage resulting in the release of substances that either sensitize (leukotrienes, prostaglandins, substance P) or stimulate (bradykinin, histamine, serotonin, potassium, norepinephrine) pain fibers.
  - *Transmission* occurs when the stimulation is great enough that the nerve generates an impulse that is transmitted from the site of injury to the spinal cord, through the brain stem and up to the thalamus and cortex.
    - The N-methyl-D-aspartate (NMDA) receptor is one of many receptors that facilitates pain transmission. When this receptor is blocked, pain transmission is blunted or inhibited.
  - *Perception* occurs once the pain impulse reaches the brain.
    - The somatosensory cortex identifies the location and character of the pain while the limbic system assigns emotional and behavioral response to the pain.
  - *Modulation* is the final process where the descending pathway from the brain through the dorsal horn of the spinal cord releases substances that moderate or inhibit pain transmission.
    - These substances include endogenous opioids such as dynorphins and enkephalins, serotonin, norepinephrine, gamma-aminobutyric acid (GABA), neurotensin and alpha 2 adrenergic substances.

Somatic pain is a subset of nociceptive pain arising from afferent nerve stimulation from bone, joint, muscle, skin or connective tissues. Somatic nociceptive pain can be either acute or chronic in nature. Although the focus here is somatic pain, most patients will experience more than one type of pain.

Clinical Characteristics

- A comprehensive and systematic assessment of pain is crucial for the development of an appropriate treatment plan.
- Since pain is a subjective symptom, both physical and humanistic factors must be considered.
- Somatic pain is usually well localized and presents as sharp, pressure-like, throbbing or aching.

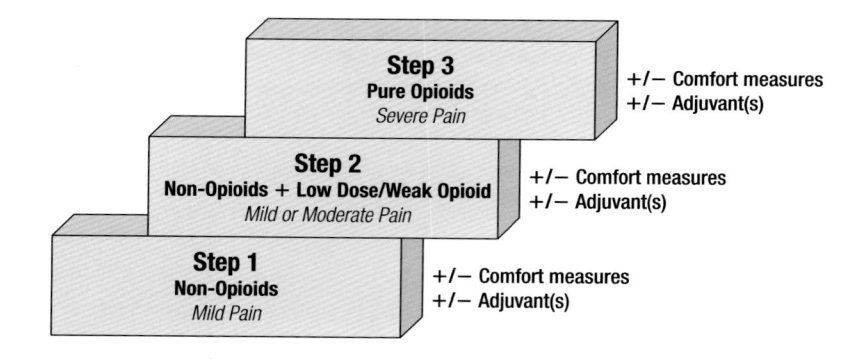

Step 3
Pure Opioids
Severe Pain

+/− Comfort measures
+/− Adjuvant(s)

Step 2
Non-Opioids + Low Dose/Weak Opioid
Mild or Moderate Pain

+/− Comfort measures
+/− Adjuvant(s)

Step 1
Non-Opioids
Mild Pain

+/− Comfort measures
+/− Adjuvant(s)

Non-Pharmacologic Treatment

- Nonpharmacologic therapies are essential in chronic pain management.
- Physical, complementary and cognitive behavioral interventions reduce the perception of pain and can decrease the dosage requirements of medication.
- Nonpharmacologic strategies include:
  - ◆ Education and information about medical treatments, (including myths and misconceptions about pain medication)
  - ◆ Massage
  - ◆ Ice and heat
  - ◆ Physical therapy
  - ◆ Music therapy
  - ◆ Imagery
  - ◆ Distraction
  - ◆ Psychotherapy, reframing and cognitive-behavioral training

Pharmacotherapy

The World Health Organization's stepladder approach to cancer pain management is appropriate for most nociceptive somatic pain, including non-cancer chronic pain in the terminally ill patient.

Pharmacologic Management of Somatic Pain

Generic Name (Brand Name)	Usual Adult Starting Dose/Range	Routes	Common Strengths and Formulations	Comments
First Line Therapy				
World Health Organization (WHO) Step 1				
Acetaminophen (Tylenol)	325–650 mg q4–6h or 500–1000 mg q6–8h	PO, PR	**Tablets/Capsules:** 325 mg, 500 mg **Suppositories:** 120 mg, 325 mg, 650 mg **Syrup:** 160 mg/5 mL	• Maximum daily dose = 4000 mg (3000 mg in geriatric patients) • Weigh risk–benefit in patients with severe liver dysfunction (e.g., cirrhosis)
NSAIDs (Especially beneficial for bone pain and inflammatory pain)				
Ibuprofen (Motrin)	400–800 mg q6–8h	PO	**Tablets:** 200 mg, 400 mg, 600 mg, 800 mg **Syrup:** 100 mg/5 mL	• Maximum daily dose = 3200 mg • Weigh risk-benefit in patients with renal insufficiency
Naproxen (Naprosyn)	250–500 mg q8–12h	PO	**Tablets:** 250 mg, 375 mg, 500 mg **Suspension:** 125 mg/5 mL	• Maximum daily dose =1250 mg/day (expressed as naproxen base, not naproxen sodium) • Aleve® (naproxen sodium) 220 mg = naproxen base 200 mg + 20 mg sodium • Weigh risk-benefit in patients with renal insufficiency
Second Line Therapy				
WHO Step 1				
NSAIDs (Especially beneficial for bone pain and inflammatory pain)				
Choline Magnesium Trisalicylate (Trilisate)	500 mg to 1.5g BID-TID	PO	**Liquid:** 500 mg/5 mL **Tablets:** 500 mg, 750 mg, 1000 mg	• Less platelet effect on aggregation than other NSAIDS • Salicylate derivative
Aspirin	325 mg–650 mg q4–6 h	PO, PR	**Tablets:** 325 mg, 500 mg, 650 mg **Suppositories:** 300 mg, 600 mg	• Maximum daily dose =4000 mg/day (3000 mg in geriatric patients) • Avoid in children due to Reyes Syndrome

Generic Name (Brand Name)	Usual Adult Starting Dose/Range	Routes	Common Strengths and Formulations	Comments
NSAIDs (Especially beneficial for bone pain and inflammatory pain)				
Ketorolac (Toradol)	**IV:** 60 mg initially, then 30 mg q6h **IM:** 30 mg q6h **PO:** 20 mg initially then 10 mg q6h	IV, IM, PO	**Injection:** 15/mL, 30 mg/mL **Tablet:** 10 mg	• Maximum daily parenteral dose = 120 mg • IV/IM administration should not exceed 5 days • Oral route not recommended due to toxicities: Maximum daily dose = 40 mg orally
First Line Therapy **WHO Step 2**				
Acetaminophen + Hydrocodone (Lortab, Vicodin)	**PO:** 5–10 mg/500 mg q6h titrate to effect	PO	**Tablets:** 2.5/500 mg, 5/325 mg, 5/400 mg 5/500 mg, 7.5/325 mg, 7.5/400 mg 7.5/500 mg, 7.5/650 mg 7.5/750 mg, 10/325 mg, 10/400 mg 10/500 mg, 10/650 mg, 10/660 mg **Capsules:** 5/500 mg **Syrup:** 7.5/500 mg/15 mL, 7.5/325 mg/15 mL	• Schedule III controlled substance • Hydrocodone also available in combination with ibuprofen • Watch acetaminophen content (MDD acetaminophen = 4000 mg; 3000 mg in geriatric patients) • Maximum daily dose = 60 mg Hydrocodone • Elderly dosing of hydrocodone is ½ starting dose
Acetaminophen + Oxycodone (Percocet)	**PO:** 5–10 mg/325 mg q4–6h titrate to effect	PO	**Tablets:** 2.5/325 mg, 5/325 mg, 5/500 mg, 7.5/325 mg, 7.5/500 mg, 10/325 mg, 10/650 mg **Capsules:** 5/500 mg **Syrup:** 5/325 mg/mL	• Schedule II controlled substance • Watch acetaminophen content (MDD acetaminophen = 4000 mg; 3000 mg in geriatric patients) • Elderly dosing of oxycodone is ½ starting dose
Second Line Therapy **WHO Step 2**				
Acetaminophen + Codeine (Tylenol #3)	**PO:** 30–60 mg/300 mg q4–6h titrate to effect	PO	**Tablets:** 15/300 mg, 30/300 mg, 60/300 mg **Suspension:** 12/120 mg/5 mL **Syrup:** 12/120 mg/5 mL	• Schedule III controlled substance (Acetaminophen + Codeine 15 mg is Schedule V) • Weak opioid • Very constipating • Watch acetaminophen content (MDD acetaminophen = 4000 mg; 3000 mg in geriatric patients)

| Acetaminophen + Propoxyphene (Darvocet N 100) | **PO:** 50–100 mg/325–650 mg q4h | PO | **Tablets:** 65/650 mg, 50/325 mg, 100/325 mg, 100/500 mg 100/650 mg, | • NOT RECOMMENDED
• Schedule IV controlled substance
• Weak, ineffective opioid
• Cardiotoxic metabolites
• Watch acetaminophen content (MDD acetaminophen = 4000 mg: 3000 mg in geriatric patients)
• Maximum daily dose = 600 mg propoxyphene |

Third Line Therapy

WHO Step 2

| Tramadol +/− Acetaminophen (Ultram, Utlracet) | **PO:** 50–100 mg q4–6h | PO | **Tablets:** 50 mg, 37.5/APAP 325 mg | • Major mechanism of action is inhibition of serotonin and norepinephrine reuptake
• VERY weak opioid activity
• Is not a controlled substance
• Maximum daily dose = 400 mg of tramadol
• Elderly, renal MDD = 200 mg |

First Line Therapy

WHO Step 3

| Morphine IR (Roxanol) | **PO:** 2.5–5 mg q4h
IV: 2 mg q3–4h
IM/SQ: 2–4 mg q3–4h
PR: 10–20 mg q3–4h | PO, PR, SL, IV, IM, SQ | **Tablets/Capsules:** 15 mg, 30 mg
Oral Solution: 10 mg/5 mL, 20 mg/5 mL,
Oral Concentrate: 20 mg/mL
Injection: 2 mg/mL, 4 mg/mL, 8 mg/mL, 10 mg/mL, 15 mg/mL, 25 mg/mL, 50 mg/mL
Suppositories: 5 mg, 10 mg, 20 mg, 30 mg | • Schedule II controlled substance
• Glucuronide metabolites accumulate in renal insufficiency and with high doses causing neurotoxicity |

Generic Name (Brand Name)	Usual Adult Starting Dose/Range	Routes	Common Strengths and Formulations	Comments
First Line Therapy (continued)				
WHO Step 3				
Morphine SR (MS Contin, Avinza, Kadian)	**PO:** Starting dose based on immediate release equivalent dose Lowest starting dose = Morphine SR 15 mg q12 h or Avinza® = 30 mg q24h Kadian® = 20 mg q24h	PO, PR	**SR Tablets:** 15 mg, 30 mg, 60 mg, 100 mg, 200 mg **SR Capsules:** 20 mg, 30 mg, 50 mg, 60 mg, 90 mg, 100 mg, 120 mg	• Schedule II controlled substance • Glucuronide metabolites accumulate in renal insufficiency and with high doses causing neurotoxicity • Do not crush • May give rectally (Unapproved route) • Avinza + Kadian capsules are 24 hour products • Avinza and Kadian capsules may be opened and the pellets may be sprinkled on food or put down feeding tube • Concurrent administration of Avinza and alcohol may disrupt extended release mechanism
Methadone (Dolophine)	see Methadone Dosing Protocol	PO,SL, PR, IV, SQ	**Tablets:** 5 mg, 10 mg **Oral Solution:** 5 mg/5 mL, 10 mg/5 mL **Oral Concentrate:** 10 mg/mL **Injection:** 10 mg/mL	• Schedule II controlled substance • Requires knowledgeable clinician to dose methadone • Long and variable half-life (Average ~25 hrs) • Multiple drug interactions & QT prolongation • Dosage adjustment needed only in severe renal insufficiency (GFR <10 mL/min)
Oxycodone IR (Oxy IR)	**PO:** 2.5–5 mg q4–6h	PO, PR, SL	**Tablets:** 5 mg, 15 mg, 30 mg **Capsules:** 5 mg **Oral Solution:** 5 mg/5 mL **Oral Concentrate:** 20 mg/mL	• Schedule II controlled substance
Oxycodone SR (OxyContin)	**PO:** 10 mg q12h (opioid naïve)	PO, PR	**CR Tablets:** 10 mg, 20 mg, 40 mg, 80 mg	• Schedule II controlled substance • Safer than morphine in severe renal insufficiency • Do not crush • May give rectally (Unapproved route)

Second Line Therapy				
WHO Step 3				
Fentanyl Patch (Duragesic)	12.5 mcg/hr in opioid naïve patients Change patch every 48–72 hrs.	Transdermal	**Transdermal:** 12.5 mcg/hr, 25 mcg/hr, 50 mcg/hr, 75 mcg/hr, 100 mcg/hr,	• Schedule II controlled substance • Matrix product may be cut • Variable absorption in geriatric and cachectic patients • Do not apply heat to patch • Some patients require every 48 hour dosing
Hydromorphone (Dilaudid)	**PO:** 2–4 mg q3–4h **IV:** 0.2–0.6 mg q2–3h **IM/SQ:** 0.5 mg/mL q4–6h **Rectal:** 3 mg q4–8h	PO, PR, SL, IV, SQ	**Tablets:** 2 mg, 4 mg, 8 mg **Oral Solution:** 1 mg/mL **Suppository:** 3 mg **Injection:** 1 mg/mL, 2 mg/mL, 4 mg/mL, 10 mg/mL	• Schedule II controlled substance • Hydromorphone 10 mg/mL injection (most potent opioid per volume) good for SQ • Less neurotoxicity than morphine • Currently not available in SR form
Fentanyl Injection	50–100 mcg q1–2h	IV	**Injection:** 0.5 mg/mL	• Schedule II controlled substance • Short duration of action
Oxymorphone (Opana, Opana ER, Numorphan Inj.)	**IR:** 10–20 mg q4–6h **ER:** 5 mg q12h **Inj:** 0.5 mg q4–6h	PO, IM, IV	**Tablets:** 5 mg, 10 mg **ER Tablets:** 5 mg, 10 mg, 20 mg, 40 mg **Injection:** 1 mg/mL	• Expensive • Administer on empty stomach, 1 hour before or 2 hours after a meal

Clinical Pearls

- Pain and patient's response to therapy should be assessed thoroughly and frequently.
- Opioids should be started at the lowest effective dose and titrated judiciously.
- If pain is constant, around the clock dosing of analgesics is preferred.
- Know equianalgesic dosing of opioids (see chart, pages 186-187).
- When titrating opioid doses, increase daily maintenance dose by 25–50% if patients are requiring 2 to 3 breakthrough doses per 24 hours.
- Breakthrough and incident pain should be treated with 5–15% of the daily maintenance dose. Frequency of breakthrough dosing depends on route of administration. Breakthrough dosing frequency should not exceed: PO = every 1–2 h, SQ = every 20–30 min. and IV = every 6–20 min.
- Use only short acting opioids for breakthrough pain (e.g., morphine IR, oxycodone IR, hydromorphone IR).
- Monitor and treat side effects. Common side effects of opioids include constipation, nausea & vomiting, itching, transient sedation.
- Constipation occurs with all opioids and should be prevented. A stimulant laxative +/− a stool softener is the most appropriate therapy for opioid induced constipation (see Constipation GEMS).
- Myoclonus, delirium, hallucinations and hyperalgesia are signs of opioid neurotoxicity and require opioid rotation.
- Respiratory depression, although uncommon with proper dosing, may occur if a patient is opioid naïve, in combination with other respiratory depressant drugs or when overdose occurs. In the case of significant respiratory depression (respirations < 6), small doses of diluted naloxone (0.1 mg/0.25 mL) may be administered SQ, IV or IM every 5 to 15 minutes until respirations are >10, without causing the patient to get out of pain control.
- Drugs NOT recommended for treatment of pain in hospice
  - Meperidine (Demerol):
    - Short (2–3 hour) duration of analgesia. Repeated administration may lead to CNS toxicity (tremor, confusion, or seizures).
  - Opioid agonist-antagonists (pentazocine (Talwin), butorphanol (Stadol), nalbuphine (Nubain))
    - Analgesic ceiling. Risk of precipitating withdrawal in opioid-dependent patients.
    - Possible production of unpleasant psychotomimetic effects (e.g., dysphoria, delusions, hallucinations).

- Partial agonist (buprenorphine (Buprenex))
  - Analgesic ceiling. May precipitate withdrawal.
- Antagonists (naloxone (Narcan), naltrexone (ReVia))
  - Precipitate withdrawal. Limit use to treatment of life-threatening respiratory depression. Give only in diluted form to opioid-tolerant patients.
- Anxiolytics alone (alprazolam (Xanax), diazepam (Valium), lorazepam, (Ativan))
  - Analgesic properties not demonstrated except for some instances of neuropathic pain. Added sedation from anxiolytics may compromise neurological assessment in patients receiving opioids.
- Sedative/hypnotic drugs alone (barbiturates, benzodiazepines)
  - Analgesic properties not demonstrated. Added sedation from sedative/hypnotic drugs limits opioid dosing.

Key References

American Pain Society: *Principles of Analgesic Use in the Treatment of Acute Pain and Cancer Pain*. 5th Ed., 2003.

Berger AM, Portenoy RK, Weissman DE: *Principles & Practices of Palliative Care & Supportive Oncology*. 2nd Ed. Philadelphia: Lippincott Williams & Wilkins., 2002.

Davis MP, Frandsen JL: *Palliative Practices: An Interdisciplinary Approach*. St. Louis: Elsevier Mosby, Inc., 2005.

http://www.cancer.gov/cancertopics/pdq/supportivecare/pain/HealthProfessional

McCaffery M, Pasero C: Pain: *Clinical Manual*. 2nd Ed. St. Louis: Elsevier Mosby, Inc., 1999.

Somatic Pain

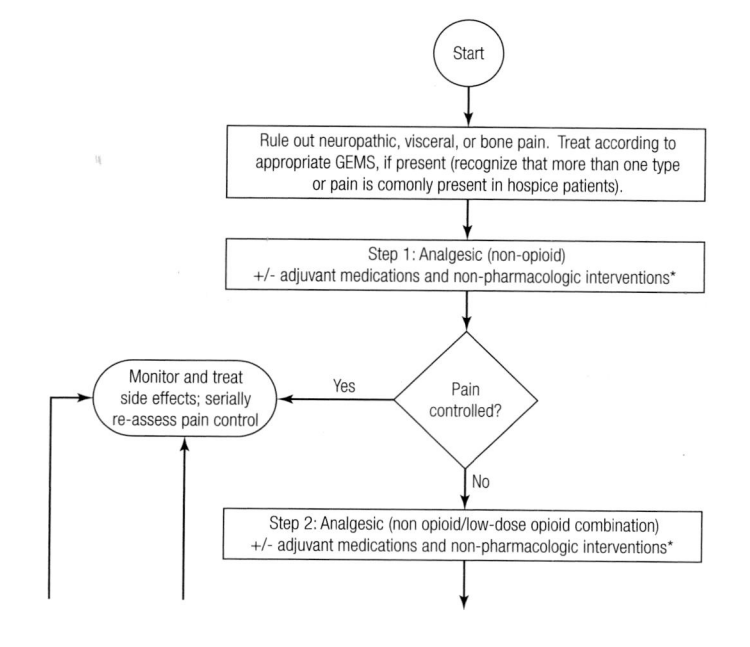

Start

Rule out neuropathic, visceral, or bone pain. Treat according to appropriate GEMS, if present (recognize that more than one type or pain is comonly present in hospice patients).

Step 1: Analgesic (non-opioid)
+/- adjuvant medications and non-pharmacologic interventions*

Pain controlled?

Yes

Monitor and treat side effects; serially re-assess pain control

No

Step 2: Analgesic (non opioid/low-dose opioid combination)
+/- adjuvant medications and non-pharmacologic interventions*

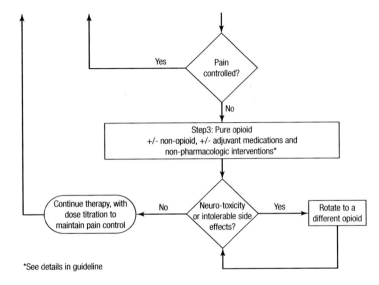

*See details in guideline

Methadone

General Considerations

Methadone, when used appropriately, is an effective analgesic and often relieves pain when other opioids and analgesics have been ineffective. By careful patient assessment, education and monitoring, adverse events can be avoided.

Consider Methadone for Patients with

- Rapidly escalating analgesic requirements
  - > 200 mg oral morphine equivalent/day
- Prominent neuropathic pain
- Renal insufficiency
  - Dosage adjustment needed only when CrCl <10 mL/min
- Dose-limiting side effects from other opioids
  - e.g., nausea, constipation,
  - Neurotoxicity–hyperalgesia, hallucinations, myoclonus.

Methadone and Neuropathic Pain

- Methadone is the most effective opioid for neuropathic pain.
- Methadone's pharmacologic properties make it unique:
  - Uniquely affects neurotransmitters in the brain (inhibits re-uptake of serotonin and nor-epinephrine).

- Active N-methyl-D-aspartate (NMDA) receptor antagonist:
  - Reduces CNS excitatory amino acid amplification of pain sensation (pain "wind-up"), thereby reducing CNS sensitization to pain/hyperalgesia.
- Methadone has reduced development of analgesic tolerance.

Methadone Patient Evaluation and Assessment

- Evaluate patient appropriateness for methadone therapy by assessing the patient and caregiver for potential non-compliance with dosing regimen.
- Educate the patient that he or she should not expect the same immediate effects (sedation or euphoria) as with other opioids such as morphine.
- Educate the caregiver about signs and symptoms of oversedation or opioid toxicity.
- Review current medications for potential adverse drug interactions.
- Assess for cardiac risk factors (e.g., QT interval prolongation).
- Determine if opioid use is for pain and/or dyspnea (methadone is not recommended for the management of dyspnea).

SAFETY CONSIDERATIONS

The Food and Drug Administration (FDA) Methadone Warning

- On November 27, 2006, the FDA issued a Public Health Advisory regarding the risk of death or life-threatening adverse events due to respiratory depression and cardiac arrhythmias in patients receiving methadone.

- These risks of adverse events with methadone are primarily related to:
  - Lack of knowledge regarding dosing and dose titration, leading to inadvertent overdose;
  - Drug interactions; and
  - Cardiac arrhythmias (e.g., Torsades de Pointes).

Methadone and Cardiac Arrhythmias

- A small number of reports describe patients taking methadone who have experienced ventricular arrhythmias (e.g., Torsades de Pointes):
  - Primarily in doses greater than 200 mg daily
  - Mostly when administered by the IV route
- Methadone may not be appropriate in patients with:
  - Known history of cardiac arrhythmias
  - Bradycardia
  - Electrolyte disturbances (particularly hypokalemia, hypomagnesemia, hypocalcemia)
  - Congenital or other pre-existing QT interval prolongation
- Methadone should be used with caution with other medications which have been associated with prolonged QT interval (such as tricyclic antidepressants, antiarrhythmics, antiemetics, antipsychotics, erythromycin, clarithromycin). (See Drugs That Prolong QT Interval chart, pg. 303)
- If QT interval prolongation is a major concern AND methadone is indicated, some clinicians choose to obtain a baseline electrocardiogram prior to initiating methadone therapy and obtain repeat EKGs periodically while on methadone (e.g. obtaining serial EKGs after each dose change).

Avoiding Problems with Methadone

- Problems arise from the cumulative effect of risk factors.
- Care should be taken to avoid concomitant use of *multiple medications, (particularly in high doses)*:
  - That can prolong the QT interval
  - In patients with predisposing clinical conditions
  - That interact with methadone
    - CYP450 metabolism (See Drugs Affected by Cytochrome P450 Enzyme Metabolism chart, pg. 324)
    - CNS depressants

DOSING/DOSE CONVERSION CONSIDERATIONS

Methadone Rotation Protocol Controversies (no literature consensus)

- Dosage conversion ratio:
  - Fixed VERSUS variable
- Discontinuation of previous opioid:
  - Abrupt VERSUS decreasing over 3–5 days
- Maintenance dosing intervals:
  - Every 6, 8, 12 or 24 hours
- Breakthrough medication:
  - Short acting opioid (morphine, oxycodone or hydromorphone) VERSUS methadone

Methadone Dosing, Titration and Monitoring Guidelines

1. Understand the pharmacokinetics of methadone:
   - Methadone has a long elimination half-life (8–59 hours)
   - Methadone has a duration of analgesia that is substantially shorter than its elimination half-life (6–12 hours–up to 24 hours in some patients with continued use)
   - Methadone is metabolized by CYP450 enzymes CYP3A4 and CYP2D6 (and, to a lesser extent, CYP1A2)
   - Dosing guidelines and equianalgesic dosage conversions vary
2. Maintain an accurate medication profile of prescription drugs and over the counter medications (including herbals and dietary supplements) taken along with methadone.
3. Avoid the use of medications known to interact with methadone. (See Drugs That Prolong QT Interval or Induce Torsades de Pointes chart, pg. 303 and Drugs Affected by Cytochrome P450 Enzyme Metabolism chart, pg. 324).
4. When co-administering methadone with potentially interacting medications, adjust methadone doses based on patient response rather than a calculated dose correction.
5. Educate the patient on the importance of adhering to the prescribed medication regimen.
6. Educate the patient and caregiver regarding signs of overmedication and opioid withdrawal.
   - *Overmedication:* Increased sedation, early respiratory depression (< than 9 breaths/minute not associated with normal dying process) and pinpoint pupils.
   - *Opioid withdrawal:* Yawning, sweating, lacrimation, rhinorrhea, anxiety, restlessness, insomnia, dilated pupils, piloerection, chills, tachycardia, hypertension, nausea/vomiting, crampy abdominal pains, diarrhea, and muscle aches and pains.

Dose Conversion Strategy 1: AAHPM Methadone Equianalgesic Dosing Ratio[1]	
24 Hour Oral Morphine Equivalent	Morphine : Methadone Ratio (per 24 hours)
< 30 mg / 24 hrs	2 :1
30–99 mg / 24 hrs	4 : 1
100–299 mg / 24 hrs	8 : 1
300–499 mg / 24 hrs	10 : 1
500–999 mg / 24 hrs	15 : 1
>1000 mg / 24 hrs	20 : 1
Divide calculated 24 hour methadone dose to administer every 8–12 hours	

[1]Storey, P Primer of Palliative Care 3rd Ed American *Academy of Hospice and Palliative Medicine Handbook,* 2004

Dose Conversion Strategy 2: Methadone Dosing Rotation[1,2]
1. Calculate 24 hour oral morphine equivalent dose based on current opioid use

2. Calculate Methadone dose equivalent
   • 20% of 24 hour oral morphine equivalent (1:5 methadone to morphine ratio)
   • **Do not exceed starting methadone dose = 60 mg PO/24hrs (30 mg IV/SC/24hrs)**

3. Consider reduction of calculated 24 hour methadone dose (administering 2/3 of calculated dose initially) IF dose of previous opioid was escalated for reasons including cross tolerance, lack of co-analgesics, non-physical pain component, neurotoxicity, hyperalgesia, etc.
4. Divide 24 hour calculated methadone dose by 2 for q12h ATC or 3 for q8h ATC

5. Calculate methadone breakthrough:
   • 1/6th the 24 hour scheduled methadone dose dosage equivalent q4h prn
   • May choose to use short acting opioid for breakthrough in certain patients

6. Monitor patients closely (daily) for the first 5 to 7 days after initiating methadone therapy.
7. Escalate doses no more frequently then every three (3) days in most cases. Doses should generally NOT be escalated in more than 25–30% increments.   • Allow the patient to use breakthrough doses in between dosage titrations.
8. In patients on high dose or parenteral opioids, consider titrating down previous opioid over 3–5 days instead of abruptly stopping drug   • Prevents opioid withdrawal & potential for psychological methadone failure

[1]*Clinical experience Grauer, PA Palliative Care Consulting Group Protocol, Unpublished*
[2]*Several effective dosing methods have been published.*

Parenteral Methadone

- Most clinicians support a methadone parenteral-to-oral conversion ratio of 1 : 2
- May give intermittently or by continuous infusion
  - Subcutaneous administration can cause local irritation
  - IV may be associated with higher risk of QT interval prolongation

References

http://www.fda.gov/medwatch/safety/2006/safety06.htm#Methadone.

Walker, Georgina; Wilcock, Andrew; Carey, Ann Marie; et al. Prolongation of QT Interval in Palliative Care Patients. Journal of Pain and Symptom Management. 2003, 26(3): 855–9.

Woosley, RL. Drugs That Prolong the QT Interval and/or Induce Torsades de Pointes, Arizona Center for Education and Research on Therapeutics. http://www.arizonacert.org/medical-pros/drug-lists/printable-drug-list.cfm Accessed 1/28/07.

Methadone for cancer pain: what have we learned from clinical studies? American Journal of Hospice and Palliative Care. 2005, 22(5):337.

Davis MP, Walsh D. Methadone for relief of cancer pain: a review of pharmacokinetics, pharmacodynamics, drug interactions and protocols of administration. Supportive Care in Cancer. 2001, 9(2):73–83.

Storey, P Primer of Palliative Care 3rd Ed AAHPM 2004.

Mercurio TC, McPherson ML. Using Methadone Effectively and Safely as Analgesic. Practical Pain Management. 2005, 7 (2):68–75.

Bone Pain

Introduction and Background

- Bone pain is a subset of somatic, nociceptive pain.
- Bone metastases cause moderate to severe pain in 70–90% of patients.
- Bone pain may be intermittent but increases with standing or walking in weight bearing bones with a persistent quality that can cause or exacerbate collateral symptoms such as:
  - Insomnia
  - Fatigue
  - Malaise
  - Loss of appetite/Anorexia
  - Depression/Anxiety

Prevalence

- Bone pain commonly occurs with multiple myeloma and from metastatic spread in lung (64%), breast (50–80%), and prostate (60–85%), bladder (42%), and kidney/thyroid (28–60%) cancers.

Causes

- Bone pain can be due to primary bone cancer or more commonly to bone metastases.
- Bone cancer pain is due in part to stretching of the periosteum as tumor size increases but also results from stimulation of nerve endings within bone structures.

Clinical Characteristics

- Severe bone cancer pain is rarely controlled with a single analgesic agent.
- As the tumor increases in size, the pain often becomes continuous and achy with sharp exacerbations. Some patients may experience continuous pain early in the disease process.
- In addition to pain from periostitis, vertebral lesions can cause neuropathic pain due to spinal cord compression. Both anti-inflammatory and neuropathic analgesics are usually needed in such cases.

Non-Pharmacologic Treatment

- Heat therapy: Heat relaxes tense surrounding muscles, acts as a counter-irritant, and may directly affect local tissues.
- Clothing: Warm clothes are beneficial as cold can worsen pain. Avoid tight fitting or heavy garments that may cause further irritation to sensitive tissues.
- Activity: Balancing activity with rest is an important factor in the control of bone pain.
- Positioning: Resting with joints extended and in good alignment, rather than flexed may reduce pain.
- Physical therapy: Light exercise can relieve general musculoskeletal discomfort associated with inactivity.
- Surgery: Sometimes necessary to stabilize the bone and reduce fracture risk. However, not commonly indicated in palliative care.

Pharmacotherapy

- Anti-inflammatory analgesics, especially nonsteroidal anti-inflammatory drugs (NSAIDs), are the most important pharmacotherapy for bone cancer lesions. NSAIDs are synergistic with and are dose sparing for opioids (and vice versa).
- Acetaminophen does NOT have peripheral anti-inflammatory effects and can be a dose limiting factor when opioid/acetaminophen combinations are used. A frequent failure in management of bone pain occurs when opioids are used exclusively or in combination with acetaminophen in place of an anti-inflammatory medication.
- Anti-inflammatory agents are first line therapy as up to 80% respond to these drugs. When NSAIDs no longer provide adequate relief as the bone involvement of disease progresses, addition, not substitution, of an opioid is indicated.
- All non-selective NSAIDs have similar efficacy. Ibuprofen and naproxen are the most cost effective choices in hospice care.
- Non-selective NSAIDs and the COX-2 selective NSAID celecoxib are also similar in efficacy. Celecoxib may be indicated in patients with impaired clotting disorders or who are receiving anticoagulants as COX-2s have less effect on platelet aggregation.
- Glucocorticosteroids are an alternative anti-inflammatory if NSAIDs cannot be used. Since steroids are not analgesics, acetaminophen (up to 4 grams per day) may be a useful adjunct to steroid therapy for bone pain. Steroids are often used in pain crises related to bone metastases in conjunction with opioids.
- Steroids, usually in combination with opioids, improve the severe pain of spinal cord compression within several hours.
- Bisphosphonates can be useful in bone pain, but are expensive. These agents are administered intravenously once a month and often lose their effectiveness over time, therefore, they may not be appropriate in the hospice setting.
- Calcitonin has also been used to treat bone pain with limited success.
- Palliative radiation is highly effective in treating pain due to localized bone lesions and may greatly reduce or eliminate the need for analgesics and their side effects. However analgesic pharmacotherapy is generally needed for several days until the radiation effect is maximized. In some cases, a single fraction of radiation may be as effective as multiple fractions administered over days to weeks.
- Systemic radionuclide therapy, e.g. strontium (Metastron)[89] has been used to provide pain relief from bone cancer for up to three to six months. This therapy might be considered when patients have multiple, remote bone metastases, a life expectancy of at least six months, and are unable to tolerate systemic pharmacotherapy.

Pharmacologic Management of Bone Pain

Generic Name (Brand Name)	Usual Adult Starting Dose/Range	Maximum Daily Dose	Common Strengths and Formulations	Comments
First Line Therapy				
Non-steroidal anti-inflammatory drugs:				
Ibuprofen (Motrin)	400 –800 mg po TID. Doses of 400 mg and 600 mg normally require a 4–6 hour dosing interval.	3200 mg/day (rarely should 2400 mg be exceeded in hospice care)	**Tablets:** 200 mg, 400 mg, 600 mg, 800 mg	• May cause an increase in systolic blood pressure and edema (all NSAIDs) • PPIs may be useful for gastric protection in selected "at risk" patients (all NSAIDs)
Naproxen (Naprosyn)	500 mg po BID	1250 mg/day (rarely should 1 gm be exceeded in hospice care)	**Tablets:** 250 mg, 375 mg, 500 mg	• Advantage over ibuprofen of BID dosing
Second Line Therapy				
Corticosteroids:				
Dexamethasone (Decadron)	2 mg–16 mg po daily	Up to 1 mg/kg of body weight	**Tablets:** 0.25 mg, 0.5 mg, 0.75 mg, 1 mg, 1.5 mg, 2 mg, 4 mg, 6 mg **Elixir:** 0.5 mg/5 mL **Oral Solution:** 0.5 mg/5 mL **Concentrated oral solution (Intensol):** 1 mg/mL	• Long term effects must be considered but the initiation of therapy should not be delayed because of undue concerns about adverse effects of prolonged use
Prednisone (Deltasone)	10 mg–20 mg po daily	60 mg/day	**Tablets:** 1 mg, 2.5 mg, 5 mg, 10 mg, 20 mg, 50 mg **Oral Solution:** 5 mg/5 mL **Concentrated Oral Solution:** 5 mg/mL **Syrup:** 5 mg/5 mL	• Long term effects must be considered but the initiation of therapy should not be delayed because of undue concerns about adverse effects of prolonged use
Opioid Choices See Somatic Pain				

NSAIDs = Non-steroidal anti-inflammatory drugs

PPIs = Proton Pump Inhibitors

Key References

Woodruff R. Palliative Medicine: Symptomatic and Supportive Care for Patients with Advanced Cancer and AIDS (2nd ed.). Victoria, Australia, 1993.

Derek D, Hanks G, MacDonald N. Oxford Textbook of Palliative Medicine. New York, Oxford University Press, 1993.

MedicineAU.net [homepage on the Internet]. Lismore: Medicine Australia; Palliation of bone pain in cancer; [about 2 screens]. Updated 12/04 [cited 2005 Feb 12]. Available from: http://www.medicineau.net.au/home.ht mL.

Phillips LL. Managing the pain of bone metastases in the home environment. The American Journal of Hospice and Palliative Care. 1998; (January/February): 32–42.

Weaver, CH. Managing side effects treatment and prevention. Cancer Consultants.com 1998–2004, last updated 05/04 [cited 2005 Feb 7]. Available from: http://patient.cancerconsultants.com/supportive_treatment.aspx?id =1001.

Kaye P. Notes on Symptom Control in Hospice and Palliative Care. Revised 1st ed. USA version. Machiasport: Hospice Education Institute; 1990.

Lacy F, Armstrong L, Goldman M, Leonard L. Lexi-Comp's Drug Information Handbook. 12th ed. Hudson; Lexi-Comp; 2004.

Emanuel LL, von Gunten CF, Ferris FD. The Education for Physicians on End-of Life Care (EPEC) curriculum, 1999. Module 4: Pain Management. EPEC Project, The Robert Wood Johnson Foundation. Page M4–19.

Killion K, ed. Drug Facts and Comparisons. Electronic edition. St. Louis; Facts and Comparisons, 2005, [Various drug monographs.]

Mundy GR. In: Bone Remodeling and Its Disorders. 1995;104–107.

Bone Pain

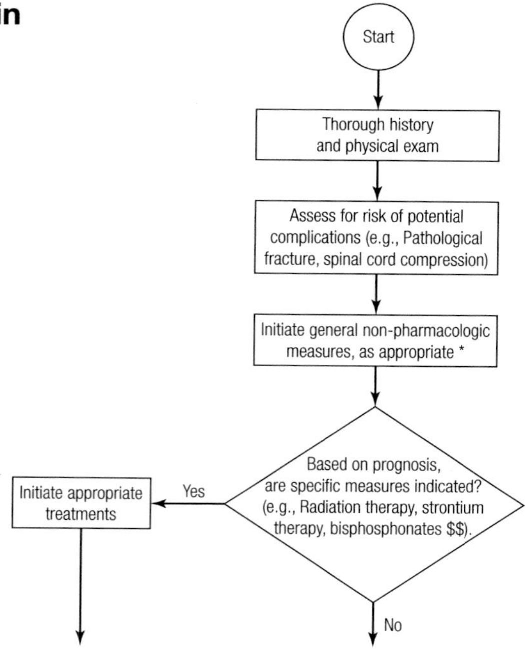

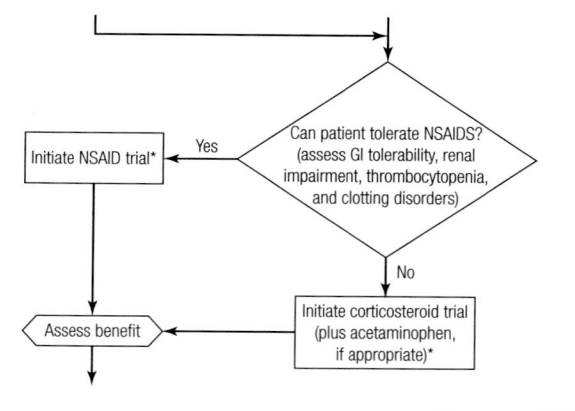

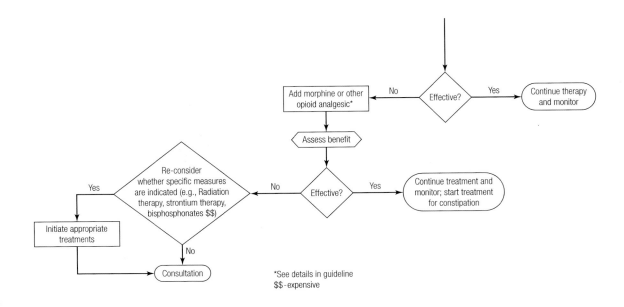

Add morphine or other opioid analgesic*

Effective? — No

Effective? — Yes → Continue therapy and monitor

Assess benefit

Effective? — Yes → Continue treatment and monitor; start treatment for constipation

Effective? — No → Re-consider whether specific measures are indicated (e.g., Radiation therapy, strontium therapy, bisphosphonates $$)

Re-consider... — Yes → Initiate appropriate treatments → Consultation

Re-consider... — No → Consultation

*See details in guideline
$$ - expensive

Visceral Pain

Introduction and Background
- Pain is defined by the International Association for the Study of Pain (IASP) as *"an unpleasant sensory and emotional experience associated with actual or potential tissue damage and described in terms of such damage"* (IASP, 1979).
- ***Visceral pain*** is a subset of nociceptive pain that arises from visceral organs such as the gastrointestinal tract, liver and pancreas. This type of pain can be further subdivided into two major categories–pain resulting from tumor involvement within the organ capsule which causes stretching, aching and is a fairly localized pain or pain resulting from obstruction of a hollow viscus which presents as intermittent cramping and is poorly localized. Visceral nociceptive pain can be either acute or chronic in nature. Although the focus here is visceral pain, most patients will experience more than one type of pain. For specific information about other types of pain, please refer to the Somatic Pain, Bone Pain, and Neuropathic Pain GEMS.

Prevalence
- Abdominal pain is a common complaint in all health care settings ranging from benign underlying conditions such as constipation and irritable bowel syndrome (IBS) to life-threatening illnesses such as pancreatic cancer.

In patients with cancer, visceral pain due to tumor invasion of a hollow viscus, with or without pleural or peritoneal involvement is the second most common type of pain.

Causes
- Visceral pain is caused by either a disease process or an abnormal function of an internal organ or its covering (peritoneum, pericardium or parietal pleura).
- Pathological causes of visceral pain may include irritable bowel syndrome, pancreatic cancer, ovarian cancer, lung cancer pain, hepatomegaly, midline retroperitoneal syndrome, chronic intestinal obstruction, peritoneal carcinomatosis, and ureteric obstruction.

Clinical Characteristics
- Visceral nociceptors are fewer in number in the primary somatosensory cortex than their somatic counterparts. However, their presence in the secondary somatosensory cortex leads to intense perception and psychological processing of visceral pain even though it is not well localized.

- Visceral nociceptors are activated by mechanical (stretching, distension, contraction, compression) and chemical (substance P, serotonin, prostaglandins, and H^+ ions) stimuli.
- Visceral nociceptive pain is gnawing, crampy, diffuse and poorly localized. Colic occurs with obstruction of a hollow viscus as a spasmodic achy, sharp or throbbing pain with internal organ capsule invasion or mesenteric infiltration. Nausea, vomiting and diaphoresis often accompany visceral pain.
- Referred pain is a common characteristic of visceral pain and occurs when visceral pain and somatic pain converge upon the same area of the dorsal horn.
- The intensity of the referred pain is a reflection of the severity of the visceral involvement.
- Visceral pain can also be referred to the skin and present as cutaneous hyperalgesia.
- Referred pain is often misdiagnosed as musculoskeletal pain due to its somatic presentation.

Non-Pharmacologic Treatment

- Non-pharmacologic therapies are essential in chronic pain management.
- Physical, complementary and cognitive behavioral interventions reduce the perception of pain and can decrease the dosage requirements of medication.
- Non-pharmacologic strategies include:
  - Education and information about medical treatments, (including myths and misconceptions about pain medication)
  - Massage
  - Ice and heat
  - Physical therapy
  - Music therapy
  - Imagery
  - Distraction
  - Reframing and cognitive-behavioral training
  - Psychotherapy

Pharmacotherapy

- Visceral pain due to organ infiltration generally responds to The World Health Organization's (WHO) stepladder approach to cancer pain management. Please refer to the Somatic Pain GEMS for details of pharmacologic treatment using these medications.
  - Step One: Nonopioids
  - Step Two: Nonopioids + Opioid Combinations
  - Step Three: Pure Opioid Agonists
- Visceral pain that is not adequately managed using the stepladder approach or presents as colic or cramping may be better managed by the following interventions either alone or in combination with opioid and nonopioid analgesics.

Pharmacologic Management of Visceral Pain

Generic Name (Brand Name)	Usual Adult Starting Dose/Range	Routes	Common Strengths and Formulations	Comments
First Line Therapy–Colicky/Cramping Visceral Pain				
Dicyclomine (Bentyl)	10–20 mg QID PRN	PO	**Capsules/Tablets:** 10 mg capsule, 20 mg tablet **Syrup:** 10 mg/5 mL **Injection:** 10 mg/mL	• Can cause constipation, confusion and dry mouth • Not recommended in the elderly • MDD–160 mg/24 h
Hyoscyamine (Levsin)	0.125–0.25 mg q4–6h ATC or prn	PO, SL	**Tablet:** 0.125 mg **SL Tablet:** 0.125 mg **Oral Concentrate:** 0.125 mg/mL	• Can cause constipation, confusion and dry mouth • Not recommended in the elderly • MDD–1.5 mg/24 h
Second Line Therapy–Colicky/Cramping Pain				
Scopolamine (Transderm Scop)	1–3 patches topically q3 days	Topical	**Transdermal Patch:** 1.5 mg	• Sedating and constipating • May cause confusion and visual disturbances
Glycopyrrolate (Robinul)	1–2 mg PO q4–6h 0.2 mg SQ, IV q4–6h	PO, SQ, IV	**Tablets:** 1, 2 mg **Injection:** 0.2 mg/mL	• Causes less confusion and visual disturbance because it is less likely to cross the blood-brain barrier
First Line Therapy–Stretching/Capsule Pain				
Prednisone (Deltasone)	10–40 mg daily-BID	PO	**Tablets:** 5,10,20,50 mg	• Less expensive than dexamethasone • More mineralocorticoid activity than dexamethasone
Dexamethasone (Decadron)	4 mg daily-QID	PO. IV. SQ, PR	**Tablets:** 0.5, 2, 4 mg **Solution:** 1 mg/mL **Injection:** 4 mg/mL	• May titrate to 48 mg/day
Second Line Therapy for Specific Visceral Pain Syndromes				
Irritable Bowel Syndrome with Constipation				
Tegaserod (Zelnorm)	6 mg BID	PO	**Tablets:** 2, 6 mg	• Withdrawn from U.S. market in 2007. Limited availability only via FDA restricted access IND (Investigational New Drug) program. Contact manufacturer, Novartis, for more information. • Expensive • Administer 30 minutes before meals • May cause diarrhea with accompanying dehydration

Bowel Obstruction Colic Pain (See Bowel Obstruction GEMS Guideline)				
Octreotide (Sandostatin)	50mcg BID-TID titrating up as needed (mean daily dosage is 300 mcg)	IV, SQ	**Ampules:** 50, 100, 500 mcg (as acetate) **Multi-dose Vials:** 200 and 1000 mcg/mL	• Expensive • Selectively inhibits secretion of fluids and electrolytes into the gut lumen • May be beneficial in patients with complete obstruction
Pancreatic Colic Pain				
Pancrelipase (Multiple brands)	30,000 IU pancreatic lipase with each meal	PO	**Tablets:** various strengths	• Use non-enteric coated products for colicky pancreatic pain

Clinical Pearls

- Although anticholinergic agents such as hyoscyamine and scopolamine effectively treat colic, they can contribute to constipation. Patients should be encouraged to drink plenty of fluids and increase their fiber intake to balance benefits and the constipating effects of these agents.
- The anti-inflammatory effects of corticosteroids make them a beneficial adjuvant to opioids in the treatment of pain that results from visceral stretching.
- Non-enteric coated pancreatic lipase enzymes are used for pain control from pancreatic disease. Enteric coated pancreatic lipase enzymes are used for the treatment of steatorrhea (fatty stool).

Key References

American Pain Society: *Principles of Analgesic Use in the Treatment of Acute Pain and Cancer Pain.* 5th Ed., 2003.

Berger AM, Portenoy RK, Weissman DE: *Principles & Practices of Palliative Care & Supportive Oncology.* 2nd Ed. Philadelphia: Lippincott Williams & Wilkins., 2002.

Davis MP, Frandsen JL: *Palliative Practices: An Interdisciplinary Approach.* St. Louis: Elsevier Mosby, Inc., 2005.

Gebhart GF: Visceral pain-peripheral sensitization. *Gut.* 47: iv54–iv55, 2000.

http://www.cancer.gov/cancertopics/pdq/supportivecare/pain/HealthProfessional. Accessed 3/30/06

Kuiken SD, Tytgat GN, Boeckxstaens GE: Drugs interfering with visceral sensitivity for the treatment of functional gastrointestinal disorders—the clinical evidence. Aliment Pharmacol Ther. 21: 633–651, 2005.

McCaffery M, Pasero C: *Pain: Clinical Manual.* 2nd Ed. St. Louis: Elsevier Mosby, Inc., 1999.

Mercadante S, Casuccio A, Agnello A, Pumo S, Kargar J, Garofalo S: Analgesic effects of nonsteroidal anti-inflammatory drugs in cancer pain due to somatic or visceral mechanisms. *J Pain Symptom Manage.* 17: 351–356, 1999.

Visceral Pain

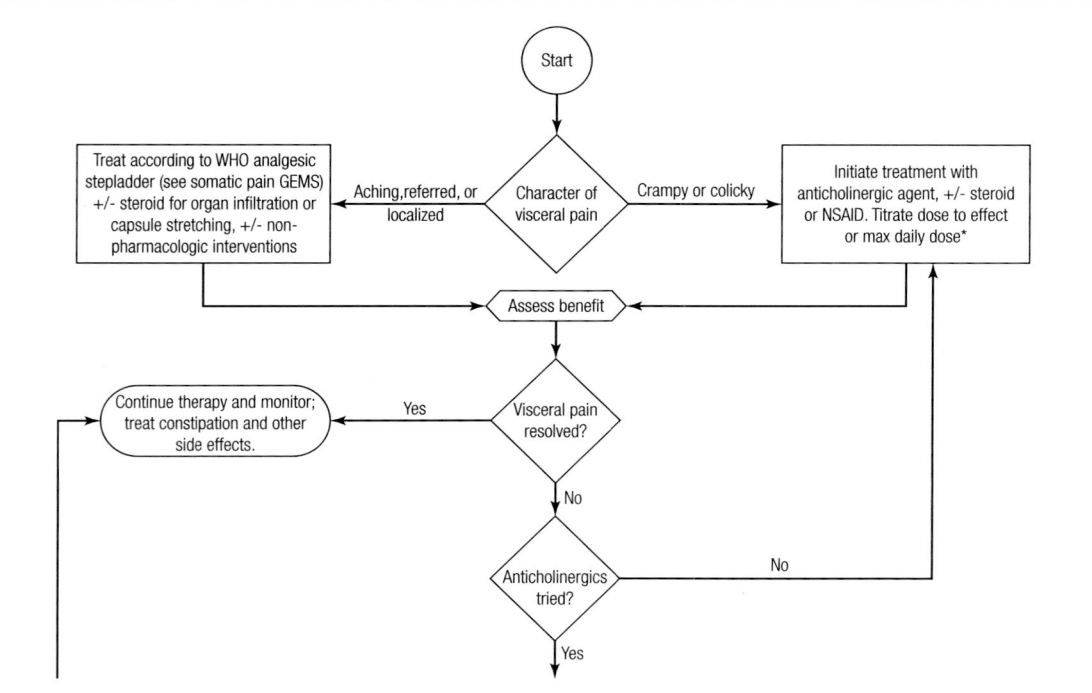

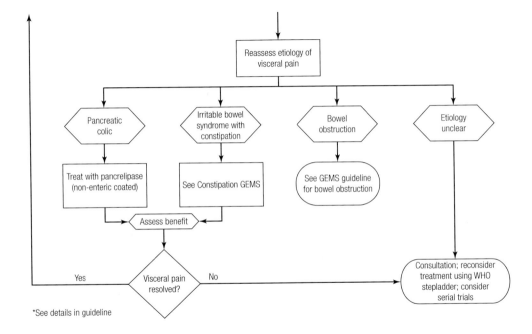

Reassess etiology of visceral pain

Pancreatic colic → Treat with pancrelipase (non-enteric coated)

Irritable bowel syndrome with constipation → See Constipation GEMS

Bowel obstruction → See GEMS guideline for bowel obstruction

Etiology unclear

Assess benefit

Visceral pain resolved?

Yes

No → Consultation; reconsider treatment using WHO stepladder; consider serial trials

*See details in guideline

Neuropathic Pain

Introduction

- Neuropathic pain is chronic pain resulting from injury to the nervous system, either to the central nervous system (brain and spinal cord) or the peripheral nervous system (nerves outside the brain and spinal cord).
- Neuropathic pain is typically more difficult to eradicate than nociceptive pain.

Prevalence

- An estimated 30% of cancer patients experience neuropathic pain at some point in their disease (usually advanced disease).

Causes

- Neuropathic pain is pain due to direct *damage* to the primary afferent nociceptive nerve fibers (axons) (not the nociceptors, *per se*) in either the peripheral or central nervous system.
- Causes of neuropathic pain seen in hospice care include:
  - Tumor invasion of nerve
  - Nerve ischemia due to impaired blood supply
  - Mechanical damage of nerve due to pathological fracture, etc.
  - Demyelination of nerves as in MS and ALS
  - HIV invasion of nerve in AIDS neuropathy

- Other causes of neuropathic pain that may be seen in hospice patients include:
  - Diabetic neuropathy
  - Microbiological injury
    - postherpetic neuralgia
  - Amputation (phantom pain)
  - Traumatic nerve damage
    - Surgery
  - Alcoholism
  - Back, leg, and hip problems
  - Chemotherapy
  - Diabetes
  - Facial nerve problems

Clinical Characteristics

- Neuropathic and nociceptive pains tend to present differently.
  - Nociceptive pain may be sharp or dull typically making the affected areas achy and sore.
  - Neuropathic pain, conversely, tends to feel like "pins and needles", electrical shocks, burning, or "creepy-crawly" (paresthetic). Both types of pain can exist concurrently.
- Acute nerve injury pain is called neuralgia.
  - Examples include acute herpes zoster neuralgia ("shingles"), traumatic neuralgia, e.g. nerve damage due to pathological fracture, and neuralgia due to acute nerve inflammation (neuritis).
  - Acute neuralgias are treated in the same manner as other acute pains, e.g. opioids, ice, heat, nerve blocks.
- Neuropathic pain is, by definition, a secondary pain that typically occurs weeks to months after an acute nerve injury has occurred, and normally has at least begun to resolve.

- Patients typically describe their neuropathic pain as a "new pain" that is different in its presentation than acute nerve injury pain.
- Unfortunately, most neuropathic pain seen in the hospice setting cannot be eliminated and must be treated symptomatically. Symptomatic treatment usually produces a marked reduction in pain.

Non-Pharmacological Treatment

- Pharmacotherapy is the primary modality to manage neuropathic pain, but non-drug measures also are indicated.
  - Management of underlying causes should always be attempted, e.g.:
    - Maintain careful glycemic control in diabetic neuropathy
    - Shrink tumors that impinge nerve, e.g.:
      - Therapeutic radiology
      - Surgical debulking of tumor
      - Palliative chemotherapy (to shrink, not destroy the tumor)

    Note: These relatively invasive and expensive approaches often are impractical with limited life expectancy.
  - When possible, physical therapy of the affected area should be done.
    - Often impractical in hospice care
  - Physical activation (movement) of the affected area may be uncomfortable initially but helps the pain to resolve. It should only be attempted as tolerated by the patient.
  - Refractory neuropathic pain, especially central neuropathic pain, may respond to spinal cord stimulation.

- Stimulator implantation is normally reserved for long-lasting (indefinite duration) pain; implantation of a spinal cord stimulator is nearly always too invasive and too expensive for hospice care and is not cost-effective if life expectancy is limited.

Pharmacotherapy

- Both systemic and topical drugs can be useful in managing neuropathic pain.
- Systemic drugs useful in neuropathic pain include tricyclic antidepressants, antiepileptic drugs, lidocaine, and opioids.
- Capsaicin cream or solution is the only consistently useful topical agent for neuropathic pain.
- Tricyclic antidepressants (TCAs)
  - TCAs are drugs of choice for neuropathic pain according to numbers needed to treat analyses and systematic literature reviews.
  - Secondary side chain TCAs, i.e. desipramine, nortriptyline, are equally effective and far better tolerated than tertiary side chain TCAs, e.g. amitriptyline.
  - TCAs can cause or exacerbate anticholinergic problems. Use with caution (if at all) in patients with severe benign prostatic hyperplasia (BPH), urinary retention, constipation, or cardiac arrhythmias.
    - If used in such patients, start at lower than normal dose, e.g. 10 mg HS, and monitor for exacerbation of underlying condition.
  - Begin dosing at 25 mg one hour before HS and increase dose by 25 mg every three days to a maximum of 100 mg HS.
  - The dose, time to onset, and side effects are typically ½ to ⅓ of those typical of TCAs when used for depression.

- Maximal effect is typically seen in two to three weeks.
- Use with caution in patients with proximal cardiac conduction system delays or prolongation of the QT interval on EKG.
- One-half to two-thirds of patients receive adequate pain relief with TCA monotherapy; additional drugs are commonly needed.
- If TCA therapy alone is insufficient, add an antiepileptic drug.
- Other Antidepressants
  - Serotonin selective reuptake inhibitor (SSRI) antidepressants are not as effective as TCAs and are not indicated to treat neuropathic pain.
    - Both norepinephrine and serotonin levels must be increased for neuropathic pain efficacy.
    - Serotonin-norepinephrine reuptake inhibitors (SNRIs) have been studied in neuropathic pain.
      - Venlafaxine (Effexor) has produced variable and often disappointing results and higher doses are typically required to achieve benefit for neuropathic pain.
      - Duloxetine (Cymbalta) is effective for both neuropathic pain and depression, but is expensive.
- Antiepileptic drugs (AEDs)
  - Epilepsy is associated with spontaneous, ectopic discharges of motor neurons; neuropathic pain is associated with spontaneous, ectopic discharges of sensory neurons.
  - Therefore it is not surprising that all AEDs have some effectiveness in neuropathic pain.
  - The best evidence is available for gabapentin (Neurontin) and carbamazepine (Tegretol).
  - An AED may be used as first line therapy in patients unable to tolerate a TCA.
  - When used as second line therapy, the AED should be ADDED TO the TCA.
  - Because carbamazepine has potential toxicities that exceed gabapentin, gabapentin often is the AED of choice.
    - Gabapentin dosing normally started at 100–300 mg TID and increased by 300 per day every three to five days.
      - Most patients who respond will do so at total daily doses between 900 and 1800 mg.
      - Three time a day dosing is necessary.
  - Pregabalin is the newest AED that has good efficacy data in neuropathic pain, is effective with BID dosing.
  - Other AEDs have been used in neuropathic pain and been effective (in at least some patients).
- Lidocaine
  - Topical lidocaine patches (Lidoderm) are FDA approved for postherpetic neuralgia but have been used successfully for other types of neuropathic pain as well. Systemic levels are very low and side effects rare. Minor local irritation at the application site can normally be managed with hydrocortisone cream.
    - Patches are normally placed directly over the painful area and left on for 12 hours a day, then removed for 12 hours before another patch is applied.
  - Up to three patches a day are FDA approved.
  - Lidocaine patches might be considered first line therapy if the neuropathic pain is in a small area of nerve distribution because one patch can be cut before the backing is removed and placed over the area of pain.

- Lidocaine patch therapy may be added to TCA and/or AED therapy. These agents all work by different mechanisms so multiple drug use is synergistic.
  - Lidocaine patches are costly.
- IV lidocaine is effective in managing neuropathic pain, but is potentially toxic and very inconvenient.
- The oral local anesthetic analogues used in cardiology have been studied for neuropathic pain, but have been disappointing.
  - Mexiletine (Mexitil) works in some patients but not in others.
  - Tocainide (Tonocard) is too toxic for routine use.
- Opioids
  - Opioids are used in neuropathic pain in the same way they are used in nociceptive pain but the doses required for neuropathic pain may be somewhat higher.
  - Opioids normally are added to one or more of the above therapies, not used in place of those therapies.
  - Methadone has the unique property among opioids of blocking the NMDA receptor. As this action is associated with the relief of neuropathic pain, methadone has been reported to be the most effective opioid for the treatment this type of pain.
  - Tramadol is a weak mu agonist and weak norepinephrine-serotonin reuptake inhibitor. Neither mechanism alone explains the effectiveness of this drug; that appears to result from synergy between these two weak effects. It is not a controlled substance.
- Capsaicin topical
  - Capsaicin depletes the pain facilitating chemical Substance P from sensory nerves.
  - It is a potentially useful adjunct to the therapies listed above; it is not a primary therapy.
  - Capsaicin requires three to four weeks to work and must be applied four times daily for full effect.
  - Initially this drug causes irritation and burning at the application site; this effect normally lessens within a few days to a week.
  - Patients/families must be instructed to use gloves or wash carefully after use; touching mucous membranes or eyes can cause severe local pain.
  - Capsaicin cream and solution are available in low (0.025%) and high (0.075%) concentrations (always use a full container of low strength before moving up to the high strength).
- Other Pharmacotherapy in neuropathic pain
  - NMDA antagonists; this class of medications has great toxicity and should be used only by experienced clinicians.
    - Ketamine (Ketalar, others)
      - This dissociative anesthetic can be injected or ingested; it has been used successfully in some hospice programs for refractory neuropathic pain.
      - Serious side effects include hallucinations and emergence reactions.
      - Ketamine can be abused; it can cause hallucinations and other adverse effects.
      - It is chemically analogous to the illegal substance phencyclidine (Angel Dust).
    - Dextromethorphan
      - This anti-tussive has been studied for neuropathic pain.
      - Controlled studies have failed to show consistent clinical usefulness.
      - Doses needed for any effect on neuropathic pain are high and produce unacceptable side effects.

Pharmacological Management of Neuropathic Pain

Generic Name (Brand Name)	Usual Adult Starting Dose/Range	Maximum Daily Dose	Route of Administration	Comments
First Line Therapy–Tricyclic Antidepressants				
Desipramine (Norpramin)	10–25 mg HS	150 mg HS	PO	• Least anticholinergic and sedative side effects of all TCAs • Optimal half life for once daily dosing
Nortriptyline (Pamelor, Aventyl)	10–25 mg HS	150 mg HS	PO	• Alternative to desipramine preferred by some clinicians due to good studies for this use
Second Line Therapy–Serotonin/Norepinephrine Re-uptake Inhibitor				
Venlafaxine (Effexor)	75 mg daily	225 mg TDD	PO	• Beneficial for both depression and neuropathic pain • Risk of discontinuation syndrome, taper dose over at least 2 weeks when discontinuing
Duloxetine (Cymbalta)	60 mg daily	60 mg BID	PO	• Beneficial for both depression and neuropathic pain
First Line Therapy–Antiepileptic Drugs				
Gabapentin (Neurontin)	100–300 mg TID	1200 mg TID*	PO	• Current AED of choice in neuropathic pain; expensive; requires > a week for effect, causes sedation and dizziness
Pregabalin (Lyrica)	75–150 mg BID	300 mg QD**	PO	• Causes considerable confusion • Onset of action in 3– 5 days
Second Line Therapy—Local Anesthetic				
Lidocaine patch 5% (Lidoderm)	Apply over affected area for 12 hours/day	Apply over affected area for 12 hours/day	Topical	• Patches may be cut before removing backing • Do not shave area; clip hair to short length before applying patch. • Expensive
Second Line Therapy—Topical Adjunctive Agent				
Capsaicin (Zostrix)	Apply small amount to painful area QID	Apply small amount to painful area QID	Topical	• Start with 0.025% cream or liquid to develop tolerance to burning • Use gloves or wash carefully after use • Apply only to intact skin • Do not allow contact with mucous membrane or eyes • Optimal effect takes up to 4 to 6 weeks with regular use

First Line Therapy–Atypical Opioid-Monoamine Reuptake Inhibitor Analgesic				
Tramadol (Ultram)	25–50 mg QID	100 mg QID	PO	• Titrate slowly to full dose to minimize side effects • Lowers seizure threshold; use with caution in patient with seizure potential • Full dose typically needed for full effect • No antiinflammatory activity
First Line Therapy–Opioids				
Methadone (Dolophine)	Variable	Variable	PO. SL. PR, IV, SC	See Methadone section, pgs. 200-203

*The labeled maximum dose for gabapentin is 3,600 mg per day although this dose has minimal additional benefit and increased side effects.

**If 300 mg daily of pregabalin is tolerated and pain is not effectively controlled in 2–4 weeks, dose can be titrated to 300 mg BID.

Clinical Pearls

- Nonsteroidal anti-inflammatory drugs (NSAIDS) have limited value in managing neuropathic pain because NSAIDs work primarily at the nociceptors and neuropathic pain begins proximal to nociceptors.
- Pharmacotherapy for neuropathic pain often makes the pain tolerable, but frequently does not eliminate the pain completely.
- New research into the use of nerve toxins and other nicotinic receptor antagonists offers promise for improved pharmacotherapy for neuropathic pain in the foreseeable future.

References

Raja SN, Haythornthwaite JA, Pappagallo M, et al. Opioids versus antidepressants in postherpetic neuralgia: a randomized, placebo-controlled trial. Neurology 2002 Oct 8;59(7):1015–21.

Max MB, Lynch SA, Muir J, Shoaf SE, Smoller B, Dubner R. Effects of desipramine, amitriptyline, and fluoxetine on pain in diabetic neuropathy. N Engl J Med. 1992 May 7;326(19):1250–6. N Engl J Med. 1992 May 7;326(19):1287–8.

Dworkin RH, Backonja M, Rowbotham MC, et al. Advances in neuropathic pain: diagnosis, mechanisms, and treatment recommendations. Arch Neurol. 2003 Nov;60(11):1524–34.

Hempenstall K, Nurmikko TJ, Johnson RW, A'Hern RP, Rice AS. Analgesic therapy in postherpetic neuralgia: a quantitative systematic review. PLoS Med. 2005 Jul;2(7):e164. Epub 2005 Jul 26.

Stacey BR. Management of peripheral neuropathic pain. Am J Phys Med Rehabil. 2005 Mar;84(3 Suppl):S4–16.

Fine PG. Analgesic issues in palliative care, furthering our understanding of pain, the stability and cost of opioid infusion therapy, and opioid effectiveness doses in nociceptive and neuropathic pain. J Pain Palliat Care Pharmacother. 2002;16(3):77–81.

Lipman AG. Analgesic drugs for neuropathic and sympathetically maintained pain. Clinics in Geriatric Medicine 1996;12:501–515.

Davies PS, Galer BS. Review of lidocaine patch 5% studies in the treatment of postherpetic neuralgia. Drugs. 2004;64(9):937–47.

Kronenberg RH. Ketamine as an analgesic: parenteral, oral, rectal, subcutaneous, transdermal and intranasal administration. J Pain Palliat Care Pharmacother. 2002;16(3):27–35.

Lucas LK, Lipman AG. Recent advances in pharmacotherapy for cancer pain management. Cancer Pract. 2002 May-Jun;10 Suppl1:S14–20.

Neuropathic Pain

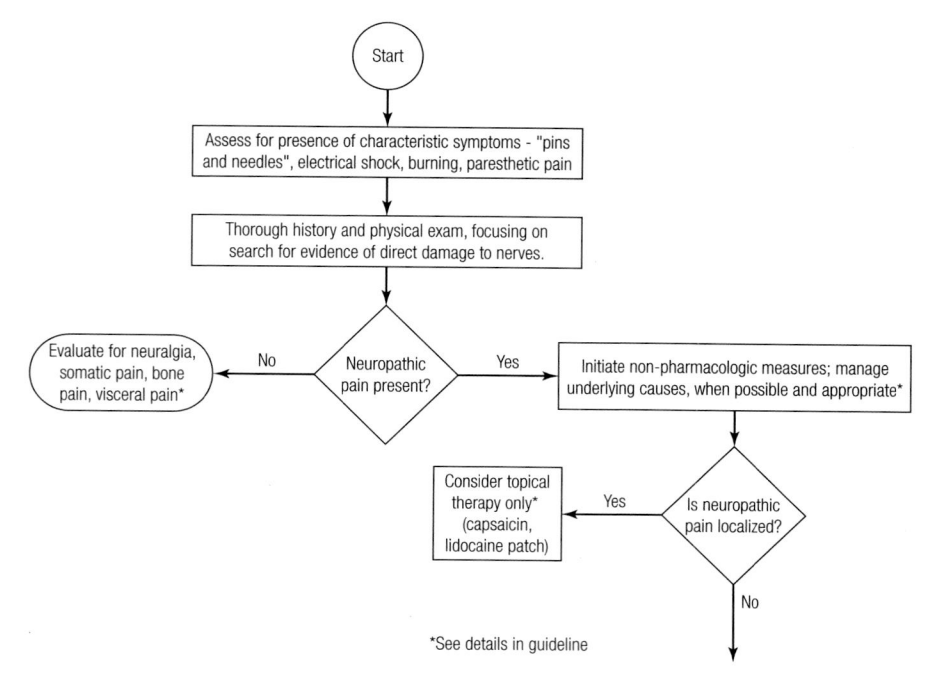

*See details in guideline

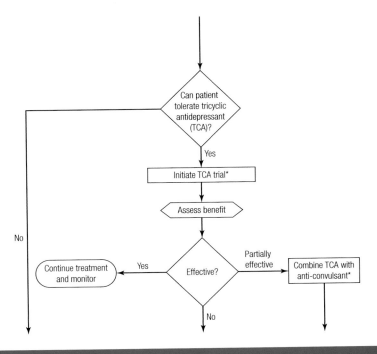

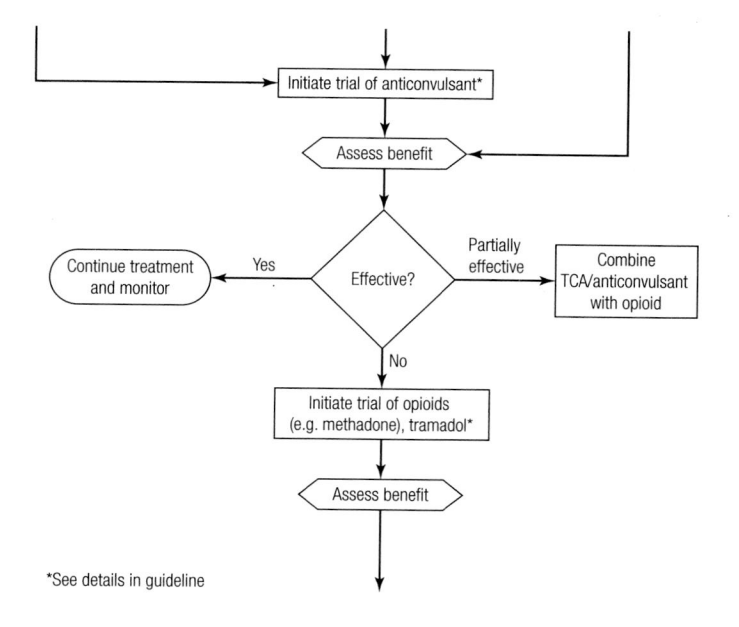

*See details in guideline

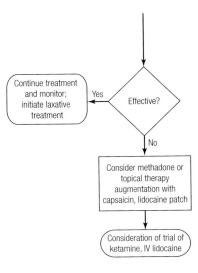

Pruritus

Introduction and Background

- Pruritus is the medical term for itching. This symptom becomes the focus of palliative treatment when the sensation of itching or the urge to scratch are frequent, generalized in distribution, or severe.
- Patients may also describe pruritus as burning, tingling, numbness, or crawling in the skin.

Prevalence

- Though itching is a common symptom, its prevalence in hospice and palliative care settings is poorly understood.
- When pruritus is constant or severe, it is a significant source of suffering and impediment to quality of life.

Causes

- In addition to chronic diseases of the skin, common causes of pruritus in hospice and palliative care include:

  - Allergens (e.g., soaps, detergents, ointments, creams)
  - Anxiety and stress
  - Carcinoid syndrome
  - Diabetes mellitus
  - Hematologic malignancies (leukemias, lymphomas, myelomas, and polycythemias)
  - Liver disease (hepatitis, cholestasis)
  - Paraneoplastic syndromes associated with a variety of cancers
  - Drug rash (drug allergies)
  - Dry skin
  - Fungal (usually Candida) or bacterial infection of the skin
  - Scratching
  - Thyroid problems (hyperthyroidism, hypothyroidism)
  - Uremia

Side Effects of Medications

- Opioid-induced pruritus is more likely with morphine, codeine, or oxycodone, than with methadone, fentanyl, hydromorphone, or oxymorphone.
- Acyclovir ointment, alprazolam, amlodipine, bicalutamide, bupropion, SSRIs, donepezil, megestrol, tramadol, and antifungal agents can also cause pruritus.

Clinical Characteristics

- Sensations of pruritus are transmitted by specific itch fibers in peripheral nerves. Itch may be mediated by peripheral histamine, serotonin, and pro-inflammatory cytokines.
- Dryness of the skin causes itch or makes it worse.
- Heat and other causes of peripheral vasodilatation worsen itching.
- Skin that is chronically damp and wet can produce pruritus.
- Though it may give immediate relief, scratching can make pruritus worse, especially if vigorous scratching produces skin injury, excoriation, or inflammation.
- Similar to pain, injury to nerve fibers that transmit itch signals can produce neuropathic pruritus.

Non-Pharmacologic Treatment

- Assessment of the patient with pruritus should begin with a thorough physical examination, focused on the skin.
- Any evidence of dry skin should be treated liberally and regularly with moisturizing lotion.
- Efforts to cool the patient's environment (and thereby cool the skin) can help reduce itching.
- Cool compresses and oatmeal baths can provide effective, though usually temporary, relief.
- Patients should be encouraged to pat or gently rub itchy areas, and not scratch (though this is easier said than done).
- Keeping nails trimmed close minimizes the injury to skin when patients do scratch. Loose fitting cotton clothes allow the skin to breathe and minimize perspiration.
- Efforts to promote relaxation can also help reduce pruritus.

Pharmacotherapy

- The first step in pharmacologic management of pruritus is to remove potentially pruritogenic medications before starting new ones to treat itch.
- It is very important to look for potential medication-related causes of itching.
- Assessment questions should include:
  - Is the onset of itching temporally related to the initiation of a new medication treatment?
  - Is the patient taking any medications commonly associated with pruritus?
  - Does the patient demonstrate a characteristic drug rash?
  - If the itching is localized, is it near the site of application of a topical medication?
- If possible, treat the underlying cause (e.g. infection, anxiety, thyroid problems).
- In general, a localized itch should initially be managed with topical measures, whereas a more generalized itch will likely require a systemic therapy.

Pharmacologic Management of Pruritus

Generic Name (Brand Name)	Usual Adult Starting Dose/Range	Routes	Common Strengths and Formulations	Comments
First Line Therapy–Topical Preparations				
Camphor/Menthol lotion (Sarna)	Applied topically several times daily	Topical	0.5% Camphor, 0.5% Menthol	• Available over-the-counter • Avoid application to excoriated, broken skin
Lidocaine Ointment	Apply topically less than three times a day	Topical	5% Lidocaine	• Frequent use can lead to significant absorption (and possible cardiac arrhythmias) • Avoid use over large surface areas or broken skin
Hydrocortisone cream (Cortaid)	Apply a thin film BID-QID	Topical	Hydrocortisone 1.0%	• May worsen skin infections (especially fungal) • Liberal use can lead to significant systemic absorption • Prolonged use will cause thinning of the skin
First Line Therapy–Antihistamines				
Diphenhydramine (Benadryl)	25 to 50 mg, BID-QID	PO	**Tablets and Capsules:** 25 mg, 50 mg	• Sedating antihistamine • Dry mouth is common
Hydroxyzine (Atarax, Vistaril)	10 to 25 mg, TID-QID	PO	**Tablets and Capsules:** 10 mg, 25 mg, 50 mg, 100 mg	• Antihistamine with some anxiolytic properties • Sedating
Second Line Therapy–Corticosteroids				
Dexamethasone (Decadron)	4–8 mg daily (in divided doses)	PO, IV, PR	**Tablets:** 0.25 mg, 0.5 mg, 0.75 mg, 1 mg, 1.5 mg, 2 mg, 4 mg, 6 mg **Solution:** 0.5 mg/5 mL, 1 mg/mL **Injection:** 4 mg/mL, 10 mg/mL	• Has less mineralocorticoid effect than prednisone
Prednisone (Deltasone)	15–60 mg daily (in divided doses)	PO	**Tablets:** 1 mg, 2.5 mg, 5 mg, 10 mg, 20 mg, 25 mg, 50 mg **Solution:** 5 mg/5 mL, 5 mg/mL	

Second Line Therapy—Antidepressants				
Doxepin (Sinequan)	10–75 mg qHS	PO, Topical	**Capsules:** 10 mg, 25 mg, 50 mg, 75 mg, 100 mg, 150 mg **Cream:** 5 %	• Tricyclic antidepressant (TCA) • Potent antihistamine (H1 and H2) activity • Often effective for pruritus at doses well below antidepressant dose • Use same general cautions as in using TCAs for depression
Paroxetine (Paxil)	10–30 mg daily	PO	**Tablets:** 10 mg, 20 mg, 30 mg, 40 mg **Suspension:** 10 mg/5 mL	• Selective Serotonin Reuptake Inhibitor (SSRI) • Antipruritic effects may wear off after a few weeks
Mirtazapine (Remeron)	7.5–30 mg qHS	PO	**Tablets:** 7.5 mg, 15 mg, 30 mg, 45 mg **Orally Disintegrating Tablets:** 15 mg, 30 mg, 45 mg	• Alpha-2 antagonist antidepressant • Histamine (H1) antagonist, 5HT2 antagonist, and 5HT3 antagonist

Clinical Pearls

- Opioids may cause pruritus, especially when administered by spinal infusion. If an opioid is the suspected cause, consider rotating to a different opioid. If opioid rotation or if other antipuritic agents have failed, the 5HT3 blocker ondansetron (and possibly mirtazapine, due to its 5HT3 inhibition) may provide relief. Treatment with NSAIDs may also be helpful.
- How to recognize a fungal skin infection: Areas that are moist are likely to be sites of fungal infections with *Candida*. Skin folds, mucous membranes, armpits, and underneath breasts are likely sites. Treatment with antibiotics and corticosteroids may increase the risk of fungal skin infections. The typical *Candida* skin rash is bright red and macular with pustules or papules at the edges of the rash ("satellite lesions"). These peripheral lesions may spread and blend in with the larger patch. Keeping affected skin clean and dry is key to healing a fungal skin infection.
- Antihistamines are particularly useful when itching is to due to allergy.
- When pruritus is a consequence of cholestasis and is resistant to other therapies, consider treatment with cholestyramine, androgens (methyltestosterone), naloxone, rifampicin, or ondansetron, all of which have been reported to be effective. Cholestyramine is the least expensive of these, but due to the high incidence of associated GI symptoms such as constipation, cholestyramine should be given with a laxative such as sorbitol $+/-$ a stimulant laxative.

Key References

Twycross R, Greaves MW, Handwerker H, Jones EA, Libretto SE, Szepietowski JC, Zylicz Z: Itch: scratching more than the surface. *QJM*. 96:7–26, 2003.

Krajnik M, Zylicz Z: Understanding pruritus in systemic disease. *J Pain Symptom Manage*. 21: 151–168, 2001.

De Conno F, Ventafridda V, Saita L: Skin problems in advanced and terminal cancer patients. *J Pain Symptom Manage*. 6: 247–256, 1991.

Zylicz Z, Krajnik M, Sorge AA, Costantini M: Paroxetine in the treatment of severe non-dermatological pruritus: a randomized, controlled trial. *J Pain Symptom Manage*. 26:1105–1112, 2003.

Katcher J, Walsh D: Opioid-induced itching: morphine sulfate and hydromorphone hydrochloride. *J Pain Symptom Manage*. 17:70–72, 1999.

Pruritus

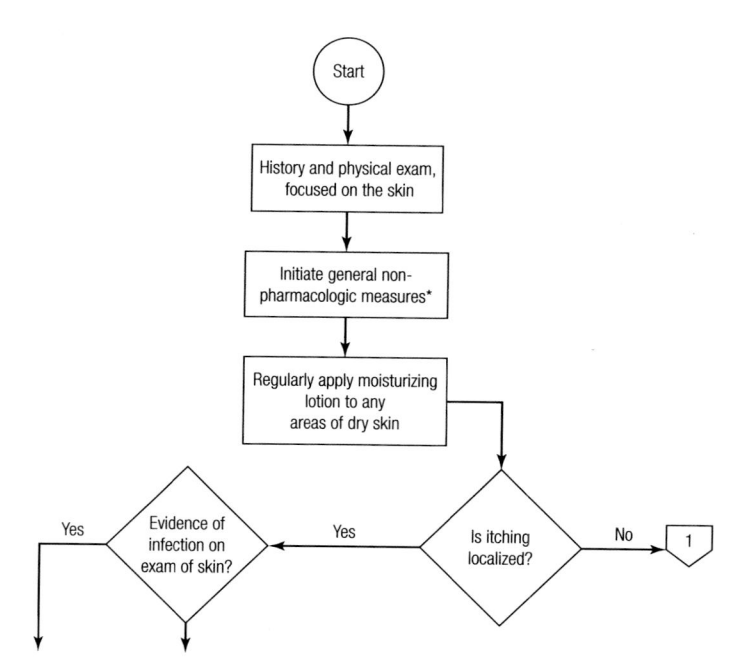

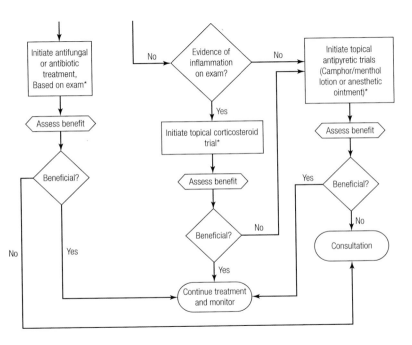

Initiate antifungal or antibiotic treatment, Based on exam*

Assess benefit

Beneficial?

No

Yes

Evidence of inflammation on exam?

No

No

Yes

Initiate topical corticosteroid trial*

Assess benefit

Beneficial?

No

Yes

Initiate topical antipyretic trials (Camphor/menthol lotion or anesthetic ointment)*

Assess benefit

Beneficial?

Yes

No

Consultation

Continue treatment and monitor

Pruritus (*continued*)

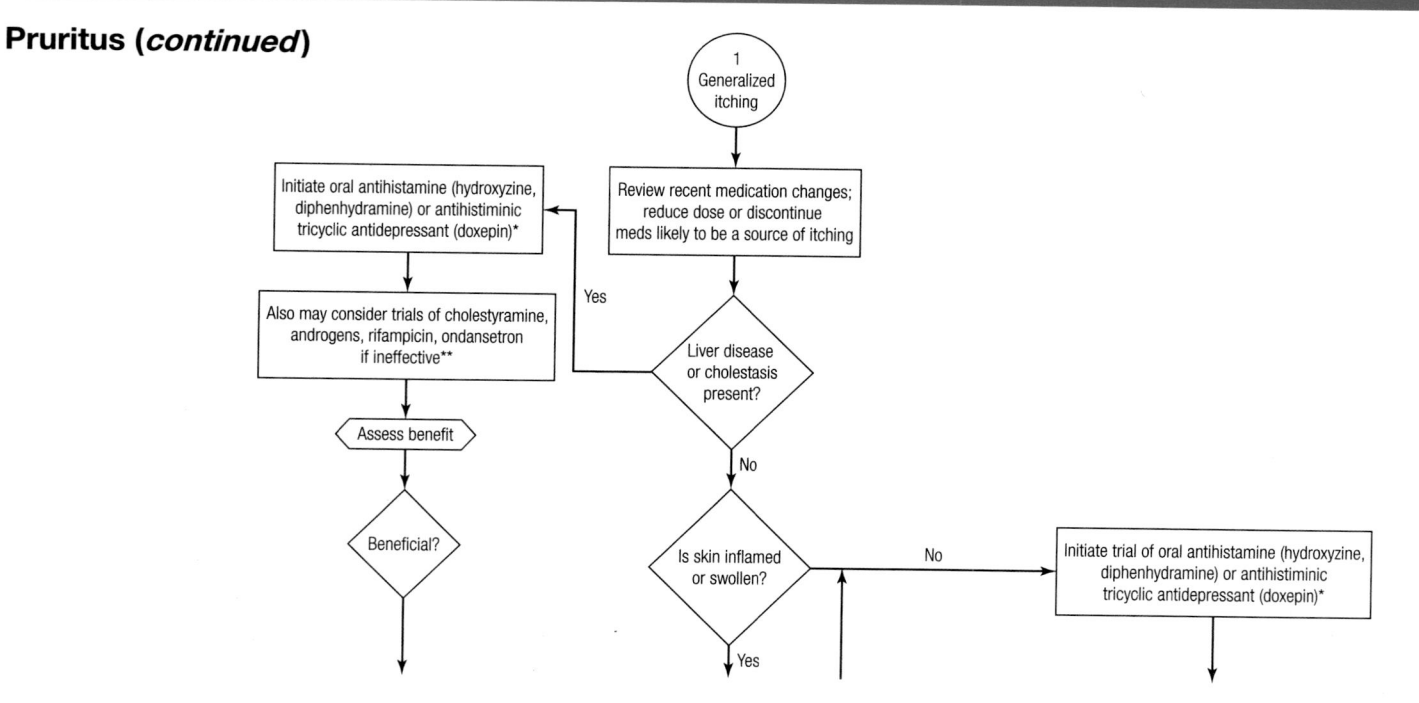

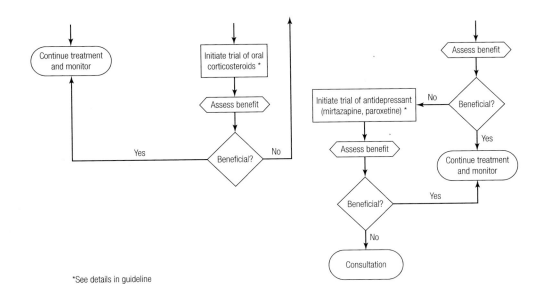

*See details in guideline

Seizures

Introduction and Background

- Seizures are caused by a brief, excessive surge of electrical activity in the brain. This surge causes changes in sensations, perceptions, and/or behaviors and is typically brief (lasting less than five minutes).
- The brain phenomenon called a seizure can be manifest in a number of ways, not just in convulsions.
- Patients may report odd physical sensations, describe strange smells (usually unpleasant ones like burning rubber or burning hair), or demonstrate brief episodes of staring into space or loss of attention or awareness.
- Patients with recurrent and unprovoked seizures are diagnosed with epilepsy.
- Since there are multiple types of seizures, it follows that there is a fairly detailed system of classifying them.
- In broad, general terms, seizures can be sorted into two groups–partial seizures and generalized seizures.
  - Partial seizures result from an abnormal electrical discharge restricted to one part of the brain (or a localized region of the brain).
  - Generalized seizures are the result of a widespread, excessive electrical discharge simultaneously involving both sides of the brain.
  - This distinction is not absolute, since an initially partial seizure can spread and become generalized.
  - Partial seizures are further subcategorized by whether consciousness is preserved (simple partial seizures) or compromised (complex partial seizures).

Prevalence

- The true prevalence of emergent seizures in the hospice setting is not well documented.
- Up to half of patients with brain tumors or metastases will develop seizures.
- Otherwise, new-onset seizures are relatively unusual overall and quite rare in the absence of one of the causes listed below.

Causes

- In the hospice and palliative care setting, the following are the most common causes of new onset seizures:
- Brain tumors (primary)
- Brain metastases (especially in patients with a diagnosis of lung cancer, breast cancer, renal cell cancer, and melanoma)
- Infections (meningitis)
- Fever
- Head injury or trauma
- Hypoglycemia
- Hypoxia
- Metabolic disturbances (e.g., uremia, hypocalcemia, hyponatremia, hypomagnesemia, multi-system failure)

- Stroke
- Withdrawal from alcohol or drugs (esp. acute withdrawal from sedative-hypnotics, anticonvulsants, or opiates)

- Drug toxicities—be alert for increasing serum levels with reductions in renal and hepatic function (e.g., some antibiotics, bupropion, meperidine, tramadol, tricyclic antidepressants)

- Conditions often confused with seizures include:
  - Anxiety (especially panic attacks)
  - Delirium (confusion and agitation)
  - Migraines
  - Myoclonus (commonly as a consequence of opiate toxicity)
  - Syncope/fainting
  - Transient ischemic attacks (TIAs)
  - Unexpected falls
- Laboratory studies may be required to detect the cause of a new onset seizure in hospice, since infectious or metabolic causes are likely.
- In patients without known central nervous system tumors, a brain imaging study should also be considered in the context of the overall goals of care.
- Electroencephalography (EEG) is the standard diagnostic test for seizures and epilepsy. In many cases, the EEG shows a widespread increase in electrical activity.
- In partial seizures, brain waves may show a localized increase in electrical activity. It is important to remember, however, that EEG tracings may be normal in between seizure episodes (or even apparently abnormal in patients who have never had a seizure).
- An EEG tracing must be interpreted by an expert experienced in the diagnosis of seizures.

Clinical Characteristics
- In a generalized, tonic-clonic seizure, the patient first becomes stiff, often uttering a cry, then loses consciousness and falls.
  - The cry results from air being forced through contracted vocal cords.
  - After this initial period of muscle stiffness, the patient's arms and legs jerk rhythmically.
  - Patients may drool, bite their tongues, or lose control of bowel or bladder during a seizure.
- The entire process (the "ictal" stage of a seizure) usually lasts from 1 to 3 minutes.
- Afterwards the person usually appears drowsy, confused, or may even fall asleep. (the "post-ictal" stage of a seizure).
- Not every seizure manifests with convulsions.
- Partial or complex partial seizures can produce troublesome and treatment refractory problems such as episodic focal pain, paresthesia, confusion, or gastrointestinal symptoms.
- Partial complex seizures can mimic psychiatric syndromes.
- A working relationship with a neurologist experienced in epilepsy to help sort out such complicated cases can be beneficial for hospice progams.

Non-Pharmacologic Treatment

- When a patient is having a generalized seizure, make sure they are not in a position from which they could fall and be injured.
- Gently move the patient to a stable position (lying down) and place the patient on one side to minimize the risk of aspiration.
- *Do not insert anything into patient's mouth.*
- Assess the patient's airway, breathing, and circulation during recovery from the seizure, recognizing that at the peak of convulsive activity there may be a brief period of apnea and asystole.

- Monitor to ensure that the seizure resolves into a post-ictal phase (cessation of seizure with somnolence), which should occur in a matter of seconds to a few minutes.
- Administer glucose (orally or parenterally), if available.
- Once seizures are controlled, search for and correct underlying abnormalities.
- Educate the patient and family about seizure precautions and what to expect and how to manage them if they recur.
- Baldwin, et al (2002) have outlined an approach to proactive screening for seizure risk in hospice, along with risk assessment templates and suggested contents of a hospice "seizure cessation kit".

Pharmacologic Management of Seizures

Generic Name (Brand Name)	Usual Adult Starting Dose/Range	Routes	Common Strengths and Formulations	Comments
First Line Therapy–Acute Management of Seizures				
Lorazepam (Ativan)	2 mg initial dose 2–20 mg daily	PO, SL, IM, IV, PR, SQ	**Tablets:** 0.5 mg, 1 mg, 2 mg **Concentrated Oral Solution:** 2 mg/mL **Injection:** 2 mg/mL, 4 mg/mL	• (ALL DRUGS IN CLASS) no ceiling dose to control acute seizures, though control may come at the cost of prolonged sedation • Well absorbed PR and SL • Better absorbed IM and SQ than diazepam. • Can repeat dose every 15 minutes until seizure subsides
Diazepam (Valium)	10 mg initial dose 10–40 mg daily	PO, SL, IV, PR	**Tablets:** 2 mg, 5 mg, 10 mg **Concentrated Oral Solution:** 5 mg/mL **Injection:** 5 mg/mL	• Well absorbed PR and SL • Can repeat dose every 15 minutes until seizure subsides • Diazepam rectal gel VERY expensive
First Line Therapy–Maintenance Management of Seizures				
Clonazepam (Klonopin)	2–10 mg daily	PO, PR	**Tablets:** 0.5 mg, 1 mg, 2 mg	• Long acting benzodiazepine • Most useful in absence seizures and myoclonus
Phenobarbital*	100–600 mg daily	PO, PR, IV	**Tablets:** 7.5 mg, 15 mg, 30 mg, 60 mg, 90 mg, 100 mg **Injection:** 30 mg/mL, 60 mg/mL, 130 mg/mL	• Barbiturate • Long half-life allows maintenance dose to be taken once daily (ideally at bedtime) • Signs of toxicity–drowsiness, nystagmus, ataxia
Phenytoin (Dilantin)*	300–400 mg daily	PO, IV	**Chewable Tablets:** 50 mg **Capsule:** 30 mg, 100 mg **Capsules, Extended Release:** 100 mg, 200 mg, 300 mg **Injection:** 50 mg/mL	• Maintenance anticonvulsant of choice in hospice • Partial/Complex & Generalized seizures • Long acting capsule formulation allows maintenance dose to be taken once daily (ideally at bedtime) • Signs of toxicity–drowsiness, diplopia, ataxia

Generic Name (Brand Name)	Usual Adult Starting Dose/Range	Routes	Common Strengths and Formulations	Comments
Maintenance Management of Seizures				
Valproic Acid, Divalproex Sodium (Depakene, Depakote ER)*	Oral: Initial: 1000–2500 mg daily in 1–3 divided doses	PO, PR, IV	**Valproic Acid** **Capsules:** 250 mg **Syrup:** 250 mg/5 mL **Injection:** 100 mg/mL **Divalproex Sodium** **Sprinkle Capsule:** 125 mg **Tablets, EC:** 125 mg, 250 mg, 500 mg **ER Tablet (24hr):** 500 mg	• Regular release and delayed release formulations are usually given in 2–4 divided doses/day, extended release formulation (Depakote ER) is usually given once daily. Conversion to Depakote ER from a stable dose may require an increase in the total daily dose between 8% and 20% to maintain similar serum concentrations • Generalized seizures, absence seizures, myoclonic seizures, partial seizures (simple and complex)
First Line Therapy–Management of Seizures Due to Brain Tumor or Metastases				
Dexamethasone (Decadron)	16–24 mg daily (in divided doses)	PO, IV, PR	**Tablets:** 0.25 mg, 0.5 mg, 0.75 mg, 1 mg, 1.5 mg, 2 mg, 4 mg, 6 mg **Injection:** 4 mg/mL, 10 mg/mL	• First line therapy in seizures related to brain tumor, metastases, or increased intracranial pressure from other causes • May give dose once daily or BID (morning and noon) to prevent insomnia

*Serum levels can be monitored to guide dosing, avoid toxicity.

Clinical Pearls

- For acute seizures, IV access is ideal and preferable, since it allows more rapid control of seizures. However, if access is unavailable, as is most often the case in the hospice setting, rectal administration of benzodiazepines is effective in controlling acute seizures.
- When discontinuing a maintenance dose of an anticonvulsant, slow taper to discontinuation minimizes the risk of withdrawal seizures. Patients and families should be advised against stopping anticonvulsants abruptly for the same reason.
- Severe or frequent seizures are rare as death approaches, but may require sedation to control.

- *Status epilepticus* is a special condition of prolonged seizure activity and is generally considered a medical emergency. Traditionally, status epilepticus is defined as a seizure lasting longer than 30 minutes or seizures recur without return of consciousness between seizures. However seizures lasting longer than 5 minutes are unlikely to self-terminate and may cause neuronal injury.
- Newer anticonvulsants with indications (Typically not initiated in hospice setting):
  - Gabapentin (Neurontin): Partial seizures (simple and complex)
  - Lamotrigine (Lamictal): Partial (simple and complex), generalized seizures
  - Levetiracetam (Keppra): Adjunctive partial and myoclonic seizures
  - Oxcarbazepine (Trileptal): Partial (simple and complex) and generalized seizures
  - Topiramate (Topamax): Partial seizures (simple and complex) and generalized seizures
  - Tiagabine (Gabitril): Partial seizures (simple and complex)
  - Zonisamide (Zonegan): Adjunctive partial seizures

Key References

Ropper AH, Brown RH, eds: *Adams and Victor's Principles of Neurology,* 8th Edition. New York: McGraw-Hill, 2005.

Eisenschenk S, Gilmore R: Strategies for successful management of older patients with seizures. *Geriatrics.* 54: 31–40 1999.

ACEP Clinical Policies Committee; Clinical Policies Subcommittee on Seizures: Clinical policy: Critical issues in the evaluation and management of adult patients presenting to the emergency department with seizures. *Ann Emerg Med.* 43: 605–625, 2004.

LaRoche SM, Helmers SL: The new antiepileptic drugs: scientific review. *JAMA.* 291: 605–614, 2004.

Sirven JI, Waterhouse E: Management of status epilepticus. Am Fam Physician. 68: 469–476, 2003.

Baldwin K, Miller L, Scott JB: Proactive identification of seizure risk improves terminal care. *Am J Hosp Palliat Care.* 19: 251–258, 2002.

Warren DE: Practical use of rectal medications in palliative care. *J Pain Symptom Manage.* 11:378–387, 1996.

Rey E, Treluyer JM, Pons G: Pharmacokinetic optimization of benzodiazepine therapy for acute seizures. Focus on delivery routes. Clin Pharmacokinet. 3: 409–424, 1999.

Seizures

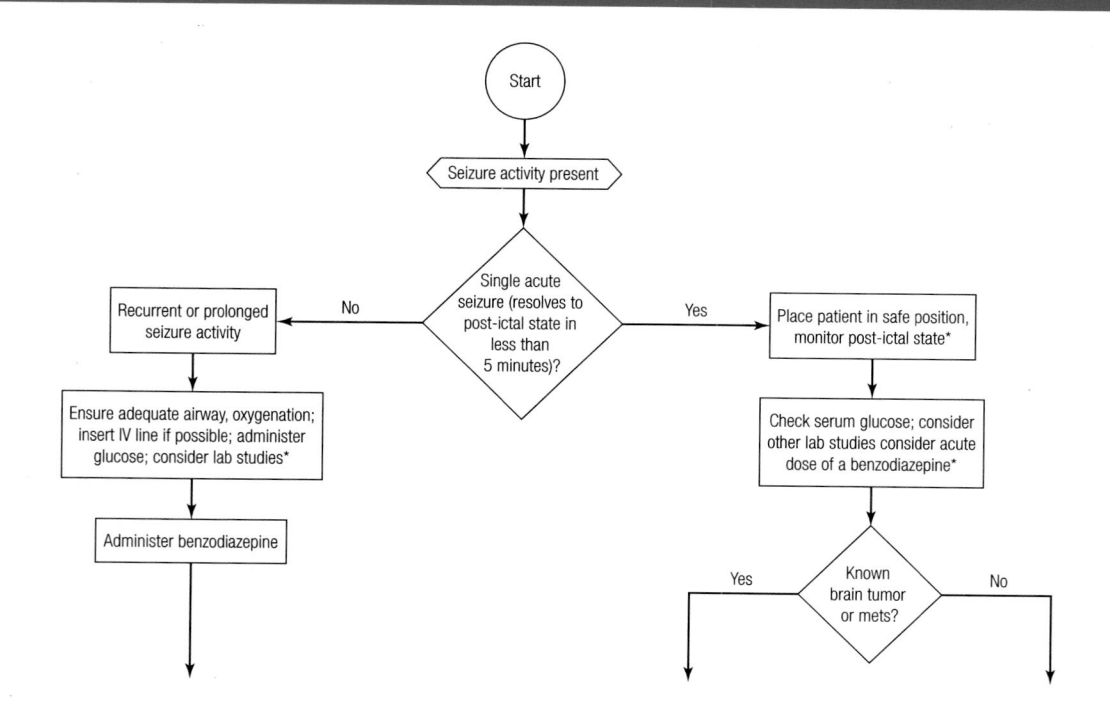

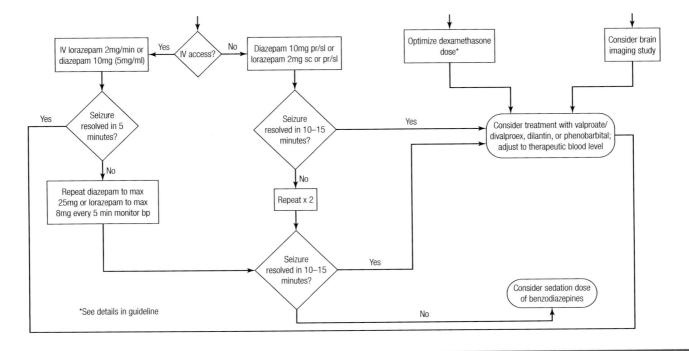

Terminal Secretions or "*Death Rattle*"

Introduction and Background

- Noisy terminal secretions (also known as "death rattle") are a common sign at the end of life. As patients lose their ability to swallow and clear oral secretions, accumulation of mucus results in a rattling or gurgling sound produced by air passing through mucus in the lungs and air passages.
- Hospice staff should advise families and caregivers that the sound does not represent discomfort for the patient. However, the sound is sometimes so distressing of the family that it should be treated.

Prevalence

- The incidence ranges from 25–92% and has been associated as a strong predictor of death within 48 hours.

Clinical Characteristics

- The noise of terminal secretions is produced by the oscillatory movements of secretions in the upper airways in association with the inspiratory and expiratory phases of respiration.
- It is typically seen only in patients who are obtunded or are too weak to expectorate.
- Drugs that decrease secretions are best initiated at the first sign of death rattle as they do not affect existing respiratory secretions.
- These agents have limited or no impact when the secretions are secondary to pneumonia or pulmonary edema.

Non-Pharmacologic Treatment

- Inform and educate the family about what to expect.
- Position the patient on his/her side or in a semi-prone position to help facilitate drainage of secretions.
- Place the patient in Trendelenburg's position (lowering the head of the bed), this allows fluids to move into the oropharynx, facilitating an easy removal. (Do not maintain this position for long, as it increases risk of aspiration.)
- Oropharyngeal suctioning is another option but may be disturbing to both the patient and visitors.
- Fluid intake can also be decreased, as appropriate.

Pharmacotherapy

- Anticholinergic drugs remain the standard of therapy for prevention and treatment of terminal secretions due to their ability to effectively dry secretions.
- Drugs used for this indication are similar pharmacologically and one can be selected by anticholinergic potency, onset of action, route of administration, alertness of patient, and cost.
- Differences among agents exist, for example, glycopyrrolate does not cross the blood brain barrier and is associated with reduced risk of central nervous system side effects.

Glycopyrrolate is a potent drying agent when compared to others discussed here, and has the potential to cause excessive dryness.

- Anticholinergic side effects are common and similar in this class and include blurred vision, constipation, urinary retention, confusion, delirium, restlessness, hallucinations, dry mouth and heart palpitations.

Pharmacologic Management of the Terminal Secretions (Death Rattle)

Generic Name (Brand Name)	Usual Adult Starting Dose/Range	Routes	Common Strengths and Formulations	Comments
First Line Therapy				
Atropine (Isopto Atropine)	1 drop SL q2h PRN or 0.4 mg IV/SC q2h PRN	SL, IV, SC	**Ophthalmic Solution:** 1% (Used SL) **Tablets:** 0.4 mg **Injection:** 0.4 mg/mL	• Administered sublingually • Use caution when administering drops to avoid potential overdose • 1 drop of atropine 1% ophthalmic sol'n delivers approximately 0.5 mg of atropine
Alternative				
Hyoscyamine (Levsin)	0.125 mg PO or SL q4h PRN **MDD:** 1.5 mg/day	PO, SL	**Tablets:** 0.125 mg **SL Tablets:** 0.125 mg **Oral Drops:** 0.125 mg/mL **Elixir:** 0.125 mg/5 mL	• Available in sublingual formulation
Second Line Therapy				
Glycopyrrolate (Robinul)	1 mg PO BID 0.2 mg SC, IV q6h	PO, SC, IV	**Tablets:** 1 mg, 2 mg **Injection:** 0.2 mg/mL	• Does not cross blood brain barrier therefore minimizes CNS side effects (e.g. sedation, confusion) • Potent drying effect; about 5 times as potent as atropine
Third Line Therapy				
Scopolamine Transdermal (Transderm-Scop)	1 patch q72h	Transdermal	**Transdermal Patch:** 1.5 mg	• Approximately 12 hours to peak effect • Patients sometimes need multiple patches (1–3) to be effective

Clinical Pearls

- Initiate therapy early to prevent secretions from accumulating.
- It is easier to prevent the accumulation of large amounts of secretions than to treat the condition. However, premature use in a patient who is still alert may lead to an unacceptable drying of oral and pharyngeal mucosa or CNS side effects (sedation, confusion).

Key References

Merriam-Webster Online Dictionary. Available at URL: http://www.m-w.com/cgi-bin/dictionary?book = Dictionary&va = death+rattle. Accessed on 01–11–05.

Bickel K, Arnold. R. Fast Facts and Concepts #109. Death rattle and oral secretions. March 2004. End-of-Life Physician Education Resource Center, wwweperc.mcw.edu. Available at URL: http://www.eperc.mcw.edu/fastFact/ff_109.htm. Accessed on 12/30/05.

Wildiers H, Menten J. Death rattle: prevalence, prevention and treatment. J Pain Symptom Manage. 2002;34:310–317.

Morita T, Tsunoda J, Inone S, Chihara S. Risk factors for death rattle in terminally ill cancer patients: a prospective exploratory study. Palliat Med. 2000;14:19–23.

Lichter I, Hunt E. The last 48 hours of life. J Palliat Care. 1990;6:7–15.

Ellershaw JE, Sutcliff JM, Saunders Cm, Dehydration and the dying patient. J Pain Symptom Manage. 1995;10:192–197.

Emanuel LL, von Gunten CF, Ferris FD, HauserJM, eds. The Education for Physicians on End-of-life Care (EPEC) Curriculum. 2003. Module 12: Last Hours of Living, Part 1.

Killion K, ed. Drug Facts and Comparisons. Electronic edition. St. Louis; Facts and Comparisons, 2005, [Scopolamine, Glycopyrrolate, Hyoscyamine, Atropine.]

Bennett M, Lucas V, Brennan M, Hughes A, O'Donnell V, Wee B. Using anti-muscarinic drugs in the management of death rattle: evidence-based guidelines for palliative care. Palliative Medicine. 2002;16:369–374.

Varkey B. Palliative Care for End-Stage Lung Disease Patients. Clin Pulm Med. 2003;10(5):269–277.

Hyson HC, Johnson AM, Jog MS. Sublingual atropine for sialorrhea secondary to parkinsonism: a pilot study. Mov Disorder. 2002;17(6):1318–20.

Terminal Secretions

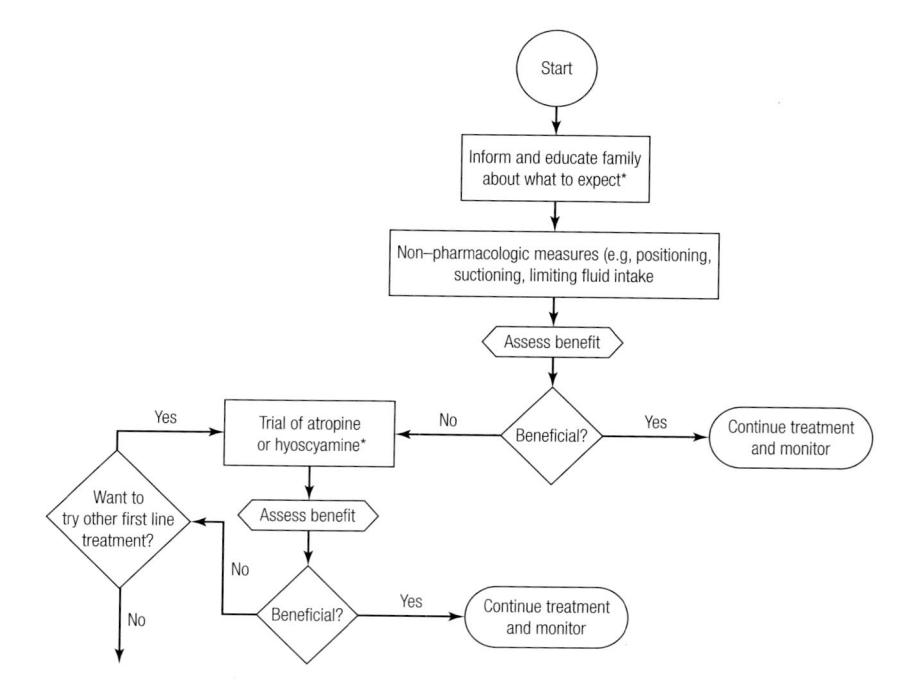

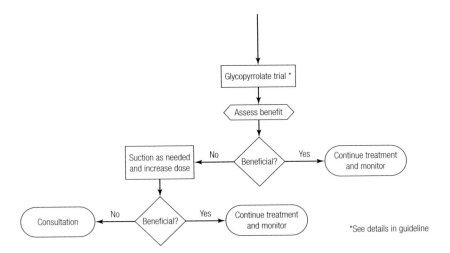

*See details in guideline

Thick Secretions

Introduction and Background
- Excessive secretions are troublesome in dying patients as secretions can partially obstruct the airway, lead to increased airway resistance and increased work of breathing.
- Secretions can also precipitate the sensation of dyspnea and can result in loss of sleep.
- Excessive secretions are common but can be managed by treating the underlying cause, non-pharmacologic therapy and pharmacologic therapy.
- Goal of treatment is to decrease morbidities associated with thick secretions such as dyspnea, insomnia and improve quality of life.

Prevalence
- Although prevalence of thick secretions is not documented, most patients will experience thick secretions as they approach the end of life.

Causes
- A thorough history and physical should be taken and possible reversible causes of thick secretions should be identified and treated, if present. Some of the possible causes are:
  - Tube feedings
  - Inability to clear secretions due to weakened condition
  - Fluid overload and edema
  - Dehydration
  - Infection–purulent sputum (Treat with antibiotic, if appropriate)

Non-Pharmacologic Therapy
- Educate family that thick secretions are common but can be effectively managed.
- Increase fluid intake when appropriate.
- Placing patients in Trendelenburg's position takes advantage of gravity to help move secretions in the appropriate direction to facilitate drainage (but prolonged placement in this position increases risk of aspiration).
- Directed cough techniques are effective in secretion removal, however in palliative care, these may be of limited utility, as significant coordination is necessary. Patients must be able to follow directions and take good deep breaths. Directed cough is a deliberate maneuver that is taught, supervised, and monitored. Consult a respiratory therapist for proper technique and advice.
- Mobilization and exercise–sometimes a challenge in palliative care patients, however any measure of activity is better than none.
- Suctioning is an option but can be uncomfortable and disturbing to patients and family.

Pharmacotherapy
- If the patient is alert but secretions are thick but the patient is able to expectorate, then pharmacological therapy that **thins mucus** can be implemented.
- If patient is unable to expectorate the emphasis of therapy is to **dry secretions.**

Pharmacologic Management When Patients Can Expectorate—These Agents Focus on Thinning Secretions

Generic Name (Brand Name)	Usual Adult Starting Dose/Range	Common Strengths and Formulations	Comments
First Line Therapy—Expectorants			
Guaifenesin Immediate Release (Robitussin)	200–400 mg PO q4h or PRN **MDD:** 2,400 mg/day	**Liquid:** 100 mg/5 mL	• If immediate release is effective converting to sustained release may increase adherence
Guaifenesin Sustained Release (Mucinex)	600–1200 mg PO q12h **MDD:** 2,400 mg/day	**Tablets, Extended-release (OTC):** 600 mg	• Do not crush, chew, or break tablet. Take with a full glass of water without regard to meals • Use of the extended release product, may increase adherence if product is needed around the clock
Second Line Therapy			
Nebulized saline	Inhale 3 mL (1 vial) with nebulizer q4h scheduled or PRN	Nebulized Saline 0.9%	

Pharmacologic Management When Patients Cannot Expectorate—These Agents Focus on Drying of Thick Secretions

Generic Name (Brand Name)	Usual Adult Starting Dose/Range	Common Strengths and Formulations	Comments
First Line Therapy			
Hyoscyamine (Levsin)	0.125 mg PO or SL q4h PRN **MDD:** 1.5 mg per day	**Tablets:** 0.125 mg **SL Tablets:** 0.125 mg **Oral Drops:** 0.125 mg/mL **Elixir:** 0.125 mg/5 mL	• Available in sublingual formulation for administration in patients that cannot swallow

Generic Name (Brand Name)	Usual Adult Starting Dose/Range	Common Strengths and Formulations	Comments
First Line Therapy (continued)			
Hyoscyamine Extended Release (Levbid, Levsinex Timecaps)	0.375 mg PO q12h **MDD:** 1.5 mg per day	**ER Tablet/Capsule:** 0.375 mg	
Atropine 1% Ophthalmic Solution (Isopto Atropine)	1 drop SL q2h PRN	**Ophthalmic Solution:** 1%	• Administered sublingually, NOT in the eye • Use caution when administering drops to avoid potential overdose • 1 drop of atropine 1% ophthalmic solution delivers approximately 0.5 mg of atropine
Second Line Therapy			
Glycopyrrolate (Robinul)	1 mg PO BID 0.1 mg SQ BID	**Tablets:** 1, 2 mg **Injection:** 0.2 mg/mL	• Does not cross blood brain barrier therefore minimizes risk of CNS side effects (e.g. sedation, confusion) • Oral absorption is erratic, SQ doses range from 0.1 mg to 0.2 mg SQ BID • Drying effect is about 5 times as potent as atropine
Third Line Therapy			
Scopolamine Transdermal (Transderm-Scop)	1 patch q72h	**Transdermal Patch:** 1.5 mg	• Onset of action is not immediate, may take 3–4 hours to begin to see effects. Peak effect is reached in approximately 12 hours • Patients sometimes need multiple patches (1–3) to be effective • Can cause CNS side effects (e.g. sedation, confusion)

Clinical Pearls

- Fluid, particularly water, administered orally or parenterally is still the best approach to thinning secretions.
- All anticholinergic drugs have similar actions and side effects. These agents should not be used in combination.
- Avoid anticholinergic agents if patients are still able to expectorate secretions.

Key References

Sorenson HM. Managing Secretions in Dying Patients. Respiratory Care. 2000. 45:11;1355–1364.

Varkey B. Palliative Care for End-Stage Lung Disease Patients. Clin Pulm Med. 2003;10(5):269–277.

Killion K, ed. Drug Facts and Comparisons. Electronic edition. St. Louis; Facts and Comparisons, 2005, [Robitussin, Mucinex, Levsin, Robinul, Transderm-Scop].

Thick Secretions

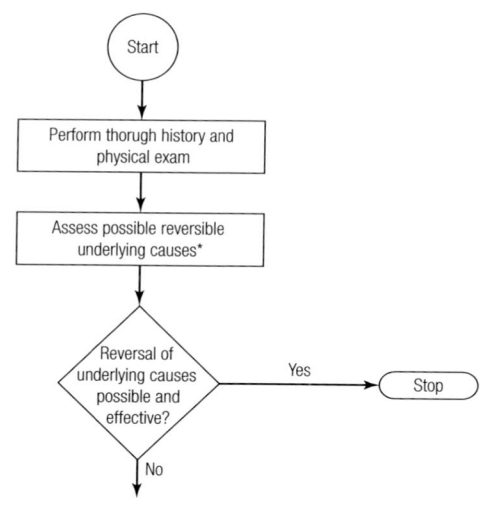

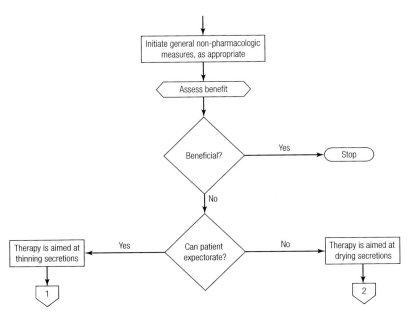

Thick Secretions (*continued*)

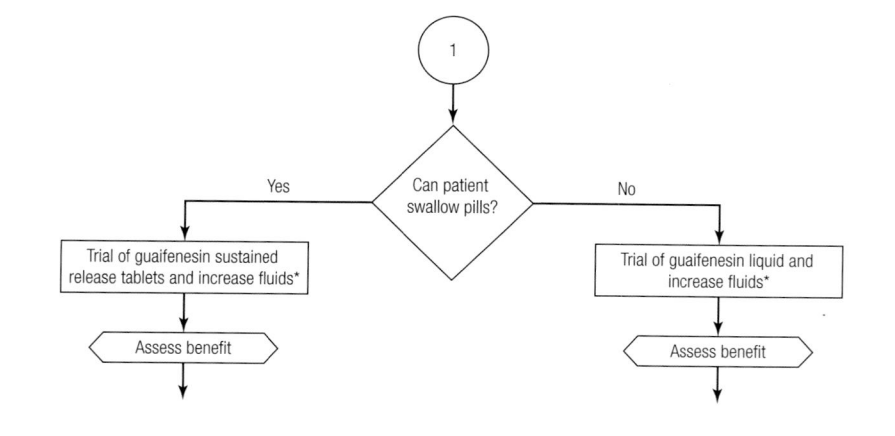

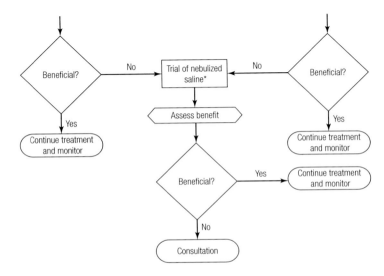

Thick Secretions (*continued*)

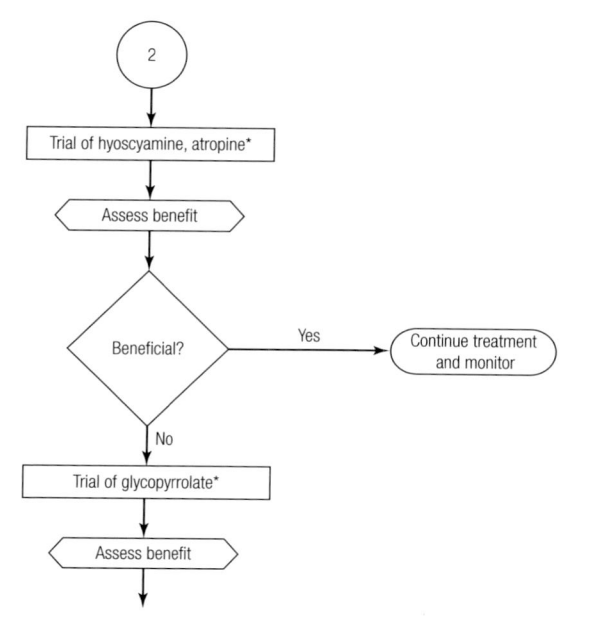

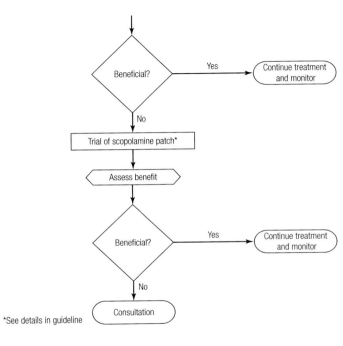

*See details in guideline

Xerostomia

Introduction and Background

- Saliva is produced by the parotid, submandibular and sublingual glands as well as by the hundreds of smaller salivary glands that are located throughout the oral cavity. These glands are innervated by both the parasympathetic and sympathetic nervous system.
- Parasympathetic stimulation produces thin, watery secretions while the sympathetic stimulation leads to less volume and more viscous saliva.
- Approximately one liter of saliva is produced daily. Flow rates fluctuate significantly due to diurnal rhythms.
- Xerostomia is a subjective, uncomfortable feeling of dry mouth related to either a decrease in the production and flow of saliva or a change in the composition of saliva.
- Saliva consists of water, electrolytes and glycoproteins.
- The major functions of saliva are to lubricate food and enhance taste, swallowing, and speech.
- The antimicrobial components and buffering activity of saliva also protect the teeth from dental caries and the upper digestive tract from oral candidiasis.

Prevalence

- The prevalence of xerostomia in the general population is about 25%. However, in patients with advanced cancer, up to 77% report xerostomia.

Causes

- Xerostomia is most commonly caused by:
  - ◆ Connective tissue disorders
  - ◆ Immunological disorders
  - ◆ Destruction of salivary glands by radiation therapy or surgery
  - ◆ Medications:
    - ° Anticholinergics: atropine, glycopyrrolate, benztropine, oxybutynin, scopolamine
    - ° Antidepressants and antipsychotics: SSRIs (particularly paroxetine), TCAs (particularly amitriptyline), venlafaxine, mirtazapine, olanzapine
    - ° Diuretics: chlorothiazide, furosemide, hydrochlorothiazide
    - ° Antihypertensives: ACE inhibitors, clonidine
    - ° Sedatives and anxiolytics: benzodiazepines
    - ° Muscle relaxants: cyclobenzaprine, tizanidine
    - ° Analgesics: opioids, tramadol, NSAIDs
    - ° Antihistamines: diphenhydramine, loratadine, meclizine
    - ° Miscellaneous medications: anticonvulsants, antidysrhythmics, anti-incontinence agents, bronchodilators, carbidopa/levodopa, ipratropium, nicotine
- Sjögren's syndrome is a condition that presents with both xerostomia and xerophthalmia (dry eyes). Sjögren's syndrome is either a primary disease, occurring predominately in women in their forties or a secondary condition associated with autoimmune or connective tissue diseases (e.g., rheumatoid arthritis, systemic lupus erythematosus, systemic sclerosis).

- Other conditions associated with xerostomia include renal dialysis, diabetes type 1 and 2, primary biliary cirrhosis, vasculitis, chronic hepatitis, HIV/AIDS, bone marrow transplantation, and graft-vs-host disease.
- Xerostomia is commonly seen in patients with fibromyalgia, chronic fatigue syndrome, and Raynaud's phenomenon.
- Patients who are anxious or depressed often complain of dry mouth.

Clinical Characteristics

- Patients with xerostomia or hyposalivation complain of dry mouth, a burning sensation, soreness of the mouth, or altered taste/loss of taste.
- Caregivers may notice increased requests for water (especially when speaking or swallowing), difficulty swallowing, or avoidance of dry or hard foods.
- As xerostomia progresses, the mouth may manifest erythematous pebbled, cobblestoned, or fissured tongue. Mucosal surfaces may become sticky to the touch.

Non-Pharmacologic Treatment

- Water or ice chips; frequent sips of water generally effective.
- Milk may be effective in moistening and lubricating, and may also buffer oral acids.
- Humidified air.
- Frozen grapes, popsicles, lemon sugar-free candy, vitamin C tablets, frozen tonic water.
- Lubricate lips.
- Stimulate salivary glands: Sour or acidic candy.
- Diet: eat foods that are soft, moist, and cool or at room temperature.
- Masticatory stimulants: sugarless gum (Biotene Dry Mouth Gum, XyliFresh) or sugarfree hard candies (Salix lozenges).

Pharmacologic Management of Xerostomia

Generic Name (Brand Name)	Usual Adult Starting Dose/Range/Directions	Common Strengths and Formulations	Comments
First Line Therapy			
Saliva Substitutes / Lubricants			
Saliva Substitute	Use PRN	**Solution**	• Sorbitol, sodium carboxymethylcellulose, methylparaben
Saliva Orthana	Use PRN	**Spray / Lozenge**	• Porcine and bovine mucin
Salivart	Spray directly into mouth for 1–2 seconds PRN	**Aerosol Spray; Preservative-free**	• Sodium carboxymethylcellulose
Chemical Stimulants			
Biotène, Oralbalance	Using clean cotton swab, apply one inch ribbon onto tongue and affected areas	**Gel, Toothpaste, Mouthwash**	• Glycerate polymer; contains anti-microbial enzymes
MouthKote	Swirl 1 or 2 tsp for 8–10 seconds, then swallow or spit	**Solution, Lemon-lime Flavor**	• Mucopolysaccharides & citric acid
Optimoist	Spray into mouth PRN; may expectorate or swallow	**Solution**	• Contains citric acid, hydroxyethylcellulose, and fluoride 2 parts per million
Second Line Therapy			
Muscarinic Agonists: (Use with caution in patients with glaucoma, cardiovascular disease or pulmonary dysfunction)			
Pilocarpine (Salagen®)	5 mg PO TID 5 gtts PO TID (equiv dose using pilocarpine 2% ophthalmic)	**Tablets:** 2.5, 5 mg **Ophthalmic Solution:** 2% (Used orally, not in eye)	• Unpleasant side effects: diarrhea, nausea, vomiting, sweating • Avoid taking with dairy products • May take up to 2 months for maximal effect • Expensive # 90 5 mg tablets~$150 • Use of ophthalmic sol'n may be easier than tabs and more cost effective Pilocarpine 2%, 30 mL ~$35
Cevimeline (Evoxac®)	30 mg TID	**Capsule:** 30 mg	• No further efficacy shown with 60 mg TID; similar side effects as pilocarpine • Expensive # 90 30 mg capsules~$150

Third Line Therapy			
Numoisyn	1 lozenge PRN (not to exceed 16 per 24 hrs)	Lozenge	• Mucopolysaccharides; must have some salivary function
Numoisyn	2 mL, rinse and swallow PRN	Liquid	• Linseed extract; must have some salivary function
Physostigmine	Apply PRN	1 mg/mL	• (Off-label use) May be applied locally in spray or as mouthwash

Clinical Pearls

- Any identifiable underlying cause of xerostomia should be rectified.
- Alternate drugs should be considered, hydration corrected if possible, and psychological factors should be addressed.
- Advise the patient to avoid use of caffeine, alcohol, and tobacco products.
- Advise the patient to avoid breathing through the mouth, if possible.
- Few data indicate superiority of any treatment; treatment selection should thus take into consideration patient preferences, cost, availability, and form of delivery.
- Patients with xerostomia have an increased risk for dental caries and oral thrush. Oral hygiene is thus very important; fluoride (alcohol-free) or chlorhexidine rinses may be used.

Key References

Davies AN, Broadley K, Beighton D: Xerostomia in patients with advanced cancer. *J Pain Sym Manage*. 22: 820–825, 2001.

Guggenheimer J, Moore PA: Xerostomia: Etiology, recognition and treatment. *JADA*. 134: 61–69, 2003.

Narhi TO, Meurman JH, Ainamo A: Xerostomia and hyposalivation: causes, consequences, and treatment in the elderly. *Drugs and Aging*. 15: 103–116, 1999.

Neiuw Amerongen AV, Veerman ACI: Current therapies for xerostomia and salivary gland hypofunction associated with cancer therapies. *Support Care Cancer*. 11: 226–231, 2003.

Doyle D, Hanks G, Cherny N, Calman K: *Oxford Textbook of Palliative Medicine*, 3rd edition. New York: Oxford University Press. 2005, pp. 674–679.

Scully C, Felix DH: Oral medicine–update for the dental practitioner. Dry mouth and disorders of salivation. *Br Dental J*. 199: 423–427, 2005.

Treatment of Drug-Induced Xerostomia. *http://www.drymouth.info/practitioner/treatment.asp*.

Yasuda H, Niki H: Review of the pharmacological properties and clinical usefulness of muscarinic agonists for xerostomia in patients with Sjögren's syndrome. *Clin Drug Invest*. 22: 67–73, 2002.

Xerostomia

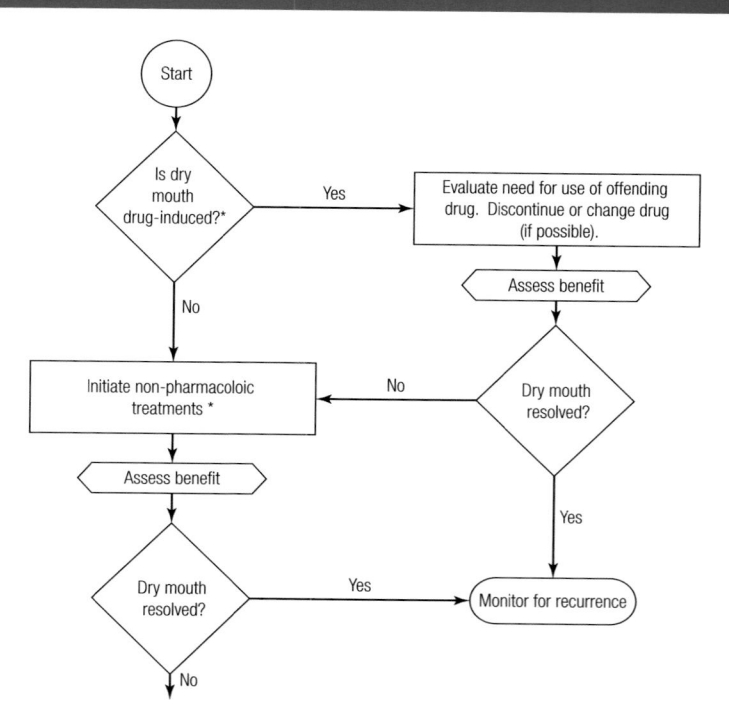

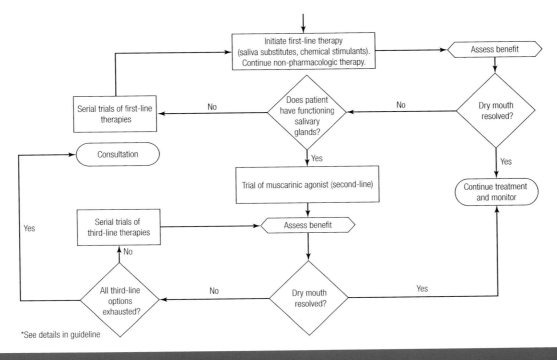

Initiate first-line therapy (saliva substitutes, chemical stimulants). Continue non-pharmacologic therapy.

Assess benefit

Dry mouth resolved?

No → Does patient have functioning salivary glands?

No → Serial trials of first-line therapies

Yes → Continue treatment and monitor

Yes → Trial of muscarinic agonist (second-line)

Assess benefit

Dry mouth resolved?

Yes → Continue treatment and monitor

No → All third-line options exhausted?

No → Serial trials of third-line therapies

Yes → Consultation

*See details in guideline

Wound Care

A recent study (Tippett, 2005) found prevalence of wounds at the end of life to be 35%, of which nearly half were pressure ulcers. Because patients and family members may not have been told that a wound probably won't heal, healthcare providers need to provide realistic assessments and advice to patients and their families on wounds, which are not likely to heal. Wound care for patients with a life-limiting illness generally focuses on comfort rather than wound healing. Treatments should include those that relieve pain and other distressing wound symptoms, rather than aggressive treatments that may be burdensome to the patient. Wound-healing becomes less likely at the end of life due to poor circulation, malnutrition and dehydration, and limited mobility of the patient. These factors predispose patients to development of new wounds and worsening of existing wounds.

Assessment of wounds should be individualized for each patient according to the patient's goals of care. This assessment includes wound physical characteristics, associated risk factors for infection and progression, effects on patient's quality of life, and caregiver/family needs. Goals of palliative wound care include: focusing on patient comfort, reducing caregiver burden, prevention of progression and infection, and maintaining the functional ability of the patient.

Wound Assessment

- Document treatments and dressings used, along with wound care education provided to patient and caregivers.
- Assess wound at regular intervals for presence of pain, location, size and shape, including depth and stage or grade.
- Wound bed assessment includes color, presence of slough, necrotic tissue, granulation tissue, epithelial tissue, undermining or tunneling.
- If exudate is present determine purulent, serous, or serosanguinous.
- Evaluate wound edges and the skin surface around the wound.
- Signs of wound infection include purulent discharge, malodor, erythema at wound edge, edema and inflammation, increasing pain, increased necrotic tissue. Wound cultures provide limited benefit in diagnosing infection because wound beds are frequently contaminated.

Wound Treatment

- Always consider pre-medication with analgesics or anxiolytics if necessary wound care may cause pain or distress to the patient.
- Debride wound via sharp instrument, enzymatic preparations, cleansing and irrigation.
- Control bacterial burden with ongoing monitoring for signs of infections, necrotic tissue debridement, use of topical silver products (silver sulfadiazine). Limit the use of systemic antibiotics to treatment of cellulitis.
- Provide a moist wound environment while controlling exudates with appropriate dressings. Negative-pressure wound therapy, such as wound vacuum-assisted closures, may be burdensome to the patient, should not be used in malignant wounds, and require specialized application and monitoring.
- Prevent further injury or progression if possible. Avoid excessive repositioning of the patient if it causes significant pain or discomfort.
- Nutritional support of wound healing has limited benefit at the end of life. Medication burden is increased when additional vitamin and mineral supplements are used in an attempt to promote wound healing.

Wound and Pressure Ulcer Products, by Drainage and Stage

Product	Drainage			Wound Stage			
	Light	Moderate	Heavy	I	II	III	IV
Transparent film	•			•	•		
Foam Island	•	•			•	•	
Hydrocolloids	•	•			•	•	
Petroleum-based nonadherent	•				•	•	
Alginate		•	•			•	•
Hydrogel	•				•	•	•
Gauze packing (moistened with saline)		•	•			•	•

Adapted from Geriatrics at Your Fingertips 2007, table 92

References

Reuben DB, Herr KA, Pacala JT, et al. Skin ulcers, chapter 32, In: *Geriatrics At Your Fingertips: 2006–2007, 8th Edition*. New York: The American Geriatrics Society; 2006.

Hughes, R.G., et al, (2005). Palliative wound care at the end of life. *Home Health Care Management & Practice*, 17(3), 196–202.

Tice, M.A. (2006). Wound care in the face of life-limiting illness. *Home Healthcare Nurse*, 24(2), 115–118.

Tippett, A.W. (2005). Wounds at the end of life. *Wounds: A Compendium of Clinical Research and Practice*, 17(4), 91–98.

Heart Failure

Introduction and Background

- Advanced heart failure (Class III-IV or Stage C and D) is defined as persistent symptoms that limit daily living despite optimal therapy with medications known to provide benefit. Patients have significant cardiac dysfunction with marked symptoms of dyspnea, fatigue, or symptoms relating to end organ hypoperfusion at rest or with minimal exertion despite optimal medical therapy.
- Expected one year mortality of patients with advanced heart failure is 30–50%. Very little clinical trial data is available to guide therapy in patients with advanced disease or to define "best practices" for end of life treatment.
- Advanced care planning should begin at the time of heart failure diagnosis. Because of the uncertainty of the disease course, discussions about quality of life and prognosis should be an ongoing part of disease management.
- Once the patient has made the decision for comfort care, deactivation of implantable defibrillators (IACD) should be considered and discussed along with other goals of care.

Symptom Management

The most common symptoms experienced in patients with end stage heart failure include breathlessness, fatigue, anxiety, pain and fluid retention. Many of the symptoms experienced are similar to terminally ill patients with cancer, including nausea, anorexia, constipation, trouble sleeping, and depression. Dyspnea and pain become the most significant symptoms reported in the last week of life in patients dying from heart failure.

Dyspnea

- Rule out cause as pulmonary congestion associated with volume overload.
  - Long term use of loop diuretics (furosemide) can lead to enhanced sodium reabsorption from the proximal and distal tubules leading to diuretic resistance.
    - The short term addition of an intermittent thiazide diuretic such as metolazone may enhance diuresis by improving sodium excretion, especially if the patient is requiring oral doses of furosemide exceeding 120 mg.
    - If large oral doses are needed to achieve euvolemia, dividing that dose over 2 to 3 times a day may be more effective.
- Morphine may be considered in patients who fail maximized diuretic and/or vasodilator therapy and other treatable causes have been ruled out.
- Nebulized furosemide for refractory dyspnea has been shown to be effective in observational studies in terminally ill patients with cancer. Though there are no English-language published reports of nebulized furosemide in patients with heart failure and refractory dyspnea, it would be reasonable to consider its use in this situation.

Pain

- In hospitalized patients with heart failure, 41% experienced moderate to severe pain in the last 3 days of life. This is comparable to patients with lung or colon cancer.
- Severe pain is second only to dyspnea in last 3 days of life.

- Etiology of pain in heart failure is not thoroughly understood but may be due to multiple factors such as:
  - Cardiac causes: angina, edema
  - Comorbid conditions: arthritis, diabetic neuropathy
- Opioids (primarily morphine) are the drugs of choice
- Avoid NSAIDs and COX2 inhibitors as they can cause fluid retention.

Medication Considerations for End-Stage Heart Failure

Medication Class	Examples	Benefit for HF symptoms	Comments
ACE Inhibitors or, Angiotensin receptor blockers	Lisinopril, Enalapril, Valsartan, Candesartan	Possibly	• Consider discontinuing or dose reduction if symptomatic hypotension is present
Aldosterone antagonists	Spironolactone, Eplerenone	No benefit	• Consider discontinuation • Primary benefit for decreased mortality only • Risk of hyperkalemia, especially with renal insufficiency
Anti-arrhythmics	Amiodarone	No benefit	• No clear indication for HF at EOL • Very long half-life, effects may persist for weeks after discontinuation
Beta blockers	Atenolol, Metoprolol, Carvedilol	Possibly	• Do not initiate or increase doses • Consider dose reduction if bradycardia (<60 bpm) • Consider discontinuing or dose reduction if hypotension still present after ACEI/ARB stopped
Calcium channel blockers	Verapamil, Amlodipine	No benefit	• No clear indication for HF at EOL • May exacerbate peripheral edema
Diuretics	Furosemide, Bumetanide, Torsemide	Probably	• Continue for symptom management • Monitor for hypovolemia, dehydration
Inotrope (oral)	Digoxin	Very limited	• Risk often outweighs benefit • Consider discontinuing if any renal insufficiency present • May exacerbate anorexia, confusion, and N/V
Inotropic (IV)	Dobutamine	Very limited	• Consider only if plan for transition to home care and therapy wean
Vasodilators	Hydralazine, Isosorbide, Nitroglycerin	Possibly	• Consider discontinuing hydralazine • Nitrates have benefit for ischemic chest pain

References

Goodlin S, Hauptman P, Arnold R, et al. Consensus statement: palliative and supportive care in advanced heart failure. *J Card Fail* 2004;10:200–209.

Stevenson L. Design of therapy for advanced heart failure. *Eur J Heart Fail* 2005;7:323–331.

Lewis W, Luebke D, Johnson N. Withdrawing implantable defibrillator shock therapy in terminally ill patients. *Am J Med* 2006;119:892–896.

Levenson J, McCarthy E, Lynn J. The last six months of life for patients with congestive heart failure. *J Am Ger Soc* 2000;48 (5 suppl): S101–109.

Nordgren L, Sorensen S. Symptoms experienced in the last six months of life in patiens with end-stage heart failure. *Eur J Card N* 2003;2:213–217.

Zambroski C, Moser D, Bhat G. Impact of symptom prevalence and symptom burden on quality of live in patients with heart failure. *Eur J Card N* 2005;4:198–206.

Zambroski C, Moser D, Roser L. Patients with heart failure who die in hospice. *Am Heart J* 2005;149: 558–564.

Davis M, Albert N, Young J. Palliation of heart failure. *Am J Hosp & Pall Med* 2005;22:211–222.

Adams K, Lindenfield J. Executive summary:HFSA 2006 comprehensive heart failure practice guidelines. *J Card Fail* 2006;12: 10–38.

Kohara H, Ueoka H, Aoe K, et al. Effect of nebulized furosemide in terminally ill cancer patients with dyspnea. *J Pain Symptom Manage* 2003;26:962–967.

Shimoyama N, Shimoyama M. Nebulized furosemide as a novel treatment for dyspnea in terminal cancer patients. *J Pain Symptom Manage* 2002;23:73–76.

Stone P, Kurowska A. Re: Nebulized furosemide for dyspnea in terminal cancer patients. *J Pain Symptom Manage* 2002;24:274–275.

Pantilat S, Steimle A. Palliative care for patients with heart failure. *JAMA* 2004;291:2476–2482.

Note: Contributions to Heart Failure section, pages 266–268, were made by Sharon Starling.

Chronic Obstructive Pulmonary Disease (COPD)

The Global Initiative for Chronic Obstructive Lung Disease (GOLD) 2006 Guidelines

I: Mild	II: Moderate	III: Severe	IV: Very Severe
• $FEV_1/FVC<0.70$	• $FEV_1/FVC<0.70$	• $FEV_1/FVC<0.70$	• $FEV_1/FVC<0.70$
• $FEV_1 \geq 80\%$ predicted	• $50\% \leq FEV_1 <80\%$ predicted	• $30\% \leq FEV_1 <50\%$ predicted	• $FEV_1<30\%$ predicted or FEV_1 $<50\%$ predicted plus chronic respiratory failure

Active reduction of risk factors: influenza vaccination ⟶
Add short-acting bronchodilator (when needed) ⟶
    Add regular treatment with one or more long-acting bronchodilators (when needed):
    Add rehabilitation
        Add inhaled glucocorticosteroids if repeated exacerbations
        Add long term oxygen if chronic respiratory failure.
        Consider surgical treatments

*Post bronchodilator FEV_1 is recommended for the diagnosis and assessment of severity of COPD

Home Management

Bronchodilators:

- Increase dose and/or frequency of existing short-acting bronchodilator therapy, preferably with β_2-agonists.
- If not already used, add anticholinergics until symptoms improve.

Glucocorticosteroids:

- If baseline $FEV_1<50\%$ predicted, add 5–40 mg oral prednisone per day for 7–10 days to the bronchodilator regimen.
- Nebulized budesonide may be an alternative to oral glucocorticosteroids in the treatment of nonacidotic exacerbations.

Antibiotics:

- Antibiotics should be given to patients:
  - With the following three cardinal symptoms: increased dyspnea, increased sputum volume, increased sputum purulence
  - Who require mechanical ventilation

Excerpts from The Global Initiative for Chronic Obstructive Lung Disease 2006 GOLD Guidelines
http://www.goldcopd.com/Guidelineitem.asp?l1=2&l2=1&intId=1116 Accessed 2–20–07.

Palliative Chemotherapy

According to NHPCO's 2006 statistics, 35–45% of all hospice patients have a primary diagnosis of cancer. Included are a subset of patients who are eligible for hospice and still receiving palliative chemotherapy. These patients represent a small but ever growing number of patients who continue ongoing palliative cancer treatments designed to provide end of life symptom management. For most hospice programs, these patients provide multi-faceted dilemmas. Patients may have had multiple treatment failures, continue to seek clinical trials, insist on continuing treatments that are likely medically futile, and desire "full code" resuscitation status. Prior to accepting palliative chemotherapy patients, each hospice organization should develop an evaluation process and well-defined admission criteria that are acceptable within the organization's culture and considers life closure issues.

Possible Admission Criteria

Past clinical treatment data—Failure of other treatment options?

Evidence that the current treatment remains palliative—Does the treatment improve symptoms?

Treatment plans and goals:

- What is the patient's goal for therapy?
- What is the treatment team's goal for therapy?
- Are there objective data that show improvements from the therapy (i.e. diagnostic tests, imaging studies, clinical performance status)?
- Clinical burden to the patient—Do the benefits/symptom management responses outweigh the risks/toxicities of the therapy?

- Flexible admission policy (including ability to admit patients whose survival is limited in relationship to desired chemotherapy).

A model that may assist in assimilating the above information is the Palliative Care Decision Model. This model is designed to provide a visual picture of all factors necessary to consider when evaluating the role of cancer treatment in hospice and palliative care.

Palliative Care Decision Model*

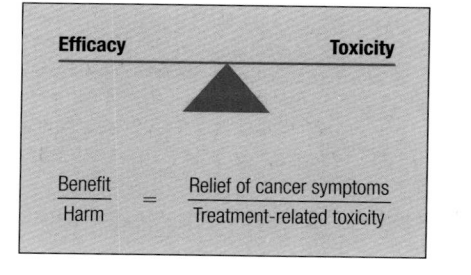

$$\frac{\text{Benefit}}{\text{Harm}} = \frac{\text{Relief of cancer symptoms}}{\text{Treatment-related toxicity}}$$

*Modified from: Seidman, A. The Evolving Role of Gencitabine in the Management of Metastatic Breast Cancer. Retrieved February 2, 2007 from http://www.medscape.com/viewarticle452532_8

Palliative Chemotherapy Support Considerations

Decisions to include cancer therapies cannot be based on the therapy alone, but also the necessary support services to provide the therapy. Additional support services which need to be considered may include the following:

- Access to the financial resources required to support a hospice palliative chemotherapy program including ongoing chemotherapy drug costs and supportive care **(Table 1)**
- Collaboration with an organization and radiation oncologist to provide possible radiation therapy services and symptom management for radiation therapy side effects
- Evaluation and ongoing diagnostic studies:
  - Lab work (including tumor marker evaluation)
  - CT and PET Scans, x-rays, MRI
- Supportive drug care management:
  - Antibiotic (oral and infusion)
  - Erythropoesis stimulating agents: Epoetin alfa(Procrit), Darbepoetin alfa (Aranesp)
  - Colony stimulating factors: Pegfilgrastim (Neulasta), Filgrastrim (Neupogen)
  - Chemotherapy Induced Antiemetic Therapy: Ondansetron (Zofran), Aprepitant (Emend), Palonosetron (Aloxi), Granisetron (Kytril), Dolasetron (Anzemet)
  - Bisphosphonate derivatives: Zolendronic acid (Zometa), Pamidronate (Aredia)
- Hospital and additional clinical support:
  - IV access, PICC line and Port maintenance
  - Sepsis Management

- Emergency room evaluation for chemotherapy-related symptoms
- Resuscitative measures for the patient who does not yet have a "Do Not Resuscitate" order
- Symptom management options

Additional Issues to Consider Related to Palliative Chemotherapy

- Hospice Medical Director with knowledge of palliative chemotherapy measurement outcomes
- Oncology advance practice nurse (APN) or certified oncology nurse resources
- Access to current drug information regarding palliative drug management
- Chemotherapy staff training and competency mechanism
- Patient education and monitoring system
- Home infusions treatment care options
- Supportive dialogue between oncology practices including communication concerning ongoing treatments plans, relevant diagnostic results, and outcomes of symptom management response
- Mechanism to review complex cases and palliative response outcomes to treatment
- Policies for admission of patients on clinical trials
- Patients who start or change palliative chemotherapy protocols after hospice admission
- Mechanism to provide financial support, symptom management, and psychosocial discharge support to treatment responsive patients

Patient/Caregiver Management Issues

- Patient and caregiver education:
  - Risks versus benefits of treatment
  - Knowledge of drugs and their related side effects
- Psychosocial and physical support:
  - Evaluate performance status, weight loss and ability to tolerate chemotherapy protocol
  - Understanding the role of cancer treatment when determining the goal of the therapy—palliative versus curative

Common Symptoms Which May Improve with Palliative Chemotherapy

Pain

Shortness of breath

Relief of bowel obstruction

Nausea/vomiting

Tumor ulceration

Lymphedema

Common Cancers Which May Benefit from End of Life Chemotherapy Treatment

Breast

Colon

Lung

Pancreas

Prostate

- All cancer sites may be appropriate for palliative chemotherapy-based current treatment failure therapy and response to symptom management.
- Most chemotherapy responses will be evaluated after two or three cycles of treatment.
- Follow-up testing may include labs and tumor specific diagnostic studies.
- Common response rates are 15–20% depending on the tumor, metastatic involvement and performance status of the patient.
- Drugs for palliation continue to evolve as new treatments and targeted therapy methods to provide symptom management relief continue to be developed.
- Symptom improvement based on tumor type or syndrome is provided in **Table 2**.
- Treatment options may be altered or discontinued related to toxic side effects (**Table 3**); patient's declining condition, or the desire to stop treatment.

Table 1 Palliative Common Chemotherapy Drugs and Drugs Cost

$ = $ 2000 or under

• Alkeran (Melphalan)	• Faslodex (Fulvestrant)	• Lupron (Leuprolide Acetate)
• Arimidex (Anastrozole)	• Femara (Letrozole)	• Nolvadex (Tamoxifen)
• Aromasin (Exemestane)	• Hydrea (Hydroxyurea)	• Zoladex (Goserelin Acetate)
• Casodex (Bicalutamide)		

$$ = $ 2000–4000

• Adriamycin (Doxorubicin, Doxil)	• Navelbine (Vinorelbine Tartrate)	• Tarceva (Erlotinib)
• Camptosar (Irinotecan)	• Novantrone (Mitoxantrone)	• Taxol (Paclitaxel)
• Cytoxan (Cyclophosphamide)	• Oncovin (Vincristine)	• Taxotere (Docetaxel)
• DTIC (Dacarbazine)	• Paraplatin (Carboplatin)	• Temodar (Temozolomide)
• Eligard (Leuprolide Acetate)	• Platinol (Cisplatin)	• Thalomid (Thalidomide)
• Emcyt (Estramustine)		• Trexall (Methotrexate)
• Fluorouracil (5FU)		• Velban (Vinblastine)
• Folinic Factor (Leucovorin Calcium)		• VePesid (Etoposide, VP–16)
• Gemzar (Gemcitabine)		• Xeloda (Capecitabine)
• Herceptin (Trastuzumab)		
• Hycamtin (Topotecan)		

$$$ = $ 4000 or above

• Abraxane (Paclitaxel, Protein Bound)	• Rituxan (Rituximab)	
• Alimta (Pemetrexed)	• Sutent (Sunitinib Maleate)	
• Avastin (Bevacizumab)	• Velcade (Bortezomib)	
• Eloxatin (Oxaliplatin)	• Vidaza (5–Azacytidine)	
• Erbitux (Cetuximab)		
• Nexavar (Sorafenib)		
• Revlimid (Lenalidomide)		

Controversial Issues Involved in Palliative Chemotherapy Include

- Palliative chemotherapy may have been offered to avoid difficult conversations as the treatment fails and disease progress.
- Ease of administration of oral chemotherapy may promote increased use of therapy with very limited benefit.
- Tumor response may be mistaken for effective symptom management.
- Cost burden of oral drugs may encourage inappropriate hospice referral in order to divert patient cost.
- Difficult family decision making along with increased access to medical information in the news and internet may encourage prolonged treatment options without clear understanding of risk versus benefit of therapies.
- The idea of palliative chemotherapy treatment may offer hope versus management of symptoms via other methods.

Table 2 Palliative Chemotherapy Symptom Management

Tumor Type	Symptoms that May Improve with Palliative Chemotherapy
Brain tumor Breast cancer Colon cancer Hematological: • Leukemia • Myelodysplastic syndrome Lung cancer Prostate cancer Lymphoma Head and neck Pancreatic cancer Ovarian cancer Other Oncology emergencies	• Headache, Nausea, Improved cognitive function • Bony metastasis, Tumor ulceration, Chest-wall pain, Lymphedema • Bowel obstruction, Pain, Lymphedema

Table 3 Common Symptoms, Toxicities, and Manifestations

Chemotherapy Agents	
• Alopecia • Anaphylaxis • Cardiac toxicity • Constipation • Diarrhea • Fluid retention • Flu-like syndrome • GI and nasal perforation • Hand-foot syndrome • Hypersensitivity • Hypertension • Liver toxicity • Marrow suppression • Mucositis	• Myalgias • Nausea • Ototoxicity • Parathesias • Leukoencephalopathy syndromes • Peripheral neuropathy • Renal toxicity • Stomatitis • Sepsis • Thromboembolism • Vesicant skin complications • Marrow suppression • Vomiting

Hormonal Agents	
• Affective disorders • Aseptic necrosis • Delirium • Gynecomastia • Hot flashes • Hyperglycemia • Infections	• Menopausal symptoms • Myopathy • Thromboembolism • Tumor flare • Ulcer disease • Weight gain

Common Disease-Specific Chemotherapy Agents

Generic drug names are listed in bold. Drugs may be given as a single agent or in combination. This drug list is not inclusive of new emerging protocols or clinical trial options (*usually not given for palliative chemotherapy).

Lung Non-Small Cell		
Cisplatin (Platinol)	**Docetaxel** (Taxotere)	**Carboplatin** (Paraplatin)
Paclitaxel (Taxol)	**Vinorelbine** Tartrate (Navelbine)	**Etoposide** (VP–16)
Gemcitabine (Gemzar)	**Erlotinib** (Tarceva)	**Bevacizumab** (Avastin)
Small Cell Lung Cancer		
Etoposide (VP–16)	***Vincristine** (Oncovin)	***Cyclophosphamide** (Cytoxan)
Paclitaxel (Taxol)	***Topotecan** (Hycamtin)	***Irinotecan** (Camptosar)
Carboplatin (Paraplatin)	***Doxorubicin** (Adriamycin)	***Ifosomide** (Mesna)
Cisplatin (Platinol)		
Breast		
Doxorubicin (Doxil)*	**Cyclophosphamide** (Cytoxan)*	**Paclitaxel** (Taxol)
Fluorouracil (5–FU)*	**Methotrexate** (Trexall)*	**Cepectibine** (Xeloda)*
Vinorelbine (Navelbine)*	**Gemcitabine** (Gemzar)*	**Paclitaxel** Protein Bound (Abraxane)
Breast (Hormonal)		
Tamoxifen (Nolvadex)	**Trastuzumab** (Herceptin)	**Anastrozole** (Arimidex)
Letrozole (Femara)	**Fulvestrant** (Faslodex)	**Tykerb** (Lapatinib)
Prostrate		
Estramustine (Emcyt)	**Mitoxantrone** (Novantrone)	**Docetaxel** (Taxotere)
Prednisone (Deltasone)		

Common Disease-Specific Chemotherapy Agents (cont'd)

Prostate Hormones		
Leuprolide Acetate (Lupron)	Flutamide (Eulexin)	Goserelin Acetate (Zoladex) Implant
Pancreatic		
Gemcitabine (Gemzar)	Capecitabine (Xeloda)	
Erlotinib (Tarceva)		
Colorectal		
Fluorouracil (5FU)	Leucovorin Calcium (Leucovorin)	Oxaliplatin (Eloxatin)
Erbitux (Cetuximab)	Irinotecan (Camptosar)	Bevacizumab (Avastin)
Ovarian		
Topotecan (Hycamtin)	*Gemcitabine (Gemzar)	*Carboplatin (Paraplatin)
Docetaxel (Taxotere)	Cisplatin (Platinol)	Regulated Liposomal Doxorubicin (Doxil)
Leukemia		
Decitabine (Dacogen)	Hydroxyurea (Hydrea)	
MDS Mylodsyplastic Syndromes		
Azacitidine (Vidaza)	Lenalidomide (Revlimid)	
Renal		
Sorafenib (Nexavar)	Sunitinib (Sutent)	
Multiple Myeloma		
Bortezomib (Velcade)	Hydroxyurea (Hydrea)	Thalidomide (Thalomid)
Brain Tumor		
Temozolomide (Temodar)		

Note: Contributions to Palliative Chemotherapy section, pages 270–276, were made by Mary Murphy.

Palliative Radiation

- Approximately 40% of radiation is delivered for palliation, however less than 3% of hospice patients receive radiation.
- Factors such as transportation issues, short life expectancy, treatment length, and therapy cost are also factors in determining the role of radiation for palliation of hospice patients.
- Radiation therapy can be given in 2 ways: as external radiation and as internal radiation.

External radiation (or external beam radiation) uses a machine that directs high-energy rays from outside the body at the cancer and some normal surrounding tissue.

- Most people receive external radiation therapy over several weeks during outpatient visits to a hospital or treatment center.
- The unit of measure of radiation therapy is called a Gray (Gy). The amount of time radiation is delivered within a treatment plan is called a fraction.

Internal radiation (brachytherapy) uses a radioactive source in the form of a wire or pellet that is usually sealed in a small container called an implant.

- The implant is placed within the body into or near the tumor.
- Radiation from an implant travels only a very short distance, so it has very little effect on normal body tissues.

Side Effects
- In general, radiation causes side effects related to the specific area irradiated.
- Fatigue may occur regardless of the site.
- Skin reactions may also occur at any site and may be treated with moisturizers, low dose topical steroids (i.e., hydrocortisone 1–2%) and normal saline soaks.
- Side effects are not immediate and usually last for a length of time similar to the course of therapy (unless single fraction).
- When palliation is the goal, the radiation oncologist must balance the need for rapid palliation with the inconvenience of therapy and potential side effects.

Oncologic Emergencies

Radiation therapy is integral in the treatment of some oncologic emergencies which can occur in hospice/palliative care patients with advanced cancer.

Spinal Cord Compression
- Most commonly patient reports a history of lung, breast, or prostate cancer.

Signs and symptoms
- Back pain, radiculopathy, paresthesias, weakness, constipation, incontinence, urinary retention.
- If ambulatory at presentation, 80% of patients retain locomotor function after external beam therapy.

- If paraparetic (partial paralysis of both legs), at presentation, 40 to 50% of patients regain function. Thus, timely diagnosis and intervention is necessary.
- Radiation should be considered if:
  - Patient's performance status is good
  - Systemic disease is controlled
  - Expected survival greater than 3 months after surgical resection
- Surgery should also be considered for patients with spinal cord compression due to renal cell carcinoma, melanoma, and sarcoma. These tumors are less radio-responsive and surgical decompression provides a more rapid decompression.
- Radiation is not effective if there is retropulsed bone in the spinal canal and surgery may be required for decompression.
- Chemotherapy +/− radiation is given for cord compressions secondary to myeloma or lymphoma.

Side effects (related to the level of the spinal cord irradiated)
- Cervical and thoracic area: a sore throat and/or esophagitis is common
  - Treat with analgesics.
- Thoracic area: temporary cough related to bronchial irritation
  - Treat with cough suppressant or narcotic.

Superior Vena Cava Syndrome

- 80% of SVC syndrome cases are related to bronchogenic carcinomas and 15% are due to lymphomas.

Signs and symptoms
- Dyspnea, truncal, extremity, and facial edema and reddish discoloration, cough, headache, light headedness, nasal stuffiness, visible collateral circulation.
- Patient may report that, "My shirt collars are too tight."
- Signs and symptoms do not come on suddenly, but are rather insidious.
- Chemotherapy is used to obtain a rapid response in lymphomas and small cell carcinoma of the lung.
- External beam radiation therapy is used for other tumor histologies or after initiation of chemotherapy in patients with lymphomas or small cell carcinoma of the lung if they do not respond to chemotherapy.
- 62–80% of small cell carcinomas experience relief of SVC syndrome with radiation compared to only 46% of non-small cell lung carcinomas.

Side effects
- Sore throat and esophagitis; treat with analgesics.

Non-emergent Indications for Palliative Radiation

Brain Metastases

- Brain metastases are most commonly found in patients who have advanced lung or breast cancers.

Signs and Symptoms

- Mental status changes, headache, nausea & vomiting, visual disturbances, numbness or tingling, paralysis, difficulties with balance or unusual gait, difficulty speaking, including slurring words or incoherent speech, seizure.
- The median survival of patients with brain metastases treated with supportive care is 1–2 months.
- The median survival with palliative radiation is 3–5 months.
- Prognostic factors have been found which correlate with survival after palliative treatment to the brain.

RPA CLASS	Prognostic Factors	Median Survival (months)
I	• KPS ≥ 70 • Age < 65 • Controlled Primary site • No extracranial mets	7.1
II	All others	4.2
III	KPS < 70	2.3

PS—Recursive partitioning analysis
KPS—Karnofsky Performance Scale

Gaspar, L., et. al IJROBP 1997;37:745

- Patients with progressive uncontrolled primary cancers, poor performance status, and limited life expectancy will not sufficiently benefit from radiation and may be treated with corticosteroids.
- Whole brain radiation therapy (WBRT) is usually the treatment of choice for palliation for patients with multiple brain metastases, progressive systemic cancer, poor performance status or who are elderly.
  - WBRT is usually delivered to a dose of 30 Gy in 10 fractions, although 20 Gy in 5 fractions may be delivered to patients with a very poor performance status and limited life expectancy.
  - 75% of patients improve symptomatically.
  - 33–50% of patients die of neurological causes after whole brain radiation.

Side Effects

- Alopecia, scalp reactions, temporary ear aches, delayed and prolonged lethargy.

Bone Metastases

- External beam is frequently used for pain control and/or prophylaxis against impending fractures or spinal cord compression.
- Increased risk of pathologic fracture from bone metastasis in weight bearing bones if:
  > 2.5 cm lytic lesion
  > 50% cortical destruction
- There are numerous fractionation schemes with similar overall responses:
  - 8 Gy/1 fraction
  - 20 Gy/5 fractions
  - 24 Gy/6 fractions
  - 30 Gy/10 fractions

- Although there is a higher re-irradiation rate after a single fraction, for patients in hospice this may not be a significant issue due to the limited life expectancy.
- The radiation oncologist must weigh the inconvenience and cost of multi-fraction palliative radiation versus the probability of the patient surviving long enough to require re-irradiation if given a single fraction for palliation.
- Improvement in pain control occurs in approximately 7–14 days.
- For wide spread blastic bone metastases with some bone marrow reserve and greater than a 3 month expected survival and the patient is not incontinent, systemic administration of radionucleotides such are Strontium-89 or Samarium-153 may provide palliation of pain.

Bleeding

- Radiation may control bleeding from advanced cancers from various primary sites.
- Sites may include bronchial, cervical/endometrial, and gastrointestinal.
- Radiation may be delivered to endobronchial or cervical tumors by means of brachytherapy.

Relief of Mass Tumor Effects and Ulcerations

- Patients may obtain relief of impending or actual obstruction with the use of radiation.
- Examples:
  - Esophageal radiation for treatment of dysphagia/odynophagia
  - External beam radiation to the chest for airway obstruction or brachytherapy for partial endobronchial obstruction
  - Chest radiation for relief of lung cancer causing chest pain
  - Pelvic radiation for partial rectal obstruction
  - If there is complete or nearly complete obstruction of the bowel, surgical intervention is usually required for a prompt resolution
  - Radiation for pain control secondary to soft tissue or nerve compression
  - Treatment of fungating or ulcerated lesions that may be bleeding or causing pain or hygiene problems may benefit from radiation

References

American Cancer Society, "Radiation Therapy Principles", http://www.cancer.org, accessed September 5, 2007.

Flounders & Ott. "Onocologic Emergencies Modules: Spinal Cord Compression." (2003). Oncology Nursing Forum, vol 30, no 1.

Lutz, S. Ohio Hospice and Palliative Care Organization-2006 annual conference. "Radiation Therapy, Hospice and Palliative Care."

Note: Contributions to Palliative Radiation section, pages 277–280, were made by Beth Delaney and Rebecca J. Paessun MD.

Centers for Medicare and Medicaid Service Department of Health & Human Service
Title 42 Chapter IV Part 418 Hospice Care

Eligibility for the Medicare Hospice Benefit

§ 418.20 Eligibility Requirements:

In order to be eligible to elect hospice care under Medicare, an individual must be:

- Entitled to Part A of Medicare; and
- Certified as being terminally ill in accordance with **§ 418.22** Certification of Terminal Illness
  - **§ 418.22** The certification of terminal illness must specify that:
    - The individual's prognosis is for a life expectancy of 6 months or less if the terminal illness runs its normal course by the medical director of the hospice or the physician member of the hospice inter-disciplinary group and the individual's attending physician if the individual has an attending physician.

Medicare Hospice Conditions of Participation Related to Provision of Medications

§ 418.96 Condition of participation—Medical supplies.

Medical supplies and appliances including drugs and biologicals, must be provided as needed for the palliation and management of the terminal illness and related conditions.

(a) *Standard: Administration.* All drugs and biologicals must be administered in accordance with accepted standards of practice.

(b) *Standard: Controlled drugs in the patient's home.* The hospice must have a policy for the disposal of controlled drugs maintained in the patient's home when those drugs are no longer needed by the patient.

Individual Participant's Coinsurance Liability for Medication

§ 418.400 Individual liability for coinsurance for hospice care.

An individual who has filed an election for hospice care in accordance with Sec. 418.24 is liable for the following coinsurance payments. Hospices may charge individuals the applicable coinsurance amounts.

(a) Drugs and biologicals. An individual is liable for a coinsurance payment for each palliative drug and biological prescription furnished by the hospice while the individual is not an inpatient. The amount of coinsurance for each prescription approximates 5 percent of the cost of the drug or biological to the hospice determined in accordance with the drug copayment schedule established by the hospice, except that the amount of coinsurance for each prescription may not exceed $5. The cost of the drug or biological may not exceed what a prudent buyer would pay in similar circumstances. The drug copayment schedule must be reviewed for reasonableness and approved by the intermediary before it is used.

http://www.access.gpo.gov/nara/cfr/waisidx_04/42cfr418_04.html Accessed 2/1/07

Guidelines for the Determination of Hospice Eligibility

Adult Failure to Thrive

The patient meets **ALL** of the following:

- Body Mass Index (BMI) below 22 kg/m^2
  - Body Mass Index (kg/m^2) = 703 × (patient's weight in pounds) ÷ (height in inches)^2
  - Online BMI Calculator http://www.nhlbisupport.com/bmi/.
- Palliative Performance Scale* equal to or less than 40% (mainly in bed and requires assistance with ADLs).
- Patient refuses enteral or parenteral nutritional support or has not responded to nutritional support, despite adequate caloric intake.

In the absence of one or more of the above criteria, rapid decline or comorbidities may also support the physician's determination of a life expectancy of less than 6 months and eligibility for hospice care, including:

- Malignancy
- Infection
- Skin or mucosa breakdown
- Aspiration
- Changes in level of consciousness or behavior

- Comorbidities of:
  - Chronic obstructive pulmonary disease
  - Congestive heart failure
  - Diabetes mellitus
  - Neurologic disease (CVA, ALS, MS)
  - Renal failure
  - Liver disease
  - Acquired immune deficiency syndrome (AIDS)
  - Dementia

Accepted ICD-9- CM Codes for Adult Failure to Thrive:
  783.4 Failure to Thrive
  799.3 Debility Unspecified
  799.9 Other unknown and unspecified causes of morbidity and mortality

*See Palliative Performance Scale (Page 297)

Amyotrophic Lateral Sclerosis

A patient with Amyotrophic Lateral Sclerosis (ALS) has:

- **Rapid disease progression** as evidenced by **ALL** of the following in the preceding 12 months:
  - Progression from independent ambulation to wheelchair or bed-bound status
  - Progression from normal to barely intelligible or unintelligible speech
  - Progression from normal to pureed diet
  - Progression from independence in most or **ALL** activities of daily living (ADLs) to needing major assistance by caretaker in **ALL** ADLS

And at least one of the following:

- **Critically impaired breathing capacity** with **ALL** of the following in the preceding 12 months:
  - Significant dyspnea at rest
  - Vital capacity less than 30%
  - Requirement for supplemental oxygen at rest
  - The patient declines artificial ventilation

OR

- **Critical nutritional impairment** demonstrated by **ALL** of the following in the preceding 12 months:
  - Oral intake of nutrients and fluids insufficient to sustain life
  - Continuing weight loss
  - Dehydration or hypovolemia
  - Absence of artificial feeding methods

OR

- **Life-threatening complications** demonstrated by one or more of the following in the preceding 12 months:
  - Recurrent aspiration pneumonia (with or without tube feedings)
  - Upper urinary tract infection (e.g. pyelonephritis)
  - Sepsis
  - Recurrent fever after antibiotic therapy

In the absence of one or more of the above criteria, rapid decline or comorbidities may also support the physician's determination of a life expectancy of less than 6 months and eligibility for hospice care.

Cancer

A patient with cancer that meets the following criteria may be eligible for hospice services:

- Clinical findings of malignancy with widespread, aggressive, or progressive disease as evidenced by increasing symptoms, worsening lab values, and/or evidence of metastatic disease
- The following information is needed:
    - Tissue diagnosis of malignancy
    - Reasons why a tissue diagnosis is not available
- Impaired performance status with a PPS* ≤ 70%
- Refuses further life-prolonging therapy OR continues to decline in spite of definitive therapy

Supporting documentation includes:

- Hypercalcemia ≥ 12
- Cachexia or weight loss of 5% in the preceding three months
- Recurrent disease after surgery/radiation/chemotherapy
- Signs and symptoms of advanced disease (e.g. nausea, requirement for transfusions, malignant ascites or pleural effusion, etc.)

In the absence of one or more of the above criteria, rapid decline or comorbidities may also support the physician's determination of a life expectancy of less than 6 months and eligibility for hospice care.

*See Palliative Performance Scale (Page 297).

Cardiovascular Disease

A patient with cardiovascular disease with:

- Poor response to optimal treatment with diuretics and vasodilators, including angiotensin converting enzyme (ACE) inhibitors, or the combination of hydralazine and nitrates *and*
- New York Heart Association (NYHA) Class IV Congestive Heart Failure with:
  - The presence of significant symptoms of recurrent congestive heart failure (CHF) and/or angina at rest
  - Inability to carry on minimal physical activity or exertion without discomfort, symptoms of heart failure (dyspnea) or angina

Supporting documentation includes:

- An ejection fraction of 20% or less
- Treatment resistant symptomatic supraventricular or ventricular arrhythmias
- History of unexplained or cardiac-related syncope
- CVA secondary to cardiac embolism
- History of cardiac arrest or resuscitation with concomitant HIV disease

In the absence of one or more of the above criteria, rapid decline or comorbidities may also support the physician's determination of a life expectancy of less than 6 months and eligibility for hospice care.

*1994 Revisions to Classification of Functional Capacity and Objective Assessment of Patients with Diseases of the Heart. The Criteria Committee of the New York Heart Association. *Nomenclature and Criteria for Diagnosis of Diseases of the Heart and Great Vessels.* 9th ed. Boston, Mass: Little, Brown & Co; 1994:253-256.

New York Heart Association (NYHA)

*Functional Classification (Class and Description)**

CLASS I

Patients with cardiac disease, but without resulting limitation of physical activity. Ordinary physical activity does not cause undue fatigue, dyspnea, palpitations or anginal pain.

CLASS II

Patients with cardiac disease resulting in slight limitation of physical activity. They are comfortable at rest. Ordinary physical activity results in fatigue, dyspnea, palpitations or anginal pain.

CLASS III

Patients with limitations of physical activity. They are comfortable at rest. Less than ordinary physical activity causes fatigue, palpitations, dyspnea or anginal pain.

CLASS IV

Patients with cardiac disease resulting in an inability to carry on any physical activity without discomfort. Symptoms of heart failure or of the anginal syndrome may be present even at rest. If any physical activity is undertaken, discomfort is increased.

Chronic Degenerative Neurologic Disease

A patient with chronic neurologic disease (e.g. Muscular Dystrophy, Myasthenia Gravis or Multiple Sclerosis) has:

- **Critically impaired breathing capacity with ALL of the following findings:**
  - Dyspnea at rest
  - The requirement of supplemental oxygen at rest
  - The patient declines artificial ventilation

OR

- **Critical nutritional impairment demonstrated by ALL of the following in the preceding 12 months:**
  - Oral intake of nutrients and fluids insufficient to sustain life
  - Continuing weight loss
  - Dehydration or hypovolemia
  - Absence of artificial feeding methods

OR

- **Rapid disease progression or complications in the preceding 12 months as demonstrated by:**
  - Progression from independent ambulation to wheelchair or bed-bound status
  - Progression from normal to barely intelligible or unintelligible speech
  - Progression from normal to pureed diet
  - Progression from independence in most or **ALL** Activities of Daily Living (ADLs) to needing major assistance by caretaker in **ALL** ADLs

- **Life-threatening complications demonstrated by one or more of the following in the preceding 12 months:**
  - Recurrent aspiration pneumonia (with or without tube feedings)
  - Upper urinary tract infection (e.g. pyelonephritis)
  - Sepsis
  - Recurrent fever after antibiotic therapy
  - Stage 3 or Stage 4 pressure ulcer(s)

In the absence of one or more of the above criteria, rapid decline or comorbidities may also support the physician's determination of a life expectancy of less than 6 months and eligibility for hospice care.

Dementia

A patient with dementia that meets the following criteria may be eligible for hospice services:

The patient has both 1 and 2:

1. Stage 7C or beyond according to the Functional Assessment Staging Scale* with **ALL** of the following:
   - Inability to ambulate without personal assistance (e.g., requires assistance from another person to ambulate)
   - Inability to dress or bathe without assistance
   - Urinary and fecal incontinence, intermittent or constant
   - No meaningful verbal communication, stereotypical phrases only, or ability to speak is limited to six or fewer intelligible words

AND

2. Has had at least one (1) of the following conditions within the past 12 months:
   - Aspiration pneumonia
   - Pyelonephritis or other upper urinary tract infection
   - Septicemia
   - Decubitus ulcers, multiple, stage 3–4
   - Fever, recurrent after antibiotics
   - Other significant event or condition that suggests a limited prognosis
   - Inability to maintain sufficient fluid and calorie intake demonstrated by either of the following:
     - 10% weight loss during the previous six (6) months

     OR
     - Serum albumin < 2.5 gm/dl

In the absence of one or more of the above criteria, rapid decline or comorbidities may also support the physician's determination of a life expectancy of less than 6 months and eligibility for hospice care, including:

- Malignancy
- Changes in level of consciousness or behavior
- Comorbidities of:
  - Chronic obstructive pulmonary disease
  - Congestive heart failure
  - Diabetes mellitus
  - Neurologic disease (CVA, ALS, MS)
  - Renal failure
  - Liver disease
  - Acquired immune deficiency syndrome (AIDS)

*See Functional Assessment Staging Scale (Page 288)

Functional Assessment Staging (FAST)

1	No difficulties, either subjectively or objectively.
2	Complains of forgetting location of objects; subjective word finding difficulties only.
3	Decreased job functioning evident to coworkers; difficulty in traveling to new locations.
4	Decreased ability to perform complex tasks (e.g., planning dinner for guests; handling finances; marketing).
5	Requires assistance in choosing proper clothing for the season or occasion.
6a	Difficulty putting clothing on properly without assistance.
6b	Unable to bathe properly; may develop fear of bathing. Will usually require assistance adjusting bath water temperature.
6c	Inability to handle mechanics of toileting (i.e., forgets to flush; doesn't wipe properly).
6d	Urinary incontinence, occasional or more frequent.
6e	Fecal incontinence, occasional or more frequent.
7a	Ability to speak limited to about half a dozen words in an average day.
7b	Intelligible vocabulary limited to a single word in an average day.
7c	Nonambulatory (unable to walk without assistance).
7d	Unable to sit up independently.
7e	Unable to smile.
7f	Unable to hold head up.

Reisburg, B. Functional assessment staging (FAST). Psychopharmacology Bulletin 1988; 24:653–659.

HIV/AIDS

Patient meets the following criteria:

- CD4+ Count < 25 cells/mcL

OR

- Persistent viral load > 100,000 copies/ mL from two (2) or more assays at least one month apart

AND

- At least one (1) of the following conditions:
  - CNS lymphoma
  - Untreated or refractory wasting (loss of > 33% lean body mass)
  - Mycobacterium avium complex (MAC) bacteremia, untreated, refractory or treatment refused
  - Progressive multifocal leukoencephalopathy
  - Systemic lymphoma with advanced HIV disease and partial response to chemotherapy
  - Refractory visceral Kaposi's sarcoma
  - Renal failure in the absence of dialysis
  - Cryptosporidium infection
  - Refractory toxoplasmosis

- Palliative Performance Scale* of ≤ 50% (requires considerable assistance and frequent medical care, activity limited mostly to bed or chair)

Supporting documentation includes:

- Chronic persistent diarrhea for one year
- Persistent serum albumin < 2.5
- Concomitant active substance abuse
- Age > 50 years
- Absence of antiretroviral chemotherapeutic and prophylactic drug therapy related specifically to HIV
- Advanced AIDS dementia complex
- Toxoplasmosis
- Congestive Heart Failure, symptomatic at rest

In the absence of one or more of the above criteria, rapid decline or comorbidities may also support the physician's determination of a life expectancy of less than 6 months and eligibility for hospice care.

Huntington's Disease

A patient with Huntington's Disease has:

- Stage 7C or beyond according to the Functional Assessment Staging Scale* with **ALL** of the following:
  - Inability to ambulate without personal assistance
  - Inability to dress without assistance
  - Urinary and fecal incontinence, intermittent or constant
  - Speech ability is limited to the use of a single intelligible word in an average day or in the course of an intensive interview (the person may repeat the word over and over)

AND

- Has had at least one (1) of the following conditions within the past twelve (12) months:
  - Aspiration pneumonia
  - Pyelonephritis or other upper urinary tract infection
  - Septicemia
  - Decubitus Ulcers, Multiple, Stage 3–4
  - Fever, recurrent after antibiotics

- Inability to maintain sufficient fluid and calorie intake with one or more of the following during the proceeding twelve (12) months:
  - 10% weight loss during the previous six (6) months
  - Serum albumin < 2.5 gm/dl
  - Significant dysphagia with associated aspiration measured objectively (e.g., swallowing test or a history of choking or gagging with feeding)

In the absence of one or more of the above criteria, rapid decline or comorbidities may also support the physician's determination of a life expectancy of less than 6 months and eligibility for hospice care.

*See Functional Assessment Staging Scale (Page 288)

Liver Disease

Patients that meet the following criteria may be eligible for hospice services:

- **End stage liver disease as demonstrated by:**
  - Prothrombin time (PT) prolonged more than 5 seconds over control or International Normalized Ratio (INR) >1.5
  - Serum albumin <2.5 gm/dl
- **End stage liver disease is present, and the patient has one or more of the following conditions:**
  - Ascites, refractory to treatment or patient is non-compliant
  - History of spontaneous bacterial peritonitis
  - Hepatorenal syndrome (elevated creatinine and BUN with oliguria [<400 mL/day]) and urine sodium concentration <10 mEq/l
  - Cirrhosis and ascites
  - Hepatic encephalopathy, refractory to treatment or patient is non-compliant with treatment
  - History of recurrent variceal bleeding despite intensive therapy or patient declines sclerosing therapy

Supporting documentation includes:
- Progressive malnutrition
- Muscle wasting with reduced strength
- Ongoing alcoholism (>80 gm ethanol/day)
- Hepatocellular carcinoma
- Hepatitis B surface antigen positive
- Hepatitis C refractory to interferon treatment

In the absence of one or more of the above criteria, rapid decline or comorbidities may also support the physician's determination of a life expectancy of less than 6 months and eligibility for hospice care.

Non-Specific Terminal Illness (Debility Unspecified/End Stage Senescence)

A patient with a non-specific terminal illness that meets the following criteria, may be eligible for hospice services:

The patient has a terminal medical condition that cannot be attributed to a single specific illness. The physician believes there is a limited prognosis of six months or less based on a constellation of signs, symptoms, test results and/or clinical decline.

The clinical impression of six months or less is based on:

- Decline is not attributable to a known primary disease process
- Rapid decline over the past 3–6 months evidenced by **ALL** of the following:
  - Progression of disease evidenced by symptoms, signs and test results
  - Decline in PPS* to 50% or lower
  - Weight loss not due to reversible causes and/or declining serum albumin levels
- **Supporting documentation includes:**
  - Aspiration pneumonia
  - Pyelonephritis or other upper urinary tract infection
  - Septicemia
  - Fever, recurrent after antibiotics
  - Inability to maintain sufficient fluid and calorie intake with > 10% weight loss during the previous six months *or*
  - Serum albumin of < 2.5 gm/dl
  - Dysphagia leading to inadequate nutritional intake or recurrent aspiration
- Measured objectively (e.g., swallowing test or history of choking/gagging with feeding)
  ° Decline in systolic blood pressure to below 90 systolic or progressive postural hypotension
  - Decline in Functional Assessment Staging (FAST)* for dementia
  - Multiple progressive Stage 3–4 pressure ulcers in spite of optimal care
- In the absence of one or more of the above criteria, rapid decline or comorbidities may also support the physician's determination of a life expectancy of less than 6 months and eligibility for hospice care.

*See the Palliative Performance Scale (Page 297) & Functional Assessment Staging Scale (Page 288)

Parkinson's Disease

A patient with Parkinson's Disease has:

- **Critical nutritional impairment demonstrated by ALL of the following in the preceding 12 months:**
  - Oral intake of nutrients and fluids insufficient to sustain life
  - Continuing weight loss
  - Dehydration or hypovolemia
  - Absence of artificial feeding methods

- **Rapid disease progression as evidenced by:**
  - Progression from independent ambulation to wheelchair or bed-bound status
  - Progression from normal to barely intelligible or unintelligible speech
  - Progression from normal to pureed diet
  - Progression from independence in most or **ALL** Activities of Daily Living (ADLs) to needing major assistance by caretaker in **ALL** ADLs

- **Supporting evidence:**
  - Dyspnea at rest
  - The requirement of supplemental oxygen at rest
  - The patient declines artificial ventilation
  - Recurrent aspiration pneumonia (with or without tube feedings)
  - Upper urinary tract infection (e.g., pyelonephritis)
  - Sepsis
  - Recurrent fever after antibiotic therapy
  - Stage 3 or Stage 4 pressure ulcer(s)

In the absence of one or more of the above criteria, rapid decline or comorbidities may also support the physician's determination of a life expectancy of less than 6 months and eligibility for hospice care.

Pulmonary Disease

A patient with severe chronic pulmonary disease that meets the following criteria, they may be eligible for hospice services:

- The patient has **ALL** of the following:
  - Disabling dyspnea at rest or with minimal exertion
  - Little or no response to bronchodilators
  - Decreased functional capacity (e.g. bed to chair existence, fatigue and cough)

And

- Progression of disease as evidenced by a recent history of increasing physician office or emergency visits and/or hospitalizations for pulmonary infection and/or respiratory failure.
- Documentation within the past 3 months of one or more of the following:
  - Hypoxemia at rest on room air (p02 < 55 mmHg by ABG) or oxygen saturation $< 88\%$

  or

  - Hypercapnia evidenced by pCO2 > 50 mmHg
- Note: A serial decrease of $FEV_1 > 40$ mL/yr is objective evidence for disease progression but is not required

Supporting documentation includes:

- Cor pulmonale and right heart failure secondary to pulmonary disease (e.g. not secondary to the left heart disease or valvulopathy)
- Unintentional progressive weight loss $> 10\%$ of body weight over the preceding six months
- Resting tachycardia > 100 bpm

In the absence of one or more of the above criteria, rapid decline or comorbidities may also support the physician's determination of a life expectancy of less than 6 months and eligibility for hospice care.

Renal Failure

A patient with acute or chronic renal failure may be eligible if:

1. The patient is not seeking dialysis or renal transplant
2. Creatinine clearance* is <10 mL/min (<15 mL/min for diabetics)
3. Serum creatinine > 8.0 mg/dl (>6.0 mg/dl for diabetics)

Supporting documentation for chronic renal failure includes:

- Gastrointestinal bleeding
- Uremia
- Oliguria (urine output is less than 400 cc in 24 hours)
- Intractable hyperkalemia (greater than 7.0) not responsive to treatment
- Uremic pericarditis
- Hepatorenal syndrome
- Intractable fluid overload, not responsive to treatment

Supporting documentation for acute renal failure includes:

- Mechanical ventilation
- Malignancy (other organ system)
- Chronic lung disease
- Advanced cardiac disease
- Advanced liver disease

In the absence of one or more of the above criteria, rapid decline or comorbidities may also support the physician's determination of a life expectancy of less than 6 months and eligibility for hospice care.

*Creatinine Clearance (CrCl) Calculation:

$$\text{CrCl} = [140\text{-age(ys)}] \times [\text{weight (kg)}] \div 72 \text{ (serum creatinine in mg/dl)} \{\times 0.85 \text{ for women}\}$$

Stroke or Coma

A patient has acute hemorrhagic or ischemic stroke evidenced by:

- Coma or persistent vegetative state secondary to stroke, beyond 3 days duration, or
- Coma or severe obtundation, secondary to post-anoxic stroke, accompanied by severe myoclonus, persisting beyond 3 days after the anoxic event, or
- Dysphagia, which prevents sufficient intake of food and fluids to sustain life in a patient who does not receive artificial nutrition and hydration

Chronic phase of hemorrhagic or ischemic stroke evidenced by:

- Poor functional status with Palliative Performance Scale* of equal to or less than 40% (mainly in bed and requires mainly assistance with ADLs)
- Poor nutritional status with inability to maintain sufficient fluid and calorie intake with at least one of the following:
  - 10% or greater weight loss over the previous six (6) months
  - 7.5% or greater weight loss over the previous three (3) months
  - Serum albumin < 2.5 gm/dl
- Current history of pulmonary aspiration without effective response to speech language pathology interventions to improve dysphagia and decrease aspiration events

Supporting documentation includes:

Coma (any etiology) with three (3) of the following on the third (3rd) day of the coma:
- Abnormal brain stem response
- Absent verbal responses
- Absent withdrawal response to pain
- Serum creatinine > 1.5 gm/dl

In the absence of one or more of the above criteria, rapid decline or comorbidities may also support the physician's determination of a life expectancy of less than 6 months and eligibility for hospice care.

*See the Palliative Performance Scale (Page 297)

Palliative Performance Scale Version 2 (PPS v2)©

%	Ambulation	Activity and Evidence of Disease	Self-Care	Intake	Conscious Level
100	Full	Normal Activity No Evidence of Disease	Full	Normal	Full
90	Full	Normal Activity Some Evidence of Disease	Full	Normal	Full
80	Full	Normal Activity with Effort Some Evidence of Disease	Full	Normal or Reduced	Full
70	Reduced	Unable to Do Normal Job/Work Some Evidence of Disease	Full	Normal or Reduced	Full
60	Reduced	Unable to Do Hobby/House Work Significant Disease	Occasional Assistance Necessary	Normal or Reduced	Full or Confusion
50	Mainly Sit/Lie	Unable to Do Any Work Extensive Disease	Considerable Assistance Necessary	Normal or Reduced	Full or Confusion
40	Mainly in Bed	Unable to Do Any Work Extensive Disease	Mainly Assistance	Normal or Reduced	Full or Drowsy or +/− Confusion
30	Totally Bed Bound	Unable to Do Any Work Extensive Disease	Total Care	Reduced	Full or Drowsy or +/− Confusion
20	Totally Bed Bound	Unable to Do Any Work Extensive Disease	Total Care	Minimal Sips	Full or Drowsy or +/− Confusion
10	Totally Bed Bound	Unable to Do Any Work Extensive Disease	Total Care	Mouth Care Only	Drowsy or Coma +/− Confusion
0	Death	—	—	—	—

References

Anderson F, Downing GM, Hill J, et al. Palliative performance scale (PPS): a new tool. J Palliat Care 1996; 12(1): 5–11.

Palliative Performance Scale Version 2 © Victoria Hospice Society 1900 Fort St, Victoria, BC, V8R 1J8, Canada.

Geriatric Depression Scale (GDS)

Choose the Best Answer for How You Felt This Past Week

CIRCLE ONE

* 1. Are you basically satisfied with your life?	yes	NO
2. Have you dropped many of your activities and interests?	YES	no
3. Do you feel that your life is empty?	YES	no
4. Do you often get bored?	YES	no
* 5. Are you hopeful about the future?	yes	NO
6. Are you bothered by thoughts you can't get out of your head?	YES	no
* 7. Are you in good spirits most of the time?	yes	NO
8. Are you afraid that something bad is going to happen to you?	YES	no
* 9. Do you feel happy most of the time?	yes	NO
10. Do you often feel helpless?	YES	no
11. Do you often get restless and fidgety?	YES	no
12. Do you prefer to stay at home, rather than going out and doing new things?	YES	no
13. Do you frequently worry about the future?	YES	no
14. Do you feel you have more problems with memory than most?	YES	no
*15. Do you think it is wonderful to be alive now?	yes	NO
16. Do you often feel downhearted and blue?	YES	no
17. Do you feel pretty worthless the way you are now?	YES	no
18. Do you worry a lot about the past?	YES	no
*19. Do you find life very exciting?	yes	NO
20. Is it hard for you to get started on new projects?	YES	no
*21. Do you feel full of energy?	yes	NO
22. Do you feel that your situation is hopeless?	YES	no
23. Do you think that most people are better off than you are?	YES	no
24. Do you frequently get upset over little things?	YES	no
25. Do you frequently feel like crying?	YES	no
26. Do you have trouble concentrating?	YES	no
*27. Do you enjoy getting up in the morning?	yes	NO
28. Do you prefer to avoid social gatherings?	YES	no

*29. Is it easy for you to make decisions?   yes   NO

*30. Is your mind as clear as it used to be?   yes   NO

*Appropriate (nondepressed) answers = YES, all others = NO
or count number of CAPITALIZED (depressed) answers

Score: _____ (Number of "depressed" answers)

Norms

Normal	5 +/− 4
Mildly depressed	15 +/− 6
Very depressed	23 +/− 5

References

Yesavage JA, Brink TL, Rose TL, et al. Development and validation of a geriatric depression rating scale: a preliminary report. J Psych Res. 1983; 17:27.

Sheikh JI, Yesavage JA. Geriatric Depression Scale: recent evidence and development of a shorter version. Clin Gerontol. 1986; 5:165–172.

The Geriatric Depression Scale may be used freely for patient assessment according to the authors.

The Mini-Mental State Examination (MMSE)

The Mini-Mental State Examination (MMSE) is a brief, quantitative assessment tool used to measure cognitive status in adults. The MMSE is a valid and reliable screen for cognitive impairment due to problems such as dementia and delirium. The MMSE is not diagnostic for any specific cognitive disorder (including Alzheimer's dementia), but is most helpful in differentiating cognitive disturbance from other psychiatric problems and in estimating the severity of cognitive disturbance when present. It can be used to follow the progression of cognitive impairment over time and to document response to treatments for impaired cognition.

The MMSE is very commonly used in clinical settings and takes 10 to 15 minutes to complete. The MMSE contains 30 items, scored at one point each, which cover the following elements of cognitive function: orientation, registration, attention and calculation, recall, and language. It is easy to administer, since the scripted instructions for administering the questions are typically integrated into the test form.

The most frequently used global cutoff score for the MMSE is 23 out of 30, with scores of 23 or lower suggesting the presence of cognitive impairment. More specifically, scores in the range of 27–30 indicate normal cognitive functioning, with scores ranging from 21–26 suggestive of mild cognitive impairment, scores ranging from 11–20 indicating moderate impairment, and scores of 10 or lower indicating severe impairment. Population-based norm scores for the MMSE decline with advancing age and increase among those with higher educational achievement.

Psychological Assessment Resources (PAR) owns the copyright to the MMSE and sells official versions of the test.

REFERENCES:

1. Folstein MF, Folstein SE, McHugh PR: "Mini-mental state". A practical method for grading the cognitive state of patients for the clinician. *J Psychiatr Res.* 12: 189–198, 1975.
2. Folstein MF, Folstein SE, McHugh PR, Fanjiang G: Mini-Mental State Examination User's Guide. Lutz, FL: Psychological Assessment Resources, Inc., 2001.
3. Crum RM, Anthony JC, Bassett SS, Folstein MF: Population-based norms for the Mini-Mental State Examination by age and educational level. *JAMA.* 269: 2386–2391, 1993.
4. Grigoletto F, Zappalà G, Anderson DW, Lebowitz BD: Norms for the Mini-Mental State Examination in a healthy population. *Neurology.* 53: 315–320, 1999.
5. http://www3.parinc.com
6. http://www3.parinc.com/uploads/pdfs/MMSE_Copyright_PermReq.pdf

Extrapyramidal Symptoms (EPS) from Medications

- Extrapyramidal symptoms, (EPS) are neurological side effects of antipsychotic medication. EPS can occur within the first few days or weeks of treatment or can appear after months and years of antipsychotic medication use.
- EPS are more common among patients taking conventional antipsychotic medications, compared to the newer atypical drugs. More than 60% of the people who take conventional antipsychotic medications experience some form of EPS.
  - Drugs which may cause extrapyramidal effects:
    - Antipsychotics
    - Haloperidol
    - Phenothiazines
    - Metoclopramide
    - Ondansetron
    - Antidepressants:
      - Tricyclics
      - SSRIs
    - Carbamazepine
    - Diltiazem
    - Fenfluramine
    - 5-Hydroxytryptophan
    - Lithium
    - Methyldopa
    - Methysergide
    - Reserpine
- EPS can present as involuntary movements, tremors and rigidity, body restlessness, muscle contractions and changes in breathing and heart rate.
- Symptoms include:
  - *Tardive dyskinesia* is a common manifestation of EPS, characterized by involuntary movements most often affecting the mouth, lips and tongue (e.g. facial tics, roll the tongue and lick the lips). Sometimes the trunk or other parts of the body are also affected. Tardive dyskinesia usually emerges after prolonged exposure to medications associated with EPS. This side effect is usually managed or minimized by reducing the medication dosage or by changing type of medication. However, the symptoms may persist (or temporarily worsen) even through the medication dose is reduced.
  - *Tremors and rigidity (Parkinsonism)* include tremors, rigidity, temporary paralysis and extreme slowness of movement. These symptoms usually appear in the first few days to weeks of medication administration.
  - *Akathisia* is a condition associated with the use of certain medications and characterized by an internal sense of motor restlessness often described as an inability to resist the urge to move. The most common form of akathisia involves pacing and an inability to sit still. This side effect is often very distressing and uncomfortable to the patient, and reduces the ability to perform everyday tasks.
  - *Acute dystonia* is characterized by spastic contraction of muscle groups. It most often affects the neck, eyes and trunk. These involuntary muscle contractions occur very suddenly and are distressing and often painful to the patient.
  - *Neuroleptic malignant syndrome* (NMS) is potentially fatal if not treated. It includes diffuse muscle rigidity, tremor, high fever, labile blood pressure, cognitive dysfunction, and autonomic disturbances. This condition can be sudden in onset and often occurs early in the course of treatment, often within the first week. NMS is treated by discontinuation of the precipitating drug along with supportive care and administration of medication aimed at reducing the source of fever and muscle rigidity (e.g., dantrolene sodium).

Medications Associated with Anticholinergic Side Effects

- Anticholinergic symptoms include constipation, restlessness, shaking, flushing, tachycardia, hallucinations, delirium, fever, dry mucous membranes, thirst, dilated pupils, blurred vision, urinary retention, nausea and difficulty speaking and swallowing.
- Anticholinergic symptoms mnemonic—"blind as a bat, dry as a bone, red as a beet, mad as a hatter, and hot as a hare."
- Medications:
  - *Antiemetics:* promethazine, prochlorperizine, trimethobenzamide, meclizine
  - *Antiparkinsonians:* benztropine, procyclidine
  - *Antidepressants:* amitriptyline, doxepin, imipramine, nortriptyline, protriptyline, amoxapine, maprotiline, clomipramine
  - *Antihistamines:* diphenhydramine, chlorpheniramine, hydroxyzine, cyproheptadine
  - *Muscle relaxants:* metaxalone, cyclobenzaprine, orphenadrine
  - *Antidiarrheal:* lomotil
  - *Urinary and GI antispasmodics:* oxybutynin, flavoxate, dicyclomine, hyoscyamine, belladonna alkaloids, propantheline
  - *Antiarrhythmics:* disopyramide, procainamide, quinidine
  - *Antipsychotics:* chlorpromazine, thioridazine, clozapine, fluphenazine, thiothixene

Generally Accepted to Have a Risk

Generic Name (Brand Name)	Drug Class/Clinical Use
Amiodarone (Cordarone®, Pacerone®)*	Antiarrhythmic
Chloroquine (Aralen®)	Anti-malarial
Chlorpromazine (Thorazine®)	Antipsychotic/antiemetic
Clarithromycin (Biaxin®)	Antibiotic
Disopyramide (Norpace®)*	Antiarrhythmic
Droperidol (Inapsine®)	Sedative/antiemetic
Erythromycin (Erythrocin®)*	Antibiotic
Haloperidol (Haldol®)	Antipsychotic/antiemetic
Methadone (Methadose®)	Opiate analgesic
Pentamidine (Pentam®)	Antibiotic-pneumocystis
Pimozide (Orap®)	Antipsychotic
Procainamide (Procan®)	Antiarrhythmic
Quinidine (Quinaglute®)	Antiarrhythmic
Sotalol (Betapace®)*	Antiarrhythmic
Sparfloxacin (Zagam®)	Antibiotic
Thioridazine (Mellaril®)	Antipsychotic

Reported to Have a Risk

Generic Name (Brand Name)	Drug Class/Clinical Use
Alfuzosin (Uroxatral®)	Alpha1 blocker/ BPH**
Amantadine (Symmetrel®)	Antiviral/dopaminergic antiparkinson's
Azithromycin (Zithromax®)	Antibiotic
Chloral Hydrate (Noctec®)	Sedative
Dolasetron (Anzemet®)	Antiemetic
Felbamate (Felbatol®)	Anticonvulsant
Flecainide (Tambocor®)	Antiarrhythmic
Foscarnet (Foscavir®)	HIV Antiviral
Fosphenytoin (Cerebyx®)	Anticonvulsant
Gatifloxacin (Tequin®)	Antibiotic
Granisetron (Kytril®)	Antiemetic
Indapamide (Lozol®)	Diuretic
Isradipine (Dynacirc®)	Antihypertensive
Levofloxacin (Levoquin®)	Antibiotic
Lithium (Eskolith®)	Bipolar Disorder
Moxifloxacin (Avelox®)	Antibiotic
Nicardipine (Cardene®)	Antihypertensive
Octreotide (Sandostatin®)	Carcinoid syndrome
Ofloxacin (Floxin®)	Antibiotic
Ondansetron (Zofran®)	Antiemetic
Quetiapine (Seroquel®)	Antipsychotic
Ranolazine (Ranexa®)	Anti-anginal
Risperidone (Risperdal®)	Antipsychotic
Tacrolimus (Prograf®)	Immunosuppressant
Tamoxifen (Novadex®)	Anti-cancer
Telithromycin (Ketek®)	Antibiotic
Tizanidine (Zanaflex®)	Muscle relaxant
Vardenafil (Levitra®)	Vasodilator
Venlafaxine (Effexor®)	Antidepressant
Voriconazole (VFend®)	Antifungal
Ziprasidone (Geodon®)	Antipsychotic

*In general, women are approximately twice as likely to develop Torsades de Pointes than are men.

**Benign prostatic hyperplasia

References

Walker, Georgina; Wilcock, Andrew; Carey, Ann Marie; et al. Prolongation of QT Interval in Palliative Care JPSM Vol 26 No 3 Sept 2003.

Woosley, RL Drugs That Prolong the QT Interval and/or Induce Torsades de Pointes. Arizona Center for Education and Research on Therapeutics. http://www.arizonacert.org/medical-pros/drug-lists/printable-drug-list.cfm. Accessed 1/28/07.

Medications That May Increase Risk of Falls

Category	Medications
Cardiovascular	
Alpha-blockers	Clonidine, doxazosin, methyldopa, prazosin, terazosin
Beta-blockers	Atenolol, betaxolol, bisoprolol, carvedilol, esmolol, labetalol, metoprolol, nadolol, penbutolol, pindolol, propranolol, sotalol, timolol
ARBs	Candesartan, irbesartan, losartan, telmisartan, valsartan
ACE-Is	Benazepril, captopril, enalapril, fosinopril, lisinopril, moexipril, perindopril, quinapril, ramipril
CCBs	Amlodipine, diltiazem, felodipine, isradipine, nicardipine, nifedipine, nimodipine, verapamil
Diuretics	Acetazolamide, amiloride, bumetanide, chlorthalidone, eplerenone, furosemide, hydrochlorothiazide, indapamide, methazolamide, metolazone, spironolactone, torsemide, triamterene
Vasodilators	Hydralazine, isosorbide, milrinone, nitroglycerin, papaverine
Antiarrhythmics	Amiodarone, bepridil, digoxin, dofetilide, flecainide, mexiletine, moricizine, nesiritide, procainamide, propafenone, quinidine
Blood Modifiers	Pentoxifylline
Antiplatelets	Aspirin, cilostazol
Statins	Atorvastatin, fluvastatin, lovastatin, pravastatin, rosuvastatin, simvastatin
CNS	
Acetylcholinesterase Inhibitors	Donepezil, galantamine, rivastigmine
Anticonvulsants/Barbiturates	Butabarbital, butalbital, carbamazepine, divalproex, ethosuximide, felbamate, fosphenytoin, gabapentin, lamotrigine, levetiracetam, mephobarbital, oxcarbazepine, phenobarbital, phenytoin, primidone, tiagabine, topiramate, valproic acid, zonisamide
Antidepressants	Amitriptyline, amoxapine, bupropion, buspirone, citalopram, clomipramine, desipramine, doxepin, fluoxetine, fluvoxamine, imipramine, maprotiline, mirtazapine, nefazodone, nortriptyline, paroxetine, phenelzine, protriptyline, sertraline, tranylcypromine, trazodone, venlafaxine

Antihistamines/Antinauseants	Meclizine, diphenhydramine
Antiparkinsons Drugs	Carbidopa/levodopa, entacapone, pergolide, pramipexole, ropinirole, selegiline, tolcapone
Antipsychotics	Aripiprazole, chlorpromazine, clozapine, fluphenazine, haloperidol, lithium, loxapine, mesoridazine, molindone, olanzapine, perphenazine, pimozide, quetiapine, riluzole, risperidone, thioridazine, thiothixene, trifluoperazine, ziprasidone
Benzodiazepines	Alprazolam, chlordiazepoxide, clonazepam, clorazepate, diazepam, flurazepam, lorazepam, midazolam, oxazepam, temazepam, triazolam
Hypnotics	Chloral hydrate, meprobomate, zaleplon, zolpidem
Narcotics/Opioid Analgesics	Bupivicaine, buprenorphine/naloxone, butorphanol, codeine, fentanyl, hydrocodone, hydromorphone, levorphanol, lidocaine, meperidine, methadone, morphine, nalbuphine, naloxone, opium, oxycodone, pentazocine, propoxyphene, tramadol
Musculoskeletal System	
Muscle Relaxants	Baclofen, carisoprodol, chlorzoxazone, cyclobenzaprine, dantrolene, metaxalone, methocarbamol, mivacurium, orphenadrine, tizanidine
NSAIDs	Celecoxib, diclofenac, diflunisal, etodolac, flurbiprofen, indomethacin, ketoprofen, ketorolac, nabumetone, naproxen, oxaprozin, piroxicam, rofecoxib, sulindac, tolmetin
Endocrine	
Antidiabetics	Acetohexamide, chlorpropamide, glimepiride, glipizide, glyburide, tolazamide, tolbutamide, metformin, insulin

References

DiPiro JT, Talbert RL, Yee GC, et al. Pharmacotherapy: a pathophysiologic approach. 6th ed. New York: McGraw-Hill Medical Publishing Division, 2005: 1647.

French DD, Campbell R, Spehar A, et al. Drugs and falls in community-dwelling older people: a national veterans study. Clin Ther 2006;28(4):619–630.

Lee JS, Kwok T, Leung PC, et al. Medical illnesses are more important than medications as risk factors or falls in older community dwellers: a cross-sectional study. Age and Ageing 2006;35:246–251.

Look-Alike and Sound-Alike Drug Names

Unfortunately, many drug names can look or sounds like other drug names, which may lead to potentially harmful medication errors. IN 2001, the Joint Commission on Accreditation of Healthcare Organization (JCAHO) published a Sentinel Event Alert on look-alike and sound-alike drug names.

Potential Problematic Drug Names	Brand Name(s) (UPPERCASE) & Generic (lowercase)
Ephedrine and epinephrine	• ADRENALIN (epinephrine) • Ephedrine
Avandia and Coumadin	• AVANDIA (rosiglitazone) • COUMADIN (warfarin)
Celebrex and Celexa and Cerebyx	• CELEBREX (celecoxib) • CELEXA (citalopram hydrobromide) • CEREBYX (fosphenytoin)
Clonidine and Klonopin	• CATAPRES (clonidine) • KLONOPIN (clonazepam)
Concentrated liquid morphine products vs. Conventional liquid morphine concentrations	• Concentrated: ROXANOL • Morphine oral liquid (conventional concentration)
Hydromorphone injection and morphine injection	• DILAUDID (hydromorphone) • ASTRAMORPH, DURAMORPH, INFUMORPH (morphine)
Insulin products Humalog and Humulin Novolog and Novolin Humulin and Novolin Humalog and Novolog Novolin 70/30 and Novolog Mix 70/30	• HUMULIN (human insulin products) • HUMALOG (insulin lispro) • NOVOLIN (human insulin products) • NOVOLOG (human insulin aspart) • NOVOLIN 70/30 (70% isophane insulin [NPH] and 30% insulin injection [regular]) • NOVOLOG MIX 70/30 (70% insulin aspart portamine suspension and 30% insulin aspart)
Lorazepam and alprazolam	• ATIVAN (lorazepam) • XANAX (alprazolam)
Metronidazole and mettormin	• FLAGYL (metronidazole) • GLUCOPHAGE (mettormin)
Topamax and Toprol XL	• TOPAMAX (topiramate) • TOPROL-XL (metoprolol)
Zyprexa and Zyrtec	• ZYPREXA (olanzapine) • ZYRTEC (cetirizine)
Acetohexamide and acetazolamide	• Acetohexamide • DIAMOX (acetazolamide)
Advicor and Advair	• ADVICOR (lovastatin + niacin) • ADVAIR (fluticasone and Salmeterol)
Amicar and Omacor	• AMICAR (aminocaproic acid) • OMACOR (omega-3-Acid Ethyl Esters)

Potential Problematic Drug Names	Brand Name(s) (UPPERCASE) & Generic (lowercase)
Avinza and Evista	• AVINZA (morphine) • EVISTA (raloxifene)
Cardura and Coumadin	• CARDURA (doxazosin) • COUMADIN (warfarin)
Darvocet and Percocet	• DARVOCET (propoxyphene + acetaminophen) • PERCOCET (oxycodone + acetaminophen)
Diabeta and Zebeta	• DIABETA (glyburide) • ZEBETA (bisoprolol)
Diflucan and Diprivan	• DIFLUCAN (fluconazole) • DIPRIVAN (propofol)
Folic acid and leucovorin calcium ("folinic acid")	• FOLVITE (folic acid) • LEUCOVORIN (folinic acid)
Heparin and Hespan	• Heparin • HESPAN (hetastarch)
Hydrocodone and oxycodone	• Hydrocodone • Oxycodone
Idarubicin and doxorubicin and daunorubicin	• IDAMYCIN (idarubicin) • ADRIAMYCIN (doxorubicin) • CERUBIDINE (daunorubicin)
Lamivudine and lamotrigine	• EPIVIR (lamivudine) • LAMICTAL (lamotrigine)
Leukeran and leucovorin calcium	• LEUKERAN (Chlorambucil) • LEUCOVORIN (folinic acid)
MS Contin and Oxycontin	• MS CONTIN (morphine SR) • OXYCONTIN (oxycodonon SR)
Mucinex and Mucomyst	• MUCINEX (guaifenesin) • MUCOMYST (acetylcysteine)
Prilosec and Prozac	• PRILOSEC (omeprazole) • PROZAC (fluoxetine)
Retrovir and Ritonavir	• RETROVIR (zidovudine) • NORVIR (Ritonavir)
Tramadol and trazadone	• ULTRAM (tramadol) • DESYREL (trazadone)
Tizanidine and tiagabine	• ZANAFLEX (tizanidine) • GABITRIL (tiagabine)
Zantac and Xanax	• ZANTAC (ranitidine) • XANAX (alprazolam)
Zantac and Zyrtec	• ZANTAC (ranitidine) • ZYRTEC (cetirizine)
Zestril and Zetia	• ZESTRIL (Lisinopril) • ZETIA (ezetimibe)
Zestril and Zyprexa	• ZESTRIL (lisinopril) • ZYPREXA (olanzepine)
Zocor and Zyrtec	• ZOCOR (simvastatin) • ZYRTEC (cetirizine)

What Prescribers Can Do

- Maintain awareness of look-alike and sound-alike drug names as published by various safety agencies.
- Clearly specify the dosage form, drug strength, and complete directions on prescriptions. These variables may help staff differentiate products.
- With name pairs known to be problematic, reduce the potential for confusion by writing prescriptions using both brand and generic name.
- Include the purpose of medication on prescriptions. In most cases drugs that sound or look similar are used for different purposes.
- Alert patients to the potential for mix-ups, especially with known problematic drug names. Advise ambulatory care patients to insist on pharmacy counseling when picking up prescriptions, and to verify that the medication and directions match what the prescriber has told them.
- Encourage inpatients to question nurses about medications that are unfamiliar or look or sound different than expected.
- Give verbal or telephone orders only when truly necessary, and never for chemotherapeutics. Include the drug's intended purpose to ensure clarity. Encourage staff to read back all orders, spell the product name, and state its indication.

What Organizations and Practitioners Can Do

- Maintain awareness of look-alike and sound-alike drug names as published by various safety agencies. Regularly provide information to professional staff.
- Whenever possible, determine the purpose of the medication before dispensing or drug administration. Most products with look or sound-alike names are used for different purposes.
- When possible, list brand and generic names on medication administration records and automated dispensing cabinet computer screens. Such redundancy could help someone identify an error.
- Encourage reporting of errors and potentially hazardous conditions with look and sound-alike product names and use the information to establish priorities for error reduction. Also maintain awareness of problematic product names and error prevention recommendations provided by ISMP (www.ismp.org), FDA (www.fda.gov), and USP (www.usp.org).

References

ISMP. What's in a name? Ways to prevent dispensing errors linked to name confusion. *ISMP Medication Safety Alert!* 7(12) June 12, 2002.

JCAHO. Sentinel Event Alert. Issue 19—May 2001.

Santell JP, Cousins DD. Medication Errors Related to Product Names. *Joint. Commission J Qual Pt. Safety* 2005; 31:649–54.

Method of Dosage Adjustment in Renal Failure

Generic Name	Brand Name	Hepatic Failure Dosage Adjustment	Method of Dosage Adjustment*	<50 mL/min	10–50 mL/min	>10 mL/min	Dialyzable	Interactions (Drug-Drug, Drug-Food)
Acetaminophen	Tylenol	C	I	q4h	q6h	q8h		
Acetaminophen with Codeine	Tylenol #2, 3, 4	Avoid chronic use in impairment	D/I	q4h, 100%	q6h, 75%	q8h, 50%		Grapefruit juice
Acyclovir	Zovirax		I	q4h	<25 q8h	q12h		
Al/Mag/Simethicone	Maalox Plus		C					Decreased absorption of multiple drugs
Albuterol/ Ipratropium	Combivent Inhaler; DuoNeb Aerosols		NR					CYP3A4—Substrate; soybean/peanut allergy
Allopurinol	Zyloprim		D/I	200 mg daily	100 mg daily	100 mg q3h	Yes	Inhibitor met of Mercaptopurine; take after meal
Alprazolam	Xanax	↓dose 50–60%	D	100%	100%	100%		CYP3A4—Substrate
Amantadine	Symmetrel		D/I	100%	50%	q7d		
Amiloride	Midamor		D	100%	50%	AVOID USE		Potassium supplements or drugs that increase potassium levels, dec Amoxicillin abs
Amiodarone	Cordarone	Decrease dose or d/c when LFts 3 × normal; decrease dose in significant impairment	NR				No	CYP3A4, 2C8—Substrate; CYP2A6, 2C9, 2D6, 3A4—Inhibitor; QT Prolongation, inc digoxin levels, grapefruit juice, Administer consistently with regard to meals
Amitriptyline	Elavil	Use with caution	D	100%	100%	100%		CYP2D6—Substrate; grapefruit juice
Amlodipine	Norvasc	For angina: 5 mg daily; For HTN: 2.5 mg daily	NR					CYP3A4—Substrate; CYP1A2—Inhibitor; grapefruit juice, Azole antifungals may inhibit metabolism
Amoxicillin	Amoxil		I	q8h	q8–12h	q24h	Yes	

*D = Dose Reduction Indicated by %; I = Dose Interval Extension; NR = No Report Found; C = Administer with Caution

Generic Name	Brand Name	Hepatic Failure Dosage Adjustment	Method of Dosage Adjustment*	<50 mL/min	10–50 mL/min	>10 mL/min	Dialyzable	Interactions (Drug-Drug, Drug-Food)
Amoxicillin/Clavulanate	Augmentin		I	q8h	q8–12h, do not use 875 mg or ER in CrCl < 30	q24h	20–50%	Take with food
Aripiprazole	Abilify	No dosage adjustment required	D	100%	100%	100%		CYP2D6, 3A4—Substrate: may need to increase or decrease dose by 50%
Aspirin	Aspirin	Avoid use in severe impairment	D	100%	100%	Avoid Use	50–100%	May displace valproic acid from binding sites, Hyperexcretion of folate
Atenolol	Tenormin		D	100%	50%	75%		Do not take with antacids
Azithromycin	Zithromax	Use with caution	C	100%	100%	Caution		Extended release suspension 1 hour before or 2 hours after meals, do not take with antacids
Baclofen	Lioresal						No, Accumulates	Avoid alcohol; take with food
Benzonatate	Tessalon Perles		NR					
Benztropine	Cogentin		NR					Increases digoxin levels due to delayed gastric emptying
Betamethasone	Diprolene	Extensively hepatic metabolism- may require adjustment	NR					
Bethanechol	Urecholine	NR	NR					1 hour before meals or 2 hours after meals
Bisacodyl	Dulcolax		NR					dairy products may disrupt enteric coating, take at least 1 hour after dairy products, take on empty stomach
Bromocriptine	Parlodel	May be necessary, but no guidelines	NR					CYP3A4—Substrate; Azole antifungals, Protease Inhibitoribitors, Telithromycin, and some macrolides are contraindicated; take with food

Drug	Brand	Adjustment	Method*	>50	10–50	<10	Supp.	Comments
Budesonide	Pulmicort Respules	Dosage reduction may be required; watch for hypercorticism	NR					CYP3A4—Substrate; grapefruit juice
Calcium Carbonate	Tums		C		Caution <25			Separate dose from levothyroxine by at least 4 hours, Avoid use with polystyrene sulfonate due to decreased potassium-binding ability, space dosing with tetracyclines, take 1–2 hours+l20 before or after iron supplementation
Captopril	Capoten		D,I	100%	75%	50%		CYP2D6—Substrate; 1 hour before or 2 hours after eating
Carbamazepine	Tegretol	C	D,I	100%	100%	100%		CYP3A4—Substrate; CYP1A2, 2B6, 2C8, 2C9, 2C19, 3A4—Ind; avoid grapefruit juice, take with food
Carisoprodol	Soma		NR				Yes	CYP2C19—Substrate
Carvedilol	Coreg	Contraindicated in severe dysfunction	D	100%	100%	100%	No	CYP2C9, 2D6—Substrate; Alcohol may cause faster release of Coreg CR—separate by at least 2 hours, take with food to minimize the risk of orthostatic hypotension
Cefaclor	Ceclor		D	100%	100–50%	50%	20–50%	
Cefpodoxime	Vantin		I		Cr <30, q24h		Yes	Take with food
Cefuroxime Axetil	Ceftin		I		Cr 10–20, q12h	q24h	25%	
Celecoxib	Celebrex	Decrease by 50% in moderate; Avoid in severe dysfunction	C				No	CYP2C9—Substrate; CYP2C8—Inhibitor; do not take with antacids
Cephalexin	Keflex		I	q8h	q12h	q12–24	Yes	
Cetirizine	Zyrtec	Use 5 mg daily in impairment			Cr 11–31, 5 mg daily	Cr <11, avoid use		

*D = Dose Reduction Indicated by %; I = Dose Interval Extension; NR = No Report Found; C = Administer with Caution

Generic Name	Brand Name	Hepatic Failure Dosage Adjustment	Method of Dosage Adjustment*	<50 mL/min	10–50 mL/min	>10 mL/min	Dialyzable	Interactions (Drug-Drug, Drug-Food)
Chloral Hydrate	Noctec	Avoid in severe impairment	C	100%	Cr <50, avoid use		50–100%	
Chlorpromazine	Thorazine	Avoid in severe dysfunction	D	100%	100%	100%	0–5%	CYP2D6—Substrate, Inhibitor; QT Prolongation, Do not take within 2 hours of antacid
Cholesterol Lowering Agents	Lipitor, Zocor, Lescol, Crestor, Mevacor, Niacin, Pravachol, Advicor	Agent dependent; in general, do not use	C					Statins: CYP3A4—Substrate, grapefruit juice; Decreased absorption with cholestyramine—separate by at least 4 hours; Niacin: Decreased absorption with bile acid sequestrants—separate by 4–6 hours
Cholestyramine	Questran							Decresed absorption of drugs/vitamins—Give other medications 1 hour before or 4–6 hours after giving cholestyramine
Choline Magnesium Trisalicylate	Trilisate	C	C					
Cimetidine	Tagamet	Reduce dose in severe	D	100%	50%	25%	5–20%	CYP1A2, 2C19, 2D6, 3A4—Inhibitor; take with meals, Avoid concurrent use w/ Amiodarone and Phenytoin; Decreased absorption of Atazanavir—separate by 12 hours
Ciprofloxacin	Cipro		I	q12h	q12–24h	q24h	<10%	CYP1A2—Inhibitor; Take 2 hours before or 6 hours after drugs with metal cations, concurrent admin w/ Tizanidine is contraindicated
Citalopram	Celexa	Reduce dose	C			C		CYP2C19, 3A4—Substrate
Clarithromycin	Biaxin	No adjustment needed if renal fxn normal	D/I		Cr <30, 50% or double the interval		No	CYP3A4—Substrate, Inhibitor; QT Prolongation, concurrent use with cisapride is contraindicated
Clindamycin	Cleocin	Recommend adjustment in severe impairment	NR					

Drug	Brand		Method					Comments
Clonazepam	Klonopin	C	D	100%	100%	100%		CYP3A4—Substrate
Clonidine	Catapres		D	100%	100%	50–75%	0–5%	
Codeine-APAP	Tylenol #2, 3, 4	Avoid chronic use in impairment	D/I	q4h, 100%	q6h, 75%	q8h, 50%		
Cyclobenzaprine	Flexeril	Mild: 5 mg 3 times daily; Mod-severe: Not recommended	NR					CYP1A2—Substrate; Do not use concomitantly or within 14 days after MAO Inhibitors
Darbepoetin	Aranesp		C					
Desipramine	Norpramin	↓daily dose 50%; avoid in severe/acute disease	D	100%	100%	100%	No	CYP2D6—Substrate; CYP2A6, 2B6, 2D6, 3A4—Inhibitor; grapefruit juice, MAO Inhibitoribitors
Desipramine	Norpramin							CYP2D6—Substrate; CYP2A6, 2B6, 2D6, 3A4—Inhibitor; grapefruit juice, MAO Inhibitors
Dexamethasone	Decadron		D	100%	100%	100%		Increased absorption of corticosteroids with antacids—separate by 2 hours
Dextroamphetamine	Dexadrine		NR					CYP2D6—Substrate; concurrent use of MAO Inhibitors or use within 14 days is contraindicated, take 30 minutes before meals
Dextromethorphan	Delsym		NR					CYP2D6—Substrate
Diazepam	Valium	↓daily dose 50%	D	100%	100%	C	0–5%	CYP2C19, 3A4—Substrate; grapefruit juice
Diclofenac	Voltaren	C	D	100%	100%	100%		CYP3A4, 1A2—Inhibitor; decreased absorption with bile acid sequestrants—separate by at least 2 hours; take with food
Dicloxacillin	Dynapen		D	100%	100%	100%	0–5%	Empty stomach 1 hour before or 2 hours after meals

*D = Dose Reduction Indicated by %; I = Dose Interval Extension; NR = No Report Found; C = Administer with Caution

Generic Name	Brand Name	Hepatic Failure Dosage Adjustment	Method of Dosage Adjustment*	<50 mL/min	10–50 mL/min	>10 mL/min	Dialyzable	Interactions (Drug-Drug, Drug-Food)
Dicyclomine	Bentyl		NR					30–60 minutes before a meal
Digoxin	Lanoxin		D or I	q24h	25–75% or q36h	10–25% or q48h	0–5%	Reduce digoxin dose by 50% with start of amiodarone, Separate administration with bile acid sequestrants
Diltiazem	Cardizem	Do not exceed 90 mg/day	C	100%	100%	100%	No	CYP3A4—Substrate, Inhibitor; may need additional potassium
Diphenhydramine	Benadryl		I	q6h	q6–12h	q12–18h	—	CYP2D6—Inhibitor
Diphenoxylate/ Atropine	Lomotil	C	C					
Dipyridamole	Persantine (Not Aggrenox)		NR				No	Administer with water 1 hour before meals
Divalproex Na	Depakote	C	D	100%	100%	73%	20%	
Donepezil	Aricept		NR				Unknown	
Doxazosin	Cardura	Use with caution in mild-mod; do not use in severe	NR				No	Take Cardura® XL with morning meal
Doxepin	Sinequan	C	D	100%	100%	100%		CYP1A2, 2D6, 3A4—Substrate; grapefruit juice, contraindicated with MAO Inhibitors, oral concentrate physically incompatible with carbonated beverages
Doxycycline Hyclate	Vibramycin		D	100%	100%	100%	0–5%	CYP3A4—Substrate, Inhibitor; sit up for at least 30 minutes after taking, take with food
Dronabinol	Marinol	C	D	100%	100%	100%		

Generic	Brand	Adjustment	Method	GFR >50	GFR 10–50	GFR <10	Dialysis	Notes
Enalapril	Vasotec	No dosage adjustment	D	100%	Cr 30–80 5 mg titrated to max 40 mg Cr < 30 2.5 mg titrated til BP controlled			CYP3A4—Substrate
Erythromycin	E-Mycin, Erytab	C	D	100%	100%	50–75%	5–20%	CYP3A4—Substrate, Inhibitor; QT Prolongation
Escitalopram	Lexapro	10 mg/day	C	100%	C	C		CYP2C19, 3A4—Substrate
Esomeprazole	Nexium	20 mg/day in severe impairment	D	100%	100%	100%	No	CYP2C19—Substrate, Inhibitor; Take at least 1 hour before meals
Estazolam	Prosom	Adjustment may be necessary	D	100%	100%	100%		Grapefruit juice
Famotidine	Pepcid		D or I	100%	50% or q36–48h	50% or q36–48h		CYP3A4—Substrate
Fentanyl	Duragesic		D	100%	100%	100%		
Filgastrim	Neupogen		NR					
Fluconazole	Diflucan		D or I	100%	50% or q48h	50% or q48h	50%	CYP2C9, 2C19, 3A4—Inhibitor; Concurrent use w/ Cisapride is contraindicated—may cause malignant arrhythmias
Fluoxetine	Prozac	Cirrhosis: lower dose or less frequent; cirrhosis with ascites: 50% of dose	C				NO	CYP2C9, 2D6—Substrate; CYP1A2, 2C19, 2D6—Inhibitor; QT Prolongation
Flurazepam	Dalmane		NR					CYP3A4—Substrate
Fosinopril	Monopril		D	100%	100%	100%	20–50%	
Furosemide	Lasix	Monitor closely	C				NO	
Gabapentin	Neurontin		D,I	400 mg tid	300 mg bid—q day	150 mg q day	YES	

*D = Dose Reduction Indicated by %; I = Dose Interval Extension; NR = No Report Found; C = Administer with Caution

Generic Name	Brand Name	Hepatic Failure Dosage Adjustment	Method of Dosage Adjustment*	<50 mL/min	10–50 mL/min	>10 mL/min	Dialyzable	Interactions (Drug-Drug, Drug-Food)
Galantamine	Reminyl	Moderate: 10 mg/day; severe: do not use	C		MAX 16 mg per day	AVOID USE	Unknown	
Glipizide	Glucotrol	Initial dose 2.5 mg/day	C			AVOID USE		Take with breakfast
Glyburide	Micronase, Diabeta	Use caution and avoid in severe disease	C		AVOID USE	AVOID USE		
Granisetron	Kytril	No dosage adjustment	D	100%	100%	100%		
Guaifenesin	Robitussin		NR					
Haloperidol	Haldol		NR					CYP2D6, 3A4—Substrate, Inhibitor; QT Prolongation
Haloperidol Metoclopramide Diphenhydramine Lorazepam +/− Dexamethasone Compounded Supp or Oral Soln	ABHR, Metaclophen, etc Ativan Benadryl Haldol Reglan +/− Decadron Supp or Oral Soln		D or I	q6h	Cr <40 50%, q6–12h	q12–18h	0–5%	
Hydralazine	Apresoline		I		q8h	q8–16h for fast acetylators and q12–24h for slow acetylators		
Hydrochlorothiazide	Oretic		C			AVOID USE		
Hydrocodone-APAP	Lortab, Vicodin	Avoid chronic use in impairment	NR					CYP2D6—Substrate
Hydromorphone	Dilaudid	C	C					

Generic	Brand	Notes	Code*	>50	10–50	<10	Dialysis	CYP / Comments
Hydroxyzine	Atarax/Vistaril	↓interval to q24h	NR				NO	
Hyoscyamine	Levsin		NR					
Ibuprofen	Motrin	Avoid in severe impairment	NR					CYP2C9—Inhibitor
Imipramine	Tofranil		NR					CYP2C19, 2D6—Substrate; CYP2D6—Inhibitor
Indomethacin	Indocin		C		AVOID USE	AVOID USE		CYP2C9—Inhibitor; take with food
Insulin Glargine	Lantus		D	100%	75%	25–50%	NO	
Insulin, Human NPH + Regular	Humulin 70/30		D	100%	75%	25–50%	NO	
Insulin, Human NPH	Humulin N		D	100%	75%	25–50%	NO	
Insulin, Human Regular	Humulin R		D	100%	75%	25–50%	NO	
Insulin, Lispro	Humalog		D	100%	75%	25–50%	NO	
Ipratropium MDI/Neb Soln	Atrovent		NR					
Irbesartan	Avapro	No dosage adjustment unless pt volume depleted	C	ONLY IF VOLUME DEPLETED	ONLY IF VOLUME DEPLETED	ONLY IF VOLUME DEPLETED	NO	CYP2C8, 2C9—Inhibitor
Isoborbide	Imdur		D	100%	100%	100%		CYP3A4—Substrate
Itraconazole	Sporanox	Use with caution	C		Cr <30 AVOID USE	AVOID USE	NO	CYP3A4—Substrate, Inhibitor; take with food
Ketamine	Ketolar	C	NR					CYP2B6, 2C9, 3A4—Substrate
Ketoconazole	Nizoral	C	D	100%	100%	100%	0–5%	CYP3A4—Substrate; CYP1A2, 2A6, 2C9, 2C19, 2D6, 3A4—Inhibitor
Ketorolac	Toradol	C	I	100%	50%	25–50% (avoid)	NO	Take with food

*D = Dose Reduction Indicated by %; I = Dose Interval Extension; NR = No Report Found; C = Administer with Caution

Generic Name	Brand Name	Hepatic Failure Dosage Adjustment	Method of Dosage Adjustment*	<50 mL/min	10–50 mL/min	>10 mL/min	Dialyzable	Interactions (Drug-Drug, Drug-Food)
Lactulose	Chronulac		NR					
Lansoprazole	Prevacid	↓dose 50%	D	100%	100%	100%	NO	CYP2C19, 3A4—Substrate; CYP2C19—Inhibitor; take before eating
Letrozole	Femara	2.5 mg every other day in severe	D	100%	100%	AVOID USE		CYP2A6—Inhibitor
Levofloxacin	Levaquin		D or I	100%	DEPENDS ON DIAGNOSIS 250–750 mg q24–48h	DEPENDS ON DIAGNOSIS 250–500 mg q48h	NO	Metal cations, QT Prolongation
Lidocaine	Xylocaine		NR				0–5%	CYP2D6, 3A4—Substrate; CYP1A2, 2D6, 3A4—Inhibitor
Lisinopril	Prinivil/Zestril		D		Cr >30 10 mg/day, Cr 10–30 5 mg/day, max 40 mg/day	2.5 mg/day, max 40 mg/day	50%	
Loratadine	Claritin	5–10 mg every other day	I		Cr <30 QOD	Cr <30 QOD	NO	CYP2C19—Inhibitor; take on empty stomach
Lorazepam	Ativan	C	D	100%	100%	100%		
Losartan	Cozaar	25 mg initial dose; divide into two dose intervals	D	100%	100%	100%	NO	CYP2C9, 3A4—Substrate; CYP2C8, 2C9—Inhibitor
Magnesium Hydroxide	Milk of Magnesia		C		Cr <25 Use with Caution	AVOID USE	YES	
Megestrol Acetate	Megace		C				Unknown	
Memantine	Namenda		C		Cr 5–29, 5 mg BID	Cr 5–29, 5 mg BID		
Meperidine	Demerol	Decrease dose	D	100%	75%	50%		
Metformin	Glucophage	Avoid use	C	AVOID USE Cr <60–70	AVOID USE	AVOID USE	YES	
Methadone	Methadose	Avoid in severe disease	D		NR	50–75%	NO	CYP3A4—Substrate; CYP2D6—Inhibitor

Metoclopramide	Reglan		I		Cr <40 50%		0–5%	
Metolazone	Zaroxolyn		NR				0–5%	
Metoprolol	Lopressor	Reduce dose	NR				YES	CYP2D6—Substrate
Metronidazole	Flagyl	C	D	100%	100%	50%	50–100%	CYP3A4—Inhibitor; take with food
Mexiletine	Mexitil	C	D	100%	100%	50–75%		CYP1A2, 2D6—Substrate; CYP1A2—Inhibitor
Midazolam	Versed		NR				NO	CYP3A4—Substrate
Mirtazapine	Remeron		D		70%	50%		CYP1A2, 2D6, 3A4—Substrate
Montelukast	Singulair	Not studies in severe impairment	D	100%	100%	100%	Unknown	CYP2C9, 3A4—Substrate
Morphine	Roxanol		D	100%	75%	50%		
Moxifloxacin	Avelox	Not recomm in severe dz	D	100%	100%	100%	9%	Metal cations, QT Prolongation
Nabumatone	Relafen		D		Cr 30–49 75%, MAX 1500 mg/DAY Cr <30 50%, MAX 1000 mg/DAY	50%, MAX 1000 mg/DAY	NO	
Naproxen	Naprosyn	↓dose 50%	D	100%	100%	100%		Take with food
Nitrofurantion	Macrodantin		C	Cr <60, Do not use	Do not use	Do not use	YES	Take with food
Nizatidine	Axid		D/I		150 mg daily	150 mg qOD		
Nortriptyline	Pamelor	C	D	100%	100%	100%		CYP2D6—Substrate
Octreotide	Sandostatin		D	100%	100%	50%		QT Prolongation
Olanzapine	Zyprexa		D	100%	100%	100%	NO	CYP1A2—Substrate
Omeprazole	Prilosec OTC, Prilosec	Use with caution	NR				NO	CYP2C19—Substrate; CYP2C9, 2C19—Inhibitor; take on empty stomach
Ondansetron	Zofran	8 mg max dose in severe	D	100%	100%	100%		CYP3A4—Substrate

*D = Dose Reduction Indicated by %; I = Dose Interval Extension; NR = No Report Found; C = Administer with Caution

Generic Name	Brand Name	Hepatic Failure Dosage Adjustment	Method of Dosage Adjustment*	<50 mL/min	10–50 mL/min	>10 mL/min	Dialyzable	Interactions (Drug-Drug, Drug-Food)
Oxycodone	Roxicodone	↓dose 1/3–1/2	NR				NO	CYP2D6—Substrate
Oxycodone + APAP	Percocet	Reduce dose in severe disease	NR				NO	CYP2D6—Substrate
Oxycodone SR	OxyContin	Reduce dose in severe disease	NR				NO	CYP2D6—Substrate
Pantoprazole	Protonix	No adjustment required	D	100%	100%	100%	NO	CYP2C19—Substrate; CYP2C9—Inhibitor
Paroxetine	Paxil	↓dose 50–75%	D	100%	50–75%	50%	NO	CYP2D6—Substrate; CYP2B6, 2D6—Inhibitor; QT Prolongation
Pentazocine	Talwin	Reduce dose or avoid use	D	100%	75%	50%		
Pentobarbital	Nembutal	Reduce dose in severe disease	NR					CYP2A6, 3A4—Inhibitors
Phenazopyridine	Pyridium		I	CR 50–80 q8–16h	AVOID USE	AVOID USE		
Phenobarbital	Luminal	Monitor levels	I			q12–16h	20–50%	CYP2C19—Substrate; CYP1A2, 2A6, 2B6, 2C8, 2C9, 3A4—Inhibitor
Phenytoin	Dilantin	Monitor levels	C					CYP2C9, 2C19—Substrate; CYP2B6, 2C8, 2C9, 2C19, 3A4—Inducer
Potassium Chloride	KlorCon		NR				YES	
Pramipexole	Mirapex		C/D/I		35% daily to BID	AVOID USE	MINIMAL	
Prazosin	Minipress		NR					
Pregabalin	Lyrica			Cr 30–60 75 mg in 2–3 divided doses or 150 mg in 2–3 divided doses or 300 mg in 2–3 divided doses	Cr 15–30 25–50 mg in once daily or in 2 divided doses or 75 mg once daily or in 2 divided doses or 150 mg once daily or in 2 divided doses	Cr <15 25 mg once daily or 25–50 mg once daily or 75 mg once daily	50%	CYP2D6—Substrate; QT Prolongation, Cisapride, moxifloxacin, take with food

Procainamide	Pronestyl/Procan SR	decrease dose by 50%	I		q6–12h	q8–24h	20–50%	CYP2D6—Substrate; QT Prolongation, Cisapride, moxifloxacin, take with food
Prochlorperazine	Compazine		NR				NO	
Promethazine	Phenergan		NR				0–5%	CYP2B6, 2D6—Substrate
Propofol	Diprovan		NR				—	CYP2B6, 2C9—Substrate; CYP1A2, 2C19, 3A4—Inhibitor
Propoxyphene-APAP	Darvocet N	No guidelines	C			AVOID USE	0–5%	
Propranolol	Inderal	Lower initial dose	NR				0–5%	CYP1A2, 2D6—Substrate
Quetiapine	Seroquel	Initial dose 25 mg/day	D	100%	100%	100%		CYP3A4—Substrate, QT Prolongation
Quinipril	Accupril	Use with caution		Cr > 60 10 mg/day	Cr 30–60; 5 mg/day Cr 10–30; 2.5 mg/day	AVOID USE		
Rabeprazole	Aciphex	Use caution in severe impairment	D	100%	100%	100%	NO	CYP2C19, 3A4—Substrate; CYP2C8, 2C19—Inhibitor
Ramelteon	Rozerem	Avoid use in severe impairment	D	100%	100%	100%	NO	CYP1A2—Substrate
Ramipril	Altace		D		Cr < 40 25%	25%	NO	
Ranitidine	Zantac	Monitor	D/I		150 mg q24h	150 mg q24h	NO	
Riluzole	Rilutek	Use of caution	C					CYP1A2—Substrate; take on empty stomach
Risperidone	Risperdal	Initial dose: 0.5 mg twice daily	C					CYP2D6—Substrate; QT Prolongation
Rivastigmine	Exelon	Interval > 2wks for dose adjustments	D	100%	100%	100%		
Salmeterol	Serevent		NR					CYP3A4—Substrate; QT Prolongation
Salmeterol/ Fluticasone	Advair		NR					CYP3A4—Substrate; QT Prolongation

*D = Dose Reduction Indicated by %; I = Dose Interval Extension; NR = No Report Found; C = Administer with Caution

Generic Name	Brand Name	Hepatic Failure Dosage Adjustment	Method of Dosage Adjustment*	<50 mL/min	10–50 mL/min	>10 mL/min	Dialyzable	Interactions (Drug-Drug, Drug-Food)
Salsalate	Disalcid		C			750 mg twice daily with an additional 500 mg after dialysis		take with food
Sertraline	Zoloft	Lower dose or less frequent dose	D	100%	100%	100%	NO	CYP2C19, 2D6—Substrate; CYP2B6, 2C19, 2D6, 3A4—Inhibitor; QT Prolongation
Spironolactone	Aldactone		I		q12–24h	AVOID USE		
Sucralfate	Carafate		C					take on empty stomach
Sulfamethoxazole/Trimethaprim	Bactrim DS				50%	AVOID USE	MODERATE	CYP2C9, 3A4—Substrate; CYP2C8, 2C9—Inhibitor; take on empty stomach
Tamoxifen	Nolvadex		NR					CYP2C9, 2D6, 3A4—Substrate; CYP2C8—Inhibitor; QT Prolongation
Tamsulosin	Flomax		D	100%	100%	AVOID USE		CYP2D6, 3A4—Substrate
Tegaserod	Zelnorm	Mod-severe: do not use	D	100%	100%	CONTRAINDICATED	NO	
Theophylline	Theodur		NR					CYP1A2, 2E1, 3A4—Substrate
Tiotropium	Spiriva		C				MINIMAL	CYP1A2—Substrate; QT Prolongation
Tizanidine	Zanaflex	Avoid use	D/I					CYP2D6, 3A4—Substrate
Tolterodine	Detrol	IR tab: 1 mg BID; ER tab: 2 mg daily	D		Cr 10–30 Immediate release tablet: 1 mg twice daily Extended release capsule: 2 mg daily			
Topiramate	Topamax	Clearance may be reduced	D				30%	
Torsemide	Demedex		NR					CYP2C9—Substrate

Drug	Brand	Dosage Adjustment	D/I	Cr > 60	Cr 40–60	Cr < 40	Dialysis	Metabolism/Comments
Tramadol	Ultram	IR: 50 mg every 12 hrs; ER: do not use	D/I		Cr <30 50–100 mg q12h, max 200 mg/day, do not use ER		NO	CYP2D6—Substrate
Trazodone	Desyrel		NR					CYP3A4—Substrate; CYP2D6—Inhibitor; take with food
Trimethobenzamide	Tigan		NR					
Vancomycin	Vancocin		D/I	Cr > 60 1 g or 10–15 mg/kg/dose every 12 hours	Cr 40–60 1 g or 10–15 mg/kg/dose every 24 hours	Cr < 40 Will need longer intervals; determine by serum concentration monitoring	NO	
Venlafaxine	Effexor	Decrease total dose by 50%	D	25%	25%	50%	NO	CYP2D6, 3A4—Substrate, QT Prolongation
Verapamil	Calan	Use 20–50% of normal dose	D			50–75%	0–5%	CYP3A4—Substrate, Inhibitor
Warfarin Sodium	Coumadin	Monitor INR	C (bleeding)					CYP2C9—Substrate, Inhibitor
Zafirlukast	Accolate	50–60% greater Cmax	D	100%	100%	100%		CYP2C9—Substrate, Inhibitor; take on empty stomach
Zaleplon	Sonata	Mild-mod: 5 mg; do not use in severe	C			AVOID USE, NOT WELL STUDIED		
Ziprasidone	Geodon	No adjustment necessary	C				NO	QT Prolongation
Zolpidem	Ambien	Ambien 5 mg; CR 6.25 mg	C				NO	CYP3A4—Substrate

*D = Dose Reduction Indicated by %; I = Dose Interval Extension; NR = No Report Found; C = Administer with Caution

Drugs Affected by Cytochrome P450 Enzyme Metabolism

SUBSTRATES

1A2	Amitriptyline, caffeine, clomipramine, clonzapine, cyclobenzaprine, estradiol, fluvoxamine, haloperidol, imipramine N-DeMe, mexilletine, naproxen, olanzapine, ondansetron, phenacetin=>, acetaminophen=>NAPQI, propranolol, riluzole, ropivacaine, tacrine, theophylline, tizanidine, verpamil, (R)warfarin, zileuton, zolmitriptan
2B6	Bupropion, cyclophosphamide, efavirenz, ifosfamide, methadone
2C8	Paclitaxel, torsemide, amodiaquine, cerivastatin, repaglinide
2C19	Proton Pump Inhibitors: lansoprazole, omeprazole, pantoprazole, rebeprazole, E-3810 Anti-epileptics: diazepam=>Nor, phenytoin(O), S-mephenytoin, phenobarbitone amitriptyline, carisoprodol, citalopram, clomipramine, cyclophosphamide, hexobarbital, imipramine N-DeME, indomethacin, R-mephobarbital, moclobemide, nelfinavir, nilutamide, primidone, progresterone, proguanil, propranolol, teniposide, R-warfarin=>8-OH
2C9	NSAIDS: diclofenac, ibuprofen, lornoxicam, meloxicam S-, naproxen=>Nor, piroxicam, suprofen Oral Hypoglycemic Agents: tolbutamide, glipizide Angiotensin II Blockers: losartan, irbesartan Sulfonylureas: glyburide/glibenclamide, glipizide, glimepiride, tolbutamide amitriptyline, celecoxib, fluoxetine, fluvastatin, glyburde, nateglinide, phenytoin=>4-OH, rosiglitazone, tamoxifen, torsemide, S-warfarin
2D6	Beta Blockers: carvedilol, S-metoprolol, propafenone, timolol Antidepressants: amitriptyline, clomipramine, desipramine, imipramine paroxetine Antipsychotics: haloperidol, perphenazine, risperidone=>90H, thioridazine, zuclopenthixol alprenolol, amphetamine, aripiprazole, atomoxetine, bufuralol, chlorpheniramine, chlorpromazine, codeine (=>O-desMe), debrisoquine, dexfenfluramine, dextromethorphan, duloxetine, encainide, flecainide, fluoxetine, fluvoxamine, lidocaine, metoclorpramide, methoxyamphetamine, mexilitine, minaprine, nebivolol, nortriptyline, ondansetron, oxycodone, perhexiline, phenacetin, phenformin, promethazine, propranolol, sparteine, tamoxifen, tramadol, venlafaxine
2E1	Anesthetics: enflurane, halothane, isoflurane, methoxyflurande, seveoflurane acetaminophen =>NAPQI, aniline, benzene, chlorzoxazone, ethanol, N,N-dimethyl, formamide, theophyline =>8-OH

3A4, 5, 7	Macrolide antibiotics: clarithromycin, erythromycin (not 3A5), NOT azithromycin, telithromycin Anti-arrhythmics: quinidein=>3-OH (not 3A5) Benzodiazepines: alprazolam, diazepam=>3OH, midazolam, triazolam Immune Modulators: cyclosporine, tacrolimus (FK506) HIV Antivirals: indinavir, nelfinavir, ritonavir, saquinavir Prokinetic: cisapride Antihistamines: astemizole, chlorpheniramine, terfenidine Calcium Channel Blockers: amlodipine, diltiazem, felodipine, lercanidipine, nifedipine, nisoldipine, nitrendipine, verpamil Hmg CoA Reductase Inhibitors: atorvastatin, cerivastatin, lovastatin, NOT pravastatin, simvastatin Steroid 6beta-OH: estradiol, hydrocortisone, progesterone, testosterone Miscellaneous: alfentanyl, aprepitant, aripiprazole, buspirone, cafergot, caffeine=>TMU, cilostazol, cocaine, codeine-N-, demthylation, dapsone, dexamethasone, dextromethorphan, docetaxel, domperidone, eplerenone, fentanyl, finasteride, gleevec, haloperidol, irinotecan, LAAM, lidocaine, methadone, nateglinide, odanestron, pimozide, propranolol, quetiapine, quinine, risperidone, NOT rosuvastatin, salmeterol, sildenafil, sirolimus, tamoxifen, taxol, terfenadine, trazodone, vincristine, zaleplon, ziprasideon, zolpidem

INHIBITORS: Inhibitors compete with other drugs for a particular enzyme thus affecting the optimal level of metabolism of the substrate drug which in many cases affect the individual's response to that particular medication, e.g. making it ineffective.

1A2	Amiodarone, cimetidine, ciprofloxacin, fluoroquinolones, fluvoxamine, furafylline, interferon, methoxsalen, mibefradil
2B6	Thiotepa, ticlopidine
2C8	Trimethoprim, quercetin, glitazones, gemfibrozil, montelukast, trimethoprim
2C19	Chloramphenicol, cimetidine, felbamate, fluoxetine, fluvoxamine, indomethacin, ketoconazole, lansoprazole, modafinil, omeprazole, oxcarbazepine, probenicid, ticlopidine, topiramate
2C9	Amiodarone, fenofibrate, fluconazole, fluvastatin, fluvoxamine, isoniazid, lovastatin, phenylbutazone, probenicid, sertraline, sulfamethoxazole, teniposide, voriconazole, zafirlukast
2D6	Amiodarone, bupropion, celecoxib, chlorpromazine, chlorpheniramine, cimetidine, citalopram, clomipramine, cocaine, diphenhydramine, doxepin, doxorubicin escitalopram, fluoxetine, halofantrine, red-haloperidol, levomepromazine, metoclopramide, methadone, mibefradil, midodrine, moclobemide, paroxetine, quinidine, ranitidine, ritonavir, sertaline, terbinafine ticlopidine, histamine H1 receptor antagonists, diphenhydramine, chlorpheniramine, clemastine, perphenazine, hydroxyzine, tripelennamine
2E1	Diethyl-dithiocarbamate, disulfiram
3A4, 5, 7	HIV Antivirals: delviridine, indinavir, nelfinavir, ritonavir amiodarone, aprepitant, NOT azithromycin, chloramphenicol, cimetidine, clarithromycin, diethl-dithiocarbamate, diltiazem, erythromycin, fluconazole, fluvoxamine, gestadene, grapefruit juice, imatinib, itraconazole, ketoconazole, mifepristone, nefazodone, norfloxacin, norfluoxetine, mibefradil, star fruit, verapamil, voriconazole

INDUCERS: Inducers stimulate the production of the enzyme thus increasing the rate of metabolism causing the substrate drug to clear out of the system faster. This will also affect the individual's response to the medication, i.e. making he drug ineffective because it has not been in the system long enough to have an effect.

1A2	Broccoli, brussel sprouts, char-grilled meat, insulin, methyl cholanthrene, modafinil, nafcillin, beta-naphthoflavone, omeprazole, tobacco
2B6	Phenobarbital, rifampin
2C8	Rifampin
2C19	Carbamazepine, norethindrone, NOT pentobarbital, prednisone, rifampin
2C9	Rifampin, secobarbital
2D6	Dexamethasone, rifampin
2E1	Ethanol, isoniazid
3A4, 5, 7	HIV Antivirals: efavirenz, nevirapine
	barbiturates, carbamazepine, efavirenz, glucocorticoids, modafinil, nevirapine, phenobarbital, phenytoin, rifampin, St. John's wort, troglitazone, oxcarbazepine, pioglitazone, rifabutin

GENETICS

1A2	Chromosome 15
2B6	Chromosome 19 Polymorphic, 3–4% Caucasians poor metabolizers
2C8	Chromosome 10
2C19	Chromosome 10 Polymorphic, 3–5% Caucasian, poor metabolizers, 15–20% Asain poor metabolizers
2C9	Chromosome 10 Polymorphic, 1–3% Caucasian poor metabolizers
2D6	Chromosome 22 Polymorphic, 5–10% Caucasian poor metabolizers
2E1	Chromosome 10
3A4, 5, 7	Chromosome 7

Adapted from: http://medicine.iupui.edu/flockhart.table.htm accessed 3/7/07.

Glucocorticoid Equivalency Table

Glucocorticoid	Equivalent Dose (mg)	Relative Potency		Half-Life (min)
		Anti-Inflammatory	Mineralocorticoid	
Short Acting				
Cortisone	25	0.8	2	30
Hydrocortisone	20	1	2	90
Intermediate Acting				
Prednisone	5	4	1	60
Prednisolone	5	4	1	200
Triamcinolone	4	5	0	300
Methylprednisolone	4	5	0	180
Long Acting				
Betamethasone	0.6–0.75	25	0	100–300
Dexamethasone	0.75	25–30	0	100–300

References

DiPiro JT, Talbert RL, Yee GC, et al. Pharmacotherapy: a pathophysiologic approach. 6th ed. New York: McGraw-Hill Medical Publishing Division, 2005: 1403.

Mager DE, Lin SX, Blum RA. Dose equivalency evaluation of major corticosteroids: pharmacokinetics and cell trafficking and cortisol dynamics. J Clin Pharmacol 2003;43:1216–1227.

Lexi-Comp Online, Hudson, Ohio: Lexi-Comp, Inc.; 2004; January 30, 2007.

Benzodiazepine Equivalency Table

Benzodiazepine		Equivalent Dose (mg)	Terminal Half-Life (hours)	Active Metabolite?*	Clinical Use
Generic	Trade				
Alprazolam	Xanax	0.5	12–15	Y**	B
Chlordiazepoxide	Librium	10	24–96	Y**	B,E
Clonazepam	Klonopin	0.25–0.5	18–50	N**	A,B,D,E
Diazepam	Valium	5	20–100	Y**	A,B,C,D
Estazolam	Prosom	0.3	10–24	N**	C
Flurazepam	Dalmane	5	40–114	Y**	C
Lorazepam	Ativan	1	10–20	N	A,B,C,E
Oxazepam	Serax	15–30	5–20	N	A,B,C,E
Temazepam	Restoril	5	10–40	N	C
Triazolam	Halcion	0.1	2–3	N**	C
Clorazepate	Tranxene	7.5	50–100	Y**	A,B,E
Quazepam	Doral	5	28–114	Y**	C

Notes

* Presence of an active metabolite may extend the pharmacological activity of the drug past the desired clinical effect, increasing the likelihood of adverse effects of confusion, lethargy, ataxia, etc.

**Undergoes oxidative metabolism. All benzodiazepines are metabolized in the liver and renally excreted. Avoid benzodiazepines that undergo oxidative metabolism in liver disease as this type of metabolism may be significantly impaired.

Clinical Use: A=anticonvulsant, B=anxiolytic, C=sedative-hypnotic, D=muscle relaxant, E=other

References

Lexi-Comp Online, Hudson, Ohio: Lexi-Comp, Inc.; 2004; January 30, 2007 (or date accessed).

Trevor, A.J. & Way, W.L. (2001). Sedative-hypnotic drugs, In *Basic and Clinical Pharmacology*, 8th ed. Lange Medical Books/McGraw-Hill: New York.

Benzodiazepine pharmacokinetics In *DrugDex Consults*. Micromedex Healthcare Series, accessed 2/8/2007.

Insulin Comparison Chart

Preparation Generic (Brand)	Onset of Action	Peak	Duration	Usual Administration Time	Cost/10 mL Vial
Rapid Acting					
Lispro (Humalog)	~15 minutes	30–90 minutes	3–4 hours	15 minutes before a meal or immediately after a meal	$79
Aspart (Novolog)	~15 minutes	1–3 hours	3–5 hours	15 minutes before a meal or immediately after a meal	$81
Glulisine (Apidra)	~15 minutes	30–90 minutes	3–4 hours	15 minutes before a meal	$53/3 mL
Short Acting					
Regular (HumulinR Novolin R)	30–60 minutes	2–4 hours	6–8 hours	30–60 minutes before a meal	$36
Intermediate-Acting					
NPH (Isophane suspension) (Humulin N, Novolin N)	1–2 hours	6–12 hours	18–24 hours	30 minutes before breakfast, 30 minutes before the evening meal	$36
Detemir (Levemir)	3–4 hours	6–8 hours	Dose dependent	Once daily: with evening meal or bedtime Twice daily: with breakfast and with evening meal or at bedtime	$78
Long-Acting					
Glargine (Lantus)	3–4 hours	Flat	~24 hours	At bedtime	$80
Mixtures					
70/30 (NPH/R) (Novolin 70/30)	30 minutes	2–12 hours	18–24 hours	~30 minutes before a meal	$37

75/25 (Lispro protamine/Lispro) (Humalog Mix 75/25)	~15 minutes	2–12 hours	18–24 hours	~15 minutes before a meal	$84
Aspart protamine susp/Insulin aspart (Novolog Mix 70/30)	~15 minutes	1–4 hours	18–24 hours	~15 minutes before breakfast,	$51/3mL

Other administration times may be designated by physician based on each patient

References

Kerscher RD. Lexi-Comp Online [database on the Internet]. Hudson (OH): Lexi-Comp Inc. c 2006–[updated 2006 Aug 11]:[cited 2006 Sept 6].
Available from: http://0-online.lexi.com.polar.onu.edu/crlsql/servlet/crlonline.

Recommended Starting Doses in Children and Adults Less than 50 kg Body Weight

	Oral Starting Dose	Parenteral Starting Dose
OPIOID AGONISTS		
Codeine	0.5–1 mg/kg q 3–4 hr	Not recommended
Hydrocodone with Acetaminophen (Vicodin)	0.2 mg/kg q 3–4 hr	
Hydromorphone (Dilaudid)	0.06 mg/kg q 3–4 hr	0.015 mg/kg q 3–4 hr
Levorphanol (Levo-Dromoran)	0.04 mg/kg q 6–8 hr	0.02 mg/kg q 6–8 hr
Methadone (Dolophine)	0.1 mg/kg q 4–8 hr	0.05 mg/kg q 4–8 hr
Morphine	0.3 mg/kg q 3–4 hr	0.05–0.1 mg/kg q 2–4 hr
Oxycodone (Roxicodone)	0.2 mg/kg q 3–4 hr	
Fentanyl (Duragesic)	Transdermal/mucosal —0.5–2 mcg/kg/h	0.5–2 mcg/kg/h as a continuous infusion
NON-OPIOIDS		
Acetaminophen (Tylenol)	10–15 mg/kg q 4–6 hr	
Aspirin	10–15 mg/kg q 4–6 hr	
Choline Mag Trisalicylate (Trilisate)	25 mg/kg q 12 hr	
Ibuprofen (Advil/Motrin)	4–10 mg/kg q 6–8 hr	
Ketorolac (Toradol)		0.5 mg/kg q 6 hr
Naproxen (Naprosyn)	5–7 mg/kg q 8–12 hr	
TRI-CYCLIC ANTIDEPRESSANTS		
Desipramine (Norpramin)	0.2 mg/kg QD (increase by 0.2–0.4 mg q 3 days)	
Nortriptyline (Pamelor)	0.2–1 mg/kg QD (increase by 0.25 mg/kg q 5–7 days to 0.2–3 mg/kg)	

Amitriptyline (Elavil)	0.2–0.5 mg/kg q HS (increase by 25% q 2–3 days to 1–2 mg/kg)	
Imipramine (Tofranil)	0.5–2 mg/kg HS (increase by 0.5 mg/kg q 5–7 days to 0.5–4 mg/kg)	
ATYPICAL ANTIPSYCHOTICS		
Risperidone (Risperdal)	0.25 mg QD (increase by 0.25 mg/day each week; max: 1.5 mg/day)	
Olanzapine (Zyprexa)	0.12–0.29 mg/kg/day	
Quetiapine (Seroquel)	1.6–5.2 mg/kg/day	

*Not recommended in the pediatric population-All opioid agonist-antagonists and partial agonists, Meperidine (Demerol), Oxymorphone (Numorphan), Propoxyphene (Darvon), Tramadol (Ultram), Celecoxib (Celebrex), Scopolamine (Transderm Scop).

All data confirmed via Lexi-Comp's Complete Reference Library, http://www.crlonline.com, accessed online: February 2007.

	Oral Starting Dose	Parenteral Starting Dose
BENZODIAZEPINES		
Alprazolam (Xanax)	0.005 mg/kg TID	
Clonazepam (Klonopin)	0.01 mg/kg q 12 hr	
Diazepam (Valium)	0.05–0.1 mg/kg q 4–6 hr	0.05–0.1 mg/kg q 4–6 hr
Lorazepam (Ativan)	0.02–0.1 mg/kg q 4–6 hr	0.02–0.1 mg/kg 4–6 hr
BARBITURATES		
Phenobarbital	2 mg/kg TID	3–5 mg/kg HS
BUTYROPHENONE		
Haloperidol (Haldol)	0.01–0.1 mg/kg q 8h	0.01–0.1 mg/kg q 8h

PHENOTHIAZINES

Chlorpromazine (Thorazine)	0.5–1 mg/kg q 4–6 hr	0.5–1 mg/kg q 6–8 hr
Prochlorperazine (Compazine)	PO/PR: 0.1 mg/kg TID-QID	IM: 0.1–0.15 mg/kg/dose

ANTI-CONVULSANTS

Divalproex Na (Depakote)	10–15 mg/kg/day in 1–3 div. doses (increase by 5–10 mg/kg/day weekly until therapeutic levels achieved; maintenance: 30–60 mg/kg/day in 2–3 divided doses)	
Gabapentin (Neurontin)	5 mg/kg HS (increase 5 mg/kg BID day 2 and 5 mg/kg TID day 3) usual dosage range: 8–35 mg/kg/day in 3 divided doses	
Carbamazepine (Tegretol)	5 mg/kg QD (increase 5 mg/kg BID day 2 and 5 mg/kg TID day 3)	

ANTI-CHOLINERGIC

Hyoscyamine (Levsin)	0.0625–0.125 mg q 4 hr	
Glycopyrrolate (Robinul)	40–100 mcg/kg TID-QID	4–10 mcg/kg q 3–4 hr
Dicyclomine (Bentyl)	5–10 mg TID-QID	

ANTI-HISTAMINE

Hydroxyzine (Atarax/Vistaril)	2 mg/kg q4–6h	0.5–1 mg/kg q4–6 h
Diphenhydramine (Benadryl)	0.5–1 mg/kg q4–6h	0.5–1 mg/kg q4–6h
Dimenhydrinate (Dramamine)	5 mg/kg/day in 4 div doses	

CORTICOSTEROIDS

Prednisone (Deltasone)	0.5–2 mg/kg QD-QID	
Dexamethasone (Decadron)	0.1 mg/kg/day in 2–4 divided doses	0.1 mg/kg/day in q6–12h

PROMOTILITY AGENTS

Metoclopramide (Reglan)	0.1–0.2 mg/kg q6–8h	0.1–0.2 mg/kg q6–8h

Pediatric Recommended Maximum Dosing

Codeine	60 mg/dose
Hydromorphone (Dilaudid)	5 mg/dose
Methadone (Dolophine)	10 mg/dose
Morphine	15 mg/dose
Oxycodone (Roxicodone)	5 mg/dose q 4–6 hrs
Acetaminophen (Tylenol)	5 doses/day of 10–15 mg/kg/dose
Aspirin	4 g/day
Ibuprofen (Advil/Motrin)	40 mg/kg/day
Ketorolac (Toradol)	Single IM dose: 30 mg Single IV dose: 15 mg
Naproxen (Naprosyn)	1000 mg/day
Desipramine (Norpramin)	5 mg/kg/day
Amitriptyline (Elavil)	3 mg/kg/day
Imipramine (Tofranil)	5 mg/kg/day in 1–4 divided doses; monitor carefully with doses 3.5 mg/kg/day
Olanzapine (Zyprexa)	20 mg/day (0.12–0.29 mg/kg/day)
Quetiapine (Seroquel)	450 mg/day
Alprazolam (Xanax)	0.02 mg/kg/dose, 0.06 mg/kg/day

Clonazepam (Klonopin)	0.2 mg/kg/day
Diazepam (Valium)	I.M, I.V.: 0.6 mg/kg within an 8-hour period
Lorazepam (Ativan)	2 mg/dose
Haloperidol (Haldol)	0.15 mg/kg/day
Chlorpromazine (Thorazine)	<5 years (22.7 kg): 40 mg/day 5–12 years (22.7–45.5 kg): 75 mg/day
Prochlorperazine (Compazine)	9–13 kg: 7.5 mg/day
	13.1–17 kg: 10 mg/day
	17.1–37 kg: 15 mg/day
Divalproex Na (Depakote)	60 mg/kg/day Larger maintenance doses may be required in younger children
Gabapentin (Neurontin)	50 mg/kg/day
Carbamazepine (Tegretol)	<6 years: 35 mg/kg/day 6–12 years: 1000 mg/day
Hyoscyamine (Levsin)	0.75 mg/day
Glycopyrrolate (Robinul)	0.2 mg/dose, 0.8 mg/day
Diphenhydramine (Benadryl)	2–5 years: 75 mg/day 6–12 years: 150 mg/day
Prednisone (Deltasone)	60 mg/day

Subcutaneous Administration of Medications Butterfly Procedure

General Information

The butterfly, wing-tip, or scalp needle is useful for providing medications via the subcutaneous (SQ) route. The SQ route of medication administration provides appropriate management of symptoms for patients who are unable to take medications through other routes of administration.

Indications

A. Circumstances that preclude or compromise oral administration:
   1. Dysphagia – due to neuromuscular weakness or mechanical obstruction
   2. Decreased level of consciousness
   3. Intestinal obstruction
   4. Nausea and vomiting
B. Symptom control crisis requiring rapid and reliable medication administration and absorption.
C. Poor or variable compliance:
   1. Dementia
   2. Agitated delirium, with paranoia and non-compliance
   3. Personality issues

Procedure for Inserting SQ Butterfly

EQUIPMENT NEEDED:
   Alcohol swabs
   Butterfly or wing-tipped catheter, 25 gauge
   Transparent adhesive dressing
   Luer-lock injection cap
   Tape
   Gloves
   Sharps container

1. Wash hands.
2. Explain the procedure to the patient/caregiver.
3. Assemble the equipment at a convenient work area.
4. Assist the patient to a comfortable position.
5. Put on gloves.
6. Attach Luer-loc to end of butterfly.
7. Draw up approximately ¼ mL of prescribed medication with syringe.
8. Inject medication into end of Leur-loc until Leur-loc and butterfly line are filled.
9. Cleanse the selected site with alcohol swabs.
10. Insert needle into subcutaneous space, with the bevel **down,** using a 45 degree angle.

11. Place a folded 2″ × 2″ gauze under the wings of the butterfly to maintain angle.
12. Secure butterfly by taping each wing of the butterfly vertically with 1½ inches of tape. Tape butterfly tubing below site of puncture. Cover site, including wings, with transparent dressing, so that the skin over the needle is visible and the Leur-loc is accessible for injections.
13. On the tape at the site, write the date of insertion and the name and concentration of the medication.
14. Discard disposable items in a plastic trash bag, and discard. Place the used needles and syringes in a sharps container.
15. Document procedure and patient's tolerance of procedure.
16. Before each medication injection, inspect the needle site for redness, or dislodgement of the needle.
17. If needle site is reddened, needle dislodged, or medication leaks from around needle, insert new butterfly in a different site.
18. Change butterfly site every 3–5 days.

Signs of Infection, Cannula Misplacement, or Overuse of Site
Leaking, redness, exudates, localized heat, localized inflammation, pain, tenderness, hardness, burning, swelling, scarring, itching, bruising, unresolved blanching, or necrosis.

If Administering More than One Medication
Establish an additional SQ site for each new medication or if there is a change in the concentration of the current medication. Label each site as to which medication is to be administered in that site.

Amount of Medication To Be Administered at One Time
The maximum amount of medication (excluding flush) to be administered at one time is 2 mL. This will allow for optimal absorption and comfort for the patient.

Instilling Medications Through SQ Butterfly (Intermittent Push)

EQUIPMENT NEEDED:
    3-mL syringes
    Alcohol swabs
    Medication
    Gloves

1. Wash hands, put on gloves.
2. Explain procedure to patient/family
3. Cleanse injection cap that is attached to butterfly tubing, with 2–3 alcohol swabs.
4. Insert the syringe needle containing medication into the injection cap. Gently draw back on the plunger. If blood appears in the tubing, remove the syringe, discard medication, and remove the SQ butterfly. Restart the SQ insertion in a different site in order to administer the medication.
5. If no blood appears in the butterfly line, instill the medication into the SQ site. Do not exceed 2 mL per administration.
6. Discard used equipment.
7. Ensure the "SQ Line" identification sticker is located by the SQ site.
8. Document medication given, any adverse effects or difficulties encountered, and patient tolerance of the procedure.

Initiating a Continuous SQ Infusion

EQUIPMENT NEEDED:
>   Alcohol swabs
>   Medication in appropriate cassette/IV bag
>   Continuous infusion pump
>   3 mL syringe with 1 mL normal saline

1. Explain procedure to patient/family.
2. Wash hands, put on gloves.
3. Prime the tubing and set the program as ordered by the physician. Insert SQ catheter or use existing site.
4. Cleanse injection site cap with 2–3 alcohol swabs.
5. Insert the syringe containing normal saline (0.5 mL) into the injection cap. Gently draw back on the plunger. If blood appears in the tubing, remove the SQ butterfly and discard. Restart the SQ insertion in a different site.
6. If no blood appears in the SQ site extension tubing, attach the primed tubing and start the infusion.
7. Discard the syringe in the appropriate container and discard the other supplies used.
8. Ensure the "SQ Line" identification sticker is located by the SQ site.
9. Document the procedure, medication that is being administered, time of initiation of infusion, rate of infusion, bolus dose information (if included in the physician's order), and patient tolerance to the procedure.

Medications That Can Be Given Via the SQ Route Per SQ Butterfly

0.9% or 0.45% Saline solution (NS or ½NS)	Ketamine
2.5% or 5% Dextrose solution (D5W)	Lorazepam
Dexamethasone	Metoclopramide
Diphenhydramine	Methadone
Fentanyl	Midazolam
Furosemide	Morphine
Glycopyrrolate	Naloxone
Haloperidol	Octreotide
Heparin	Phenobarbital
Hydromorphone	Ranitidine

Medications Not Recommended for SQ Route Per SQ Butterfly

Chlorpromazine	Hypertonic solutions
Diazepam	Prochlorperazine
Hydroxyzine	

Hydration Therapy Via SQ Route (Hypodermoclysis)

EQUIPMENT NEEDED:
- Alcohol swabs
- Medication in appropriate cassette/IV bag
- Continuous infusion pump, or gravity assist
- 3 mL syringe with 1 mL normal saline

1. Explain procedure to patient/family.
2. Wash hands, put on gloves.
3. Prime the tubing and set the program as ordered by the physician. Insert SQ catheter or use existing site.
4. Cleanse injection site cap with 2–3 alcohol swabs.
5. Insert the syringe containing normal saline (0.5 mL) into the injection cap. Gently draw back on the plunger. If blood appears in the tubing, remove the SQ butterfly and discard. Restart the SQ insertion in a different site.
6. If no blood appears in the SQ site extension tubing, attach the primed tubing and start the infusion.

   If using infusion pump: suggested rate 75–125 mL/H, (*max* 125 mL/H)
   If using gravity: Do not adjust flux, allow flow to freely adjust to gravity and rate of tissue absorption
   Hyaluronidase: It is not necessary to use hyaluronidase if infusion rate is <125 mL/H

7. Alternating the infusion site with each one liter of solution is recommended. Infusion of more than three liters in 24 hours has not been studied.
8. Discard the syringe in the appropriate container and discard the other supplies used.
9. Ensure the "SQ Line" identification sticker is located by the SQ site.
10. Document the procedure, medication that is being administered, time of initiation of infusion, rate of infusion, and patient tolerance to the procedure.

Advantages of SQ Hydration

- Can prevent hospitalization of patients with dehydration
- Procedure is safe, simple, and less expensive than intravenous (IV) hydration
- May be performed in patients with collapsed, fragile, or thrombosed veins
- Low risk of fluid overload
- Patients experience a low incidence or pain or discomfort during administration
- Low risk of infection or thrombophlebitis

Disadvantages of SQ Hydration

- Limitation of solutions used (see chart p. 338)
- Not recommended for patients with coagulopathies
- Will not correct severe electrolyte abnormalities
- Amount of fluid to be infused in 24 hours is limited (3L max)
- Slight risk of pain and infection at infusion site

References

Dickerson, E.D., et al (2001). *Palliative Care Pocket Consultant*. 2nd ed. Kendall/Hunt Publ: Dubuque, IA.

Fonzo-Christe, C., et al, (2005), Subcutaneous administration of drugs in the elderly: survey of practice and systematic literature review. *Palliative Medicine*, 19(3), 208–219.

Frisoli, A., et al, (2000). Subcutaneous hydration by hypodermoclysis: a practical and low cost treatment for elderly patients. *Drugs and Aging*, 16(4), 313–319.

Letizia, M., et al (2000). Intermittent subcutaneous injections for symptom control in hospice care: a retrospective investigation. Hospice Journal, 15(2), 1–11.

Possible SQ Insertion Sites (Shaded Areas Below)

- Outer arm (do not use for hypodermoclysis)
- Abdomen (avoid in presence of tense abdominal distention such (as ascites)
- Thigh
- Subclavicular area (avoid when patient has lung disease or is active [risk of pneumothorax])
- Upper back (use when other sites are unsuitable and/or when patient is confused)

Avoid the Following Areas for SQ Insertion

- Areas with lymphedema or edema
- Areas that have too little SQ tissue
- Areas with broken skin
- Skin sites that have recently been irradiated
- Sites with infection or inflammation present
- Area with bony prominences
- Tumor sites
- Skin folds

Drug Information Table

Generic (Example of Trade)*	Indication/Drug Class	Dosage Range (MDD**)	2007 Avg. Cost/Day for Therapy (Dose for Cost Comparison)***	Adverse Effects	Onset to Peak	T1/2	Comments
Acetaminophen (Tylenol)	Nociceptive Pain, Fever/Non-opioid	325–650 mg q4h (4000 mg/day; geriatrics 3000 mg/day)	$0.50 (650 mg po q6h)	Rash, hepatoxicity, nephrotoxicity	< 1 h	1–3 h	Good first agent or adjuvant for musculoskelatal pain. Decrease maximum dose to 3gms/day in geriatric patients. Contraindicated in severe liver failure. Opioid sparing. Maximum dose in 24 hours is 4000 mg (4 grams). Weigh risk-benefit in patients with severe liver dysfunction (eg cirrhosis).
Acetaminophen and hydrocodone (Lortab, Vicodin)	Nociceptive Pain/Non-opioid/Opioid Combination	5–10/500 q6h titrate to effect (Acetaminophen 4000 mg/day; geriatrics 3000 mg/day)	$1.50 (5/500 mg po q4h)	Pruritus, rash, drowsiness, euphoria, constipation, nausea, vomiting, respiratory depression	10–20 min	3–4 h	Schedule III controlled substance. Hydrocodone also available in combination with ibuprofen. Watch acetaminophen content. Elderly dosing of hydrocodone is 1/2 adult starting dose.
Acetaminophen with Codeine (Tylenol#3,4)	Nociceptive Pain, Cough, Diarrhea/Non-opioid/Opioid Combination	15-60 mg QID (Acetaminophen 4000 mg/day; geriatrics 3000 mg/day)	$1.05 (15 mg QID)	Lightheadedness, dizziness, sedation, nausea, vomiting, dyspnea, constipation, euphoria, pruritus	30–60 h	2.5–3.5 h	Can use Acetaminophen with Codeine as a less expensive and more accessible alternative to plain codeine (CII).
Acetylcysteine (Mucomyst)	Expectorant/Mucolytic	Nebulize diluted 10–20% q2–6h	$19.00/vial	Hypotension, pruritus, rash, diarrhea, nausea, vomiting, angioedema, anaphylactoid reaction	1–2 h	5.5 h	Not first line therapy. Must be compounded. Foul odor.

*Drugs in Italics: Not generally recommended in hospice patients
**MDD = Maximun Daily Dose
***BOLD-not available as a generic

Drug Information Table

Generic (Example of Trade)*	Indication/Drug Class	Dosage Range (MDD**)	2007 Avg. Cost/Day for Therapy (Dose for Cost Comparison)***	Adverse Effects	Onset to Peak	T1/2	Comments
Acyclovir (Zovirax)	Infection/Antiviral	800 mg q4h (5 times/day) for 7–10 days	$41.50/ Course (800 mg 5 times/day for 10 days)	Malaise, headache, nausea, vomiting, diarrhea, injection site phlebitis, burning sensation, acute renal failure	1.5–2 h	3 h	
Al/Mg /+/– Simethicone (Maalox/ Maalox Plus	Gastritis/Antacid	15–30mL q4h (500 mg/day)	$1.20 (30mL q6h)	Chalky taste, stomach cramps, constipation, nausea, vomiting, discoloration of feces, hemorrhoids	Rapid	Unknown	Frequent use leads to rebound hyperacidity.
Albuterol/Ipratropium (Combivent Inhaler; DuoNeb Aerosols)	Bronchoconstriction/ Short Acting Beta Agonist Bronchodilator	2 puffs q4h; 3mL (1 unit) q4–6h (12 inhalations/day MDI; 6 doses/day inhalation solution)	$98.45/inhaler; $13.80 nebs (2 puffs q4h; 1 unit)	Upper respiratory infection, bronchitis, tahcycardia, nervousness, dyspnea, nausea	0.5–3 h	3.5–5 h	Not appropriate for lung cancer, only COPD. As patient declines, change to nebulizer for better drug delivery. Albuterol alone probably sufficient.
Albuterol Aerosol/MDI (Proventil/Ventolin	Bronchoconstriction/ Short Acting Beta Agonist Bronchodilator	1 neb unit q4h; 1–4 puffs q4h (12 inhalations/day MDI)	$4.50/$40/MDI unit (1 unit q4h; 2 puffs q4h)	Tremor, nervousness, heartburn, nausea & vomiting, dry mouth, bronchospasms	5 min–2 h	5–6 h	Overutilization leads to shakiness and tachycardia.; As patient declines, change inhaler to nebulizer for better drug delivery.
Allopurinol (Zyloprim)	Gout/Uricosuric	100–300 mg daily-BID (800 mg/day)	$0.15 (300 mg daily)	Rash, nausea, vomiting, renal impairment	1–2 weeks	1–3 h; oxipurinol 18–30 h	Generally only covered by hospice in patients with hyperuricemia related to cancer or tumor kill.

Drug	Indication	Dose (MDD)	Cost	Side Effects	Onset	Duration	Comments
Alprazolam (Xanax)	Anxiety, Nausea & Vomiting, Dyspnea, Insomnia/ Benzodiazepine	0.25–0.5 mg q4–6h; Max dose: 2 mg QID (10 mg/day)	$1.10 (0.25 mg q6h)	Drowsiness, hypotension, lightheadedness, blurred vision	30 min	12–15 h	Benzodiazepines are drugs of choice for anxiety. Alprazolam is less expensive alternative to lorazepam. Beneficial for panic attacks. Also used for other symptoms-anxiety, insomnia, dyspnea; Intensol not available generically and very expensive; Short-acting; may produce "rebound" anxiety between doses as tolerance develops; Highest risk for withdrawl if tolerant patient abruptly stops medication. Probably the least sedating drug in the class. May not be helpful for sleep maintenance concerns due to short duraction of action.
Aluminum Hydroxide (Amphogel)	Diarrhea, Bile Salt Binder/Antacid	30mL po QID (caution with end stage renal) (5400 mg/day)	$1.20 (30 mL q6h)	Constipation, hypophosphatemia, abdominal cramps	20–40 min	< 2 h	Moderately effective.
Amantadine (Symmetrel)	Parkinson's/Antiviral	100–200 mg BID (400 mg/day)	$0.65 (100 mg BID)	Orthostatic hypotension, peripheral edema, insomnia, depression, anxiety, irritability, dizziness, hallucinations, ataxia, headache, somnolence, nervousness, dream abnormality, agitation, fatigue, confusion, livedo reticularis, nausea, anorexia, constipation, diarrhea, xerostomia, dry nose	1/4–4 h	2–8 h	Generally not effective in end stage Parkinson's.

*Drugs in Italics: Not generally recommended in hospice patients
**MDD = Maximun Daily Dose
***BOLD-not available as a generic

Drug Information Table

Generic (Example of Trade)*	Indication/Drug Class	Dosage Range (MDD**)	2007 Avg. Cost/Day for Therapy (Dose for Cost Comparison)***	Adverse Effects	Onset to Peak	T1/2	Comments
Amiloride (Midamor)	Fluid Retention/ K+ Sparing Diuretic	5–10 mg daily-BID (20 mg/day)	$0.65 (10 mg daily)	Headache, fatigue, dizziness, hyperkalemia, nausea, diarrhea, vomiting, abdominal pain, gas pain, appetite changes, constipation, impotence, muscle cramps, cough, dyspnea	2–10 h	6–9 h	No advantage over spironolactone.
Amiodarone (Cordarone)	Cardiovascular/ Antiarrhythmic	400 mg daily after loading dosage regimen	$0.95 (400 mg daily)	Hypotension, abnormal gait/ataxia, dizziness, fatigue, headache, malaise, impaired memory, involuntary movement, insomnia, poor coordination, peripheral neuropathy, sleep disturbances, tremor, photosensitivity, nausea, vomiting, anorexia, constipation, liver dysfunction, hypothyroidism, hyperthyroidism, corneal deposits	1 week to 5 months	26–107 days	Can usually discontinue as patient declines. Duration of effect lasts for up to 5 months after drug is discontinued. Can cause pulmonary fibrosis and hypothyroidism.
Amitriptyline (Elavil)	Neuropathic Pain, Secretions, Depression/ Tricyclic Antidepressant	10–150 mg QHS or in divided doses (400 mg/day)	$0.15 (150 mg QHS)	Constipation, dry mouth, urinary retention, drowsiness	2–4 h	10–25 h	Do not use as first line agent. Can increase dose for antidepressant effect if using for other indications. Optimal effect in 4–6 weeks. Most severe side effects of all tricyclic antidepressants. Also used for other symptoms- nerve pain, depression, insomnia, excessive secretions. All tablet strengths cost the same.

Drug	Indication/Class	Dose	Cost	Side Effects	Onset	Half-life	Comments
Amlodipine (Norvasc)	Hypertension/Calcium Channel Blocker	2.5–10 mg daily (10 mg/day)	**$1.80 (5 mg daily)**	Edema, headache, fatigue, palpitations, dizziness, nausea, flushing	30 min to 12 h	30–50 h	Expensive. Constipating. Suggest discontinuing as patient declines.
Amoxicillin (Amoxil)	Infection (Respiratory, Skin, UTI)/Penicillin	250–500 mg TID × 10–14 days-skin; 7 day—UTI	$8.00/course (500 mg TID × 10 days)	Nausea, vomiting, diarrhea, rash	4 h	1–3 h	
Amoxicillin/Clavulanate (Augmentin)	Infection (Respiratory, Skin, UTI)/Penicillin	250–500 mg po q 8h or 875 mg q 12h	$77.00/course (875 mg BID × 10 days)	Nausea, vomiting, diarrhea, rash, vaginal mycosis	4 h	1–3 h	Expensive.
Anastozole (Arimidex)	Breast Cancer/Antineoplastic Aromatase Inhibitor	1 mg daily	**$7.60/day (1 mg daily)**	Hot flashes, asthenia, pain, nausea, vomiting, constipation, diarrhea, cough, edema, dyspnea, rash, weight gain	24 h	50 h	Not generally appropriate in hospice patients.
Aripiprazole (Abilify)	Delirium, Agitation/Atypical Antipsychotic	10–30 mg daily (30 mg/day)	**$10.75 (15 mg daily)**	Headache, agitation, anxiety, insomnia, extrapyramidal symptoms, akathisia, nausea, dyspepsia, vomiting, weight gain, constipation	Initial: 1–3 weeks	75 h	Expensive.
Artificial Saliva (Salivart)	Xerostomia/Lubricant	PRN	$10.00/btl (1 spray prn)	Allergic reaction	Immediate	—	May also try sour candy if patient has functioning salivary glands.
Artificial Tears (Lytears)	Dry Eyes/Lubricant	PRN	$3.60/btl (2 gtts prn)	Eye irritation, blurred vision	Immediate	—	
Aspirin (Aspirin)	Antiplatelet, Nociceptive Pain, Fever/Salicylate	81–325 mg po daily-cardiac;325–650 mg q4-6h (4000 mg/day)	$0.05 (81 mg po daily)	GI irritation, rash, bleeding, nausea, vomiting	5–40 min	2–3 h	Enteric coated preferred. Watch for signs of bleeding. Avoid in children: can cause Reyes Syndrome
Atenolol (Tenormin)	Cardiovascular/Beta Blocker	25–100 mg daily	$0.15 (100 mg daily)	Hypotension, chest pain, dizziness, confusion, cold extremities, Raynaud's phenomenon, impotence, constipation, diarrhea, nausea	2–4 h	6–9 h	Abrupt discontinuation can cause rebound hypertension.

*Drugs in Italics: Not generally recommended in hospice patients
**MDD = Maximun Daily Dose
***BOLD-not available as a generic

Drug Information Table

Generic (Example of Trade)*	Indication/Drug Class	Dosage Range (MDD**)	2007 Avg. Cost/Day for Therapy (Dose for Cost Comparison)***	Adverse Effects	Onset to Peak	T1/2	Comments
Atropine (Isopto Atropine)	Secretions, Bowel Obstruction/ Anticholinergic	2–4 drops q2–4h; 0.3–1.2 mg IV/IM/SQ q4h prn (3 mg/day)	$9.00/15mL (0.4 mg q4h)	Dry mouth, blurred vision, mydriasis, constipation, dry skin, headache, restlessness, delirium, tachycardia	Rapid	2–3 h	First line therapy for terminal secretions. Ophthalmic solution given SL acts rapidly and can be titrated easily. Sal-Tropine tablets expensive. Administered sublingually. Use caution when administering drops to avoid potential overdose.
Azithromycin (Zithromax)	Infection (Respiratory)/ Macrolide	500 mg on day 1, then 250 mg × 4 days	$48.35/ course (500 mg day 1, 250 mg daily × 4 days)	Diarrhea, headache, nausea, vomiting, abdominal pain	2–5 h	59–72 h	Most common bacteria not sensitive to Z Pak.
Baclofen (Lioresal)	Hiccups, Muscle Spasms/Muscle Relaxant	10–20 mg BID-TID (60 mg/day)	$1.10 (10 mg TID)	Drowsiness, vertigo, ataxia, hypotonia, weakness, confusion, hypotension, rash	15–45 min	20–50 h	Can cause considerable drowsiness. When muscle relaxation is needed. Antispastic class. Most commonly used agent.
Beclomethasone (Vanceril, Qvar)	Respiratory/Inhaled Corticosteroid	1–4 puffs BID (8 puffs/day)	$78.75/MDI (2 puffs BID)	Headache, rhinitis, sinusitis, cough, pharyngitis, URI, oral candidiasis	1–2 h	36–54 h	Oral corticosteroids provide greater symptom relief in end stage disease. Use with caution in diabetics. (Also used for other symptoms-inflammation, pain, mood, breathing, brain metastases, N/V, anorexia).
Belladonna + Opium (B & O Suppositories)	Bladder Spasms/ Anticholinergic/Opioid Combination	1 supp q6–12h (4 doses/day)	$13.00 (16A supp q6h)	Palpitation, dizziness, drowsiness, pruritus, urinary retention, blurred vision, nausea, vomiting, constipation, dry mouth	—	—	Expensive. Hard to find. Use an oral anticholinergic and opioid as an alternative.
Benzonatate (Tessalon Perles)	Cough Suppressant/ Anesthetic	100–200 mg po TID or 100 mg q4h prn (600 mg/day)	$3.40 (200 mg TID)	Sedation, headache, dizziness, brochospasm	15–20 min	—	Do not pierce capsules. Swallow whole, do not crush or chew.

Drug	Indication/Class	Dose	Cost	Side Effects	Onset	Half-life	Comments
Benztropine (Cogentin)	Parkinson's, EPS Symptoms/ Anticholinergics	0.5–2 mg daily-BID (6 mg/day)	$0.45 (1 mg BID)	Dry mouth, constipation, urinary retention, tachycardia, confusion, nausea, vomiting	po 1 h; I.V. 15 min	—	Second line to diphenhydramine for treatment of EPS.
Betamethasone (Diprolene)	Pruritus, Rash/Topical Corticosteroid	Apply BID-QID	$10.00/tube (Apply BID)	Allergic dermatitis, burning, dry skin, striae, pruritus, irritation, hypertrichosis, skin atrophy	10–36 min	6.5 h	More expensive than hydrocortisone cream.
Bethanechol (Urecholine)	Urinary Retention/ Cholinergic	10–50 mg BID-QID	$4.00 (10 mg QID)	Abdominal cramps, nausea, diarrhea, changes in vision, watery eyes, headaches, sweating, flushing, or increased saliva	30–90 min	Unknown	Can cause excessive salivation.
Bicalutamide (Casodex)	Prostate Cancer/ Antineoplastic	50–150 mg daily	**$14.15 (50 mg daily)**	Hot flashes, pain, edema, constipation, nausea, diarrhea, abdominal pain, nocturia, hematuria, weakness, anemia, dyspnea, infection	31 h	6 days	Generally not appropriate in hospice patients. Must be palliating a symptom and have monitoring guidelines (PPS). Recommend discontinuing when out of current supply.
Bisacodyl (Dulcolax)	Constipation/Stimulant Laxative	5–30 mg daily (30 mg/day)	$1.20 (10 mg daily)	Diarrhea, nausea, vomiting, abdominal cramps, alkalosis, electrolyte disorders	6–8 h	Unknown	Use suppository as a supplement to oral route. May be used with a stool softener. Suppositories may be poorly effective if rectum full of stool.
Bismuth Subsalicylate (Kaopectate)	Diarrhea/Absorbent	30–120mL po after each loose stool (2096 mg/day)	$2.40 (30mL QID)	Blackened tongue, grayish black stools, constipation, tinnitus	Variable	Variable	Give 1 hr before or 2 hours after other medications. Caution with concomitant aspirin; impaction may occur in debilitated patients. May turn stool dark or black in color. Do not use in immunocompromised patients due to risk of bismuth encephalopathy.
Bromocriptine (Parlodel)	Parkinson's/Dopamine Agonist	1.25–5 mg BID-TID	$4.10 (2.5 mg BID)	Hypotension, headache, dizziness, nausea, vomiting, constipation, drowsiness, GI bleeding, nasal congestion	1–2 h	Initial: 6–8 h; terminal: 50 h	

*Drugs in Italics: Not generally recommended in hospice patients
**MDD = Maximum Daily Dose
***BOLD-not available as a generic

Drug Information Table

Generic (Example of Trade)*	Indication/Drug Class	Dosage Range (MDD**)	2007 Avg. Cost/Day for Therapy (Dose for Cost Comparison)***	Adverse Effects	Onset to Peak	T1/2	Comments
Budesonide (Pulmicort Respules)	Dyspnea/Inhaled Corticosteroid	250 mcg/2mL BID (1440 mcg/day)	$11.00 (250 mcg/2mL BID)	Headache, nausea, respiratory infection, oral candidiasis, nausea, vomiting, diarrhea	0.5–10 h	2–3.6 h	Oral corticosteroids provide greater symptom relief in end stage disease Use with caution in diabetics. Oral corticosteroids can also be used for other symptoms-inflammation, pain, mood, breathing, brain metastases, N/V, anorexia.
Bumetanide (Bumex)	Fluid Retention/Loop Diuretic	0.5–5 mg daily-BID (10 mg/day)	$0.65 (2 mg daily)	Hyperuricemia, hypochloremia, hypokalemia, azotemia, hyponatremia, hyperglycemia	0.5–1 h	1–1.5 h	More complete oral absorption than furosemide.
Calcium Carbonate (Tums)	Gastritis/Antacid	1–2 tabs q4h (7000 mg/day)	$0.20 (1 tab q4h)	Headache, hypophosphatemia, hypercalcemia, constipation, abdominal pain	—	—	Frequent use leads to rebound hyperacidity.
Calcium polycarbophil (Fibercon)	Constipation/Bulking Agent	2 tablets (1 gm) daily-QID (6 gm/day)	$0.25 (2 caps)daily	Bloating, diarrhea, nausea, abdominal cramps	—	—	Epigastric pain and bloating may occur with large doses.
Camphor/Menthol (Sarna)	Pruritus/Emollient	Apply as needed	$10.00 /bottle	Burning sensation	—	—	Good for pruritus due hepatic failure, renal failure, and opioids. Available over the counter.
Capecitabine (Xeloda)	Cancer/Antineoplastic Antimetabolite	2500 mg/m2 × 2 weeks	$45.90 (2gms daily)	Edema, fatigue, pain, palmar-plantar erythodysesthesia, dermatitis, diarrhea, vomiting, stomatitis, lymphopenia, anemia, thrombocytopenia, neutropenia, parasthesia, eye irritation, dyspnea	1.5 h	0.5–1 h	Generally not appropriate in hospice patients.

Drug	Classification/Use	Dosage	Cost	Side Effects	Onset	Half-life	Comments
Capsaicin (Zostrix)	Neuropathic Pain/Topical Analgesic	Apply as needed	$16.00/tube	Itching, stinging, erythema	14–28 days, peak effect 4–6 weeks	—	Start with 0.025% cream or liquid to develop tolerance to burning. Use gloves or wash carefully after use. Apply only to intact skin. Do not allow contact with mucous membrane or eyes.
Captopril (Capoten)	Cardiovascular/ACE Inhibitors	6.25–50 mg TID (450 mg/day)	$0.55 (25 mg TID)	Hypotension, rash, hyperkalemia, tahcycardia	1–1.5 h	Renal and cardiac dependent	Best if short acting agent is desired. Dry cough and angioedema side effects. No significant difference between ACE Inhibitors.
Carbamazepine (Tegretol)	Neuropathic Pain, Seizures, Hiccups/Anticonvulsant.	200–400 mg TID-QID; 600–1200 mg/day (1600 mg/day)	$0.95 (200 mg QID)	Dizziness, drowsiness, nausea/vomiting/blurred vision, rash	Unpredictable	12–17 h	Sustained release forms not available genereically. Well absorbed rectally.
Carisoprodol (Soma)	Muscle Spasm/Muscle Relaxant	350 mg QID (1400 mg/day)	$1.40 (350 mg TID)	Drowsiness, dizziness, hypotension, irritability, flushing, angioedema	30 min	2.4 h	Sedative/hyponotic class; Reports of increased abuse potential with this agent.
Carvedilol (Coreg)	Cardiovascular/Beta Blocker	3.125–50 mg BID (100 mg/day)	$3.20 (6.25 mg daily)	Hypotension, dizziness, hyperglycemia, weight gain, fatigue, bradycardia	1–2 h	7–10 h	Expensive. All dosage strengths cost the same. Abrupt discontinuation can cause rebound hypertension.
Cefaclor (Ceclor)	Infection (Respiratory)/Cephalosporin	250–500 mg q8h × 10–14 days	$42.00/course (500 mg q8h × 10 days)	Rash, diarrhea, vaginitis, eosinophilia, moniliasis, transaminases increased	45–60 min	0.5–1 h	Sustained release forms not available genereically.
Cefpodoxime (Vantin)	Infection (Respiratory)/Cephalosporin	200 mg q12h × 14 days	$69.00/course (200 mg q12h × 7 days)	Rash, diarrhea, nausea, vomiting, vaginal infection	1 h	2.2 h	Expensive.
Cefuroxime Axetil (Ceftin)	Infection (Respiratory)/Cephalosporin	250–500 mg q12h × 10 days (6 gms/day)	$120/course (500 mg q12h × 10 days)	Alkaline phosphatase increased, eosinophilia, transaminases increased, anemia	I.M.: 15–60 min; I.V.: 2–3 min	1–2 h	Expensive.
Celecoxib (Celebrex)	Nociceptive, Bone Pain/COX II NSAID	100–400 mg daily-BID (400 mg/day)	$5.35 (200 mg BID)	Headache, dyspepsia, diarrhea, abdominal pain, edema, URI, MI	10 min–3 h	6–9 h	Expensive. Potential sulfa allergy contraindication. Renal toxicity equal to mixed Cox II agents.

*Drugs in Italics: Not generally recommended in hospice patients
**MDD = Maximun Daily Dose
***BOLD-not available as a generic

Drug Information Table

Generic (Example of Trade)*	Indication/Drug Class	Dosage Range (MDD**)	2007 Avg. Cost/Day for Therapy (Dose for Cost Comparison)***	Adverse Effects	Onset to Peak	T1/2	Comments
Cephalexin (Keflex)	Infection (Skin, UTI)/Cephalosporin	250–1000 mg QID × 10–14 days; 250–500 mg po TID -QID × 7 days (4 gms/day)	$15.00/course (500 mg TID × 10 days)	Diarrhea, nausea, vomiting, rash, dizziness, headache	1 h	0.5–1.2 h	
Cetirizine (Zyrtec)	Pruritus/Antihistamine	5–10 mg daily (10 mg/day)	$2.00 (10 mg daily)	Headache, somnolence, insomnia, dry mouth, fatigue	15–60 min	8 h	Expensive. Minimal sedation.
Cevimeline (Evoxac)	Xerostomia/Cholinergic	30 mg TID (90 mg/day)	$5.85 (30 mg TID)	Nausea, vomiting, diarrhea, URI, diaphoresis, UTI, myalgia	1.5–2 h	5 h	No further efficacy shown with 60 mg TID; similar side effects as pilocarpine. Expensive #90 30 mg capsules ~$150.
Chloral Hydrate (Noctec)	Insomnia/Hypnotic	250–2000 mg QHS (2 gms/day)	$0.20 (500 mg QHS)	GI problems, rash, sedation, lightheadedness, confusion, eosinophilia, paradoxical excitation	0.5–1 h	8–11 h	Alternative to typical hypnotic agents. Use caution not to exceed recommended dose.
Chlorpromazine (Thorazine)	Anxiety, Delirium, Agitation, Nausea & Vomiting (Chemoreceptor Trigger Zone), Hiccups/Neuroleptic	10–50 mg q4–8h (600 mg/day)	$1.20 (25 mg q6h)	Drowsiness, dizziness, nasal congestion, blurred vision, dry mouth, or constipation, inability to move eyes; muscle spasms of face, neck, or back; difficulty swallowing; mask-like face; tremors of hands; restlessness; tension in legs; shuffling walk or stiff arms or legs; puffing of cheeks; lip smacking or puckering; twitching or twisting movements; or weakness of arms or legs	10–20 min	8–35 h	Use when sedation is desired. More sedating than haloperidol. Also used for other symptoms- N/V, agitation, delirium, hallucinations. Use with caution in ambulatory patients. Orthostatic hypotension. Centrally mediated hiccups. Only drug with FDA indication for hiccups. May cause EPS.

Drug	Indication/Class	Dose (MDD**)	Cost	Side Effects			Comments
Chlorzoxazone (Parafon forte)	Muscle Spasm/Muscle Relaxant	500 mg QID (3000 mg/day)	$0.70 (500 mg QID)	Drowsiness, dizziness, GI upset, paradoxical stimulation, malaise	1 h	—	Sedative/hypnotic class; Not routinely recommended; Rare hepatotoxicity.
Cholesterol Lowering Agents (Lipitor, Zocor, Lescol, Crestor, Mevacor, Niacin, Pravachol, Advicor	Cardiovascular/ Hyperlipidemia	Various	Average cost for all products $4.00	Muscle pain, liver toxicity	—	—	Never appropriate for hospice to cover these agents. Can cause muscle pain.
Cholestyramine (Questran)	Diarrhea, Pruritus, Hyperlipidemia/Bile Salt Binder	4gm daily-QID (24 gms/day)	$1.00 (4gms BID)	Constipation, heartburn, nausea, vomiting, stomach pain, bloating, diarrhea, headache	21 days	—	Constipating. Recommend giving sorbitol concomitantly; Effective in controlling chologenic (bile salt) or radiation-induced diarrhea.
Choline Magnesium Trisalicylate (Trilisate)	Nociceptive, Bone Pain/Salicylate	750–1500 mg bid (4.5 gms/day)	$2.40 (750 mg BID)	Nausea, vomiting, diarrhea, heartburn, dyspepsia, epigastric pain, constipation, tinnitus	5–40 min	2–3 h	Not as effective as other NSAIDS but less GI upset Can use with coumadin. Monitor for tinnitus. Less platelet aggregation than other NSAIDS. Salicylate derivative.
Cimetidine (Tagamet)	Gastritis/H2 Antagonist	150–400 mg BID-QID (1600 mg/day)	$.0.60 (300 mg BID)	Headache, dizziness, somnolence, agitation, gynecomastia, diarrhea	1 h	2 h	Not recommended due to high incidence of drug interactions.
Ciprofloxacin (Cipro)	Infection (Skin, UTI, Respiratory)/Quinolone	250–750 mg q12h 7–14 days, UTI—100–500 mg po bid × 3–14 days	$99.35/course (500 mg q12h × 10 days); $10.44/ course (100 mg daily × 3 days)	Nausea, diarrhea, QT prolongation,tremor, restlessness, confusion	0.5–2 h	2.5 h	Expensive. Adjust dose and frequency for renal insufficiency; Uncomplicated UTI—100 mg daily × 3 days usually sufficient.

*Drugs in Italics: Not generally recommended in hospice patients
**MDD = Maximun Daily Dose
***BOLD-not available as a generic

Drug Information Table

Generic (Example of Trade)*	Indication/Drug Class	Dosage Range (MDD**)	2007 Avg. Cost/Day for Therapy (Dose for Cost Comparison)***	Adverse Effects	Onset to Peak	T1/2	Comments
Citalopram (Celexa)	Depression, Anxiety/ Serotonin Reuptake Inhibitor	20–60 mg daily (60 mg/day)	$2.25 (40 mg daily)	GI upset, insomnia, headache, jitteriness, sexual dysfuntion	4 h	24–48 h	Onset of effect in 3–4 weeks. May be especially useful if expected survival is more than a few weeks; Slow onset of action for anxiety (like time course for antidepressant effects). May worsen anxiety in the first few days to a week of therapy-consider co-administration of a benzodiazepine in the short term. Read prescribing information for Cytochrome P-450 system mediated drug interactions. Not constipating; low liability for precipitating delirium.
Clarithromycin (Biaxin)	Infection (Respiratory)/ Macrolide	250–500 mg BID or 1000 mg XL daily × 7–14 days,	**$76.00/course (500 mg BID × 10 days)**	Headache, rash, dyspepsia, nausea, vomiting, diarrhea, BUN increased, metalic taste	2–3 h	3–7 h	
Clindamycin (Cleocin)	Infection (Respiratory)/ Lincosamide	300–600 mg q8h × 7–10 days (1.8 gms/day)	$56.00/course (300 mg q8h × 7 days)	Diarrhea, abdominal pain, hypotension, rash, Stevens-Johnson syndrome, Pseudomembranous colitis	1–3 h	2–3 h	
Clonazepam (Klonopin)	Anxiety, Seizures/ Benzodiazepine	0.5–1 mg q8–12h Max dose: 2 mg TID (20 mg/day)	$1.15 (0.5 mg q8h)	Drowsiness, ataxia, confusion, impaired memory, rash, visual changes	20–60 min	19–50 h	Longer acting than alprazolam or lorazepam. No oral solution available. Alternative to diazepam for maintenance therapy; Active metabolites may accumulate and contribute to sedation; Can split 0.5 mg tablet in half for 0.25 mg dose. Most useful in absence of seizures and myoclonus.

Drug	Indication/Class	Dose	Cost	Side Effects	Onset	Half-life	Comments
Clonidine (Catapres)	Hypertension/Alpha 2 Agonist	0.1 mg BID; 0.1 mg/day transdermal q7 days (0.8 mg/day 40 mcg/hr)	$0.40 (0.1 mg po BID)	Dry mouth, drowsiness, dizziness, constipation, sedation, weakness, orthostatic hypotension, headache	1–5 min	9±2 h	Avoid transdermal patch. Tablets more cost effective and titratable. Useful as prn for episodes of elevated BP> Monitor for hypotension.
Clopidogrel (Plavix)	Cardiovascular/ Antiplatelet	75 mg daily	**$3.60 (75 mg daily)**	Abdominal cramps, vomiting, gastritis, constipation, bleeding events, chest pain, general pain, rash, pruritus, dizziness, URI	2 h—2 days depending on dose	8 h	No significant benefits in prevention of thromboembolic events over aspirin 325 mg alone in end stage disease.
Clortrimazole 1% (Lotrimin)	Fungal Rash/Topical/ Antifungal	Apply BID	$9.50/tube (Apply BID)	Irritation, burning, stinging	8–24 h	—	
Clotrimazole (Mycelex)	Infection(Thrush)/ Antifungal	Dissolve one toche(10 mg) bucally 5 times daily for 10–14 days	$73.60/course (5x a day for 10 days)	Abnormal LFTs, nausea, vomiting, abdominal cramps	3–4 h	—	Not first line.
Codeine	Diarrhea, Cough, Nociceptive Pain/Opioid	10–60 mg BID-QID		Drowsiness, sedation, constipation, nausea, vomiting, sweating, rash, disorientation	0.5–1.5 h	2.5–3.5 h	Not recommended in patients with bacterial diarrhea. Acetaminophen with codeine may be used instead of pure codeine (CII) for cost and ease of prescribing. Codeine is more constipating than other opioids and may cause more CNS and GI side effects.
Codeine-APAP (Tylenol #2, 3, 4)	Nociceptive Pain/ Opioid/Non-opioid Pain Combination	1–2 tabs q4h (Acetaminophen 4000 mg/day; geriatrics 3000 mg/day)	$3.20 (#3 2 tabs q4h)	Constipation, nausea & vomiting, confusion, sedation	See individual agents	See individual agents	More constipating than oxycodone or hydrocodone combinations. Do not exceed 4 grams of acetaminophen per day. Avoid other medications, including OTCs that contain acetaminophen. Schedule III controlled substance (Acetaminophen + Codeine 15 mg is Schedule IV). Weak opioid.

*Drugs in Italics: Not generally recommended in hospice patients
**MDD = Maximun Daily Dose
***BOLD-not available as a generic

Drug Information Table

Generic (Example of Trade)*	Indication/Drug Class	Dosage Range (MDD**)	2007 Avg. Cost/Day for Therapy (Dose for Cost Comparison)***	Adverse Effects	Onset to Peak	T1/2	Comments
Cyclobenzaprine (Flexeril)	Muscle Spasm/Muscle Relaxant	5–10 mg TID (60 mg/day)	$0.80 (10 mg TID)	Drowsiness, dizziness, dry mouth	15–45 min	20–50 h	Not recommended. Extremely sedating and less effective than diazepam. Sedative/hypnotic class; Similar to tricyclic antidepressants.
Cyproheptidine (Periactin)	Anorexia, Pruritus/ Antihistamine	2–20 mg PO daily; Initial 4–8 mg PO TID; (0.5 mg/kg/day)	$0.99 (4 mg TID)	Drowsiness, thickening of bronchial secretions, dry mouth, dizziness, fatigue, nausea, abdominal pain	—	—	For anorexia if corticosteroids not appropriate. Clinical efficacy not established.
Dantrolene (Dantrium)	Fever, Muscle Spasms/ Muscle Relaxant	1–2.5 mg/kg IV every 6 hours or 4 to 8 mg/kg/day orally, in four divided doses should be administered for 1–3 days following a malignant hyperthermia crisis (400 mg/day)	$5.90 (100 mg QID)	Drowsiness, dizziness, fatigue, rash, nausea, vomiting, diarrhea, nervousness, chills, blurred vision, respiratory depression	—	8.7 h	For fever > 41.5°C (106°F) unresponsive to NSAIDs or acetaminophen.
Darbepoetin (Aranesp)	Anemia/Colony Stimulating Factor	200–300 mcg/kg every 2–4 weeks	**$1000/dose (200 mcg)**	HTN, hypotension, edema, fatigue, fever, headache, dizziness, diarrhea, constipation, vomiting, nausea, myalgia, arthralgia, infection	24–72 h; Cancer: 71–90 h	I.V.: 21 h; SubQ: 49 h Cancer SubQ: 74 h	Recommend prior authorization by medical director. Generally not appropriate in hospice patients. Must be palliating a symptom and have monitoring guidelines.

| Desipramine (Norpramin) | Neuropathic Pain, Depression/Tricyclic Antidepressant | 25–150 mg QHS or in divided doses (150 mg/day) | $0.45 (150 mg QHS) | Drowsiness, jaundice, hypotensin, agitation, dry mouth, constipation, urinary retention, tachycardia | 4–6 h | 7–60 h | Onset of analgesia in about 7 days. Less severe side effects compared to amitriptyline. Start low & titrate slowly. Greater side effect burden compared to Serotonin Reuptake Inhibitors. Effective for neuropathic pain. Can be used to stimulate appetite. Desipramine is the least sedating tricyclic. Can increase dose for antidepressant effect if on for other indications. Optimal effect in 4–6 weeks. |
| Dexamethasone (Decadron) | Bone Pain, Visceral Pain, Pruritus, Seizures, Respiratory Inflammation, Increased Intracranial Pressure, Bowel Obstruction/ Corticosteroid | 4–8 mg daily-QID (32 mg/day) | $1.20 (8 mg BID) | GI upset, adrenal insufficiency, steroid psychosis, hyperglycemia | 1–2 h | 36–54 h | Doses may be titrated up to 32 mg/day; the most comprehensively studied of the corticosteroids in palliative care; Indicated when short term therapy may be beneficial; also useful in the conditions of bone pain or broncospasms. Long term effects must be considered but the initation of therapy should not be delayed because of undue concerns about adverse effects of prolonged use. Given over 5–10 minutes, rapid IV bolus associated with perianal pain. Has less mineralocorticoid effect than prednisone. First line therapy in seizures related to brain tumor, metastases, or increased intracranial pressure from other causes. May give dose once daily or BID (morning and noon) to prevent insomnia. |

*Drugs in Italics: Not generally recommended in hospice patients
**MDD = Maximun Daily Dose
***BOLD-not available as a generic

Drug Information Table

Generic (Example of Trade)*	Indication/Drug Class	Dosage Range (MDD**)	2007 Avg. Cost/Day for Therapy (Dose for Cost Comparison)***	Adverse Effects	Onset to Peak	T1/2	Comments
Dextroamphetamine (Dexadrine)	Depression, Excessive Sedation/ Psychostimulants	2.5–10 mg qAM—BID (last dose before 2pm) (60 mg/day)	($0.75) 5 mg BID	Palpitations restlessness, insomnia, tachycardia, hypertension, hallucinations	1–3hrs	10–13 h	Good choice for depression if patient has less than 2–3 weeks to live. Onset of action immediately. Can use in combination with Serotonin Reuptake Inhibitor. Depression is an off-label indication. Drug of choice in hospice (among patients who can tolerate stimulants) due to no lag time to effect. Counteract opiate-induced sedation. May worsen/precipitate delirum. May induce tolerance, withdrawl depression with prolonged use. Exhibits synergistic analgesia with opiates.
Dextromethorphan (Delsym)	Cough/Antitussive	30 mg q6–8h 120 mg/day	$1.20 (30 mg q6h)	Sedation, dizziness, rash, serotonin syndrome	15–30 m	—	If dextromethorphan is not effective, use hydrocodone cough preparation instead.
Diazepam (Valium)	Seizures/Acute; Anxiety, Muscle Spasms, Dyspnea/Benzodiazepine	2–10 mg q6–12h ;10 mg q15min up to 40 mg/ seizure episode (60 mg/day)	$1.00 (10 mg × 4 doses-seizure abortive dose; 5 mg q8h)	Drowsiness, ataxia, fatigue, confusion, depression	15–45 min	20–50 h; active metabolite 50–100 h	Diastat Rectal Gel unnecessary and extremely expensive. Diazepam has the quickest onset of action among benzodiazepines. Tablets well absorbed PO/SL/PR. Most cost effective benzodiazepine Intensol. Long t 1/2. Dose no more frequently than every 6–8 hours and every 12–24 hours in geriatric patients. Not generally accepted in LTC facilities. Useful for other symptoms anxiety, insomnia, seizures, dyspnea. Tablets or oral liquid well absorbed PO/SL/PR; Benzodiazepines not

first line in delirium and can worsen delirium. Use only in combination with neuroleptics; Long-acting; active metabolites may accumulate and contribute to sedation. Benzodiazepines can decrease anxiety associated with breathlessness, however should be reserved as second line after opioids. Begin with low doses and titrate to effect. Breakthrough doses may be necessary to settle dyspnea. Can be used together with opioids with careful titration of each agent. Longer acting agents are preferred for the treatment of dyspnea to avoid pronounced peak and trough effects that could lead to rebound anxiety. Can repeat dose every 15 minutes until seizure subsides.

Diclofenac (Voltaren)	Nociceptive, Bone Pain/ Mixed COX NSAID	50 mg BID-TID: (150 mg/day)	$2.85 (50 mg BID)	Dyspepsia, nausea, abdominal pain, fluid retention, tinnitus, rash, GI bleed, acute renal failure, constipation, headache, dirrhea, flatulance	1–2 hrs	—	No benefit over ibuprofen.
Dicloxacillin (Dynapen)	Infection (Respiratory, Skin)/Penicillin	250–500 mg q6h 10–14 days	$17.60/course (500 mg q6h × 10 days)	Nausea, diarrhea, abdominal pain	1 h	0.75–1.5 h	
Dicyclomine (Bentyl)	Nausea & Vomiting, GI Spasm, Cramping, Visceral Pain/ Anticholinergic	10–40 mg q6h (160 mg/day)	$1.20 (20 mg q6h)	Constipation			Only PO available. Not recommended in the elderly.

*Drugs in Italics: Not generally recommended in hospice patients
**MDD = Maximun Daily Dose
***BOLD-not available as a generic

Drug Information Table

Generic (Example of Trade)*	Indication/Drug Class	Dosage Range (MDD**)	2007 Avg. Cost/Day for Therapy (Dose for Cost Comparison)***	Adverse Effects	Onset to Peak	T1/2	Comments
Digoxin (Lanoxin)	Cardiovascular/Cardiac Glycosides	0.125–0.25 mg QOD-daily (0.5 mg/day)	$0.30 (0.125 mg daily)	Heart block, visual disturbances, headache, dizziness, confusion, anxiety, hallucinations, rash, nausea, vomiting, diarrhea, weakness	2–8 hrs	38–48 hrs	Monitor for toxicity (Nausea, visual changes yellow halos). Narrow therapeutic index. Consider discontinuing as patient declines.
Diltiazem (Cardizen)	Cardiovascular/Calcium Channel Blocker	30–120 mg QID (360 mg/day)	$0.70 (60 mg QID)	Edema, headache, heart block, dizziness, nervousness,	2–4 hrs	3–4.5 hrs	Do not crush sustained release form. Constipating. Suggest discontinuing.
Diphenhydramine (Benadryl)	Anxiety, Parkinsonianism, Pruritus, Insomnia/Antihistamine	25 mg–100 mg q 4–6h (400 mg/day)	$0.60 (25 mg q4h)	Somnolence, dry mouth, headache, dizziness	1/4–4 h	2–8 h	Sedating antihistamine. Use cautiously in ambulatory geriatric patients. Also used for other symptoms—anxiety, insomia, itch, EPS reversal.
Diphenoxylate/Atropine (Lomotil)	Diarrhea/Hypomotility	2 tabs now then 1 tab after each loose stool (max 8 tabs/day) (20 mg/day)	$2.95 (1 tab qid)	Tachycardia, confusion, depression, dizziness, edema, dry skin, urinary retention, numbness, abdominal discomfort	2 hrs	2.5 hrs/12–14 hrs	May be more effective than loperamide if stools are watery. Not recommended in patients with bacterial diarrhea.
Dipyridamole (Persantine—Not Aggrenox)	Cardiac/Antiplatelet	25–100 mg TID-QID (60 mg/day)	$0.40 (25 mg TID)	Dizziness, headache, abdominal distention	2–2.5 hrs	10–12 hrs	Aggrenox approx = dipyridamole 50 mg QID + Aspirin 81 mg daily: Efficacy alone questionable.
Divalproex Na (Depakote)	Neuropathic Pain, Agitation, Seizures/Anticonvulsant	500–1000 mg daily (60 mg/kg/day)	$7.20 (1000 mg daily)	Somnolence, dizziness, insomnia, nervousness, alopecia, nausea, vomiting, diarrhea, abdominal pain, anorexia, tremor, weakness	2–4 h	10–25 h	Can give once daily. Also beneficial for aggressive behavior. Sprinkle dosage form may be desirable.

Drug	Indication/Class	Dose (MDD**)	Cost	Side Effects	Onset	Half-life	Notes
Docusate (Colace)	Constipation/Stool Softener	100–200 mg daily-QID (500 mg/day)	$0.60 (100 mg BID)	Bitter taste, abdominal cramps diarrhea	24–72 h	Unknown	Not sufficient without stimulant if patient is on an opioid. Must be used with adequate fluid intake to maximize benefit.
Docusate Sodium 50 mg/senna 187 mg tablet (Senokot-S)	Constipation/Stool Softener/Stimulant Combination	1–2 PO daily to BID (500 mg/100 mg/day)	$0.60 (1 BID)	Nausea, diarrhea, abdominal pain	—	—	Combination is more expensive than dosing components separetely.
Dolasetron (Anzemet)	Nausea & Vomiting/ 5HT3 Antagonist Antiemetic	50–100 mg daily	**$55.00/50 mg tab**	Headache, diarrhea	IV: 0.6hr, PO: 1hr	10 min. & 4–6 hrs (metabolite)	Expensive. Recommended alternative: Metoclopramide 20 mg q4–6h + Haloperidol 1 mg q4hprn. Primarily beneficial for chemotherapy-induced Nausea & Vomiting, not as effective in other types of Nausea & Vomiting.
Donepezil (Aricept)	Dementia/ Cholinesterase Inhibitors	5–10 mg daily (10 mg/day)	**$5.00 (10 mg daily)**	Insomnia, nausea, diarrhea, headache, dizziness, abnormal dreams, hostility	3–4 hrs	70 hrs	May not be beneficial in end-stage dementia. Can cause GI side effects.
Doxazosin (Cardura)	Cardiac, Urinary Hesitancy/Alpha Blocker	Cardiac: 1–16 mg daily; GU: 1 mg daily (Cardiac: 16 mg/daily; GU: 8 mg/day)	$1.20 (4 mg daily)	Dizziness, orthostasis, edema, flushing, fatigue, UTI, impotence	2–3 hrs	15–22 hrs	Only covered for GU in patients with prostate cancer who are not catheterized. Monitor for hypotension.
Doxepin (Sinequan)	Pruritus, Depression, Neuropathic Pain/ Tricyclic Antidepressant	10–50 mg QHS or in divided doses; 25–300 mg QHS or in divided doses; 25–150 mg QHS or in divided doses (150 mg/day)	$0.30 (25 mg QHS)	Hypo/hypertension, tachycardia, drowsiness, dizziness, headache, disorientation, alopecia, urinary retention, blurred vision	7–8 1/2 h	28–31 h	Not first line agent. Can increase dose for antidepressant effect if taking for other indications. Optimal effect in 4–6 weeks. Onset of analgesia in about 7 days. Less severe side effects compared to amitriptyline. Start low & titrate slowly. Potent antihistamine (H1 and H2) activity. Often effective for puritus at doses well below antidepressant dose.

*Drugs in Italics: Not generally recommended in hospice patients
**MDD = Maximun Daily Dose
***BOLD-not available as a generic

Drug Information Table

Generic (Example of Trade)*	Indication/Drug Class	Dosage Range (MDD**)	2007 Avg. Cost/Day for Therapy (Dose for Cost Comparison)***	Adverse Effects	Onset to Peak	T1/2	Comments
Doxycycline Hyclate (Vibramycin)	Infection (Respiratory)/ Tetracycline	100 mg BID 7–14 days	$9.00/course (100 mg BID × 10 days)	Photosensitivity, diarrhea, vomiting	1.5–4 hrs	12–15 hrs	
Dronabinol (Marinol)	Anorexia, Nausea & Vomiting/Cannabinoid	2.5–10 mg 1h ac BID; initial 2.5 mg PO daily; (20 mg/day)	$23.70 (5 mg TID)	Dysphoria	1/2–4 h	25–36 h	Clinical superiority not established in end-of-life care; Sometimes causes intolerable CNS side effects such as dysphoria or euphoria.
Enalapril (Vasotec)	Cardiovascular/ACE Inhibitors	2.5–20 mg BID	$0.75 (5 mg BID)	Hypotension, chest pain, headache, dizziness, fatigue, abnormal taste, increased creatinine	0.5–1.5 hrs	2–6 hrs	Dry cough and angioedema side effects. No significant difference between ACE Inhibitors.
Epoetin (Procrit, Epogen)	Anemia/Colony Stimulating Factor	40,000–60,000 Units weekly	$550.00/weekly (40,000 Units weekly)	Hypertension, fever, dizziness, insomnia, headache, nausea, vomiting, diarrhea	5–24 hrs	—	Recommend prior authorization by medical director. Generally not appropriate in hospice patients. Must be palliating a symptom and have monitoring guidelines.
Erlotinib (Tarceva)	Lung Cancer/ Antineoplastic	150 mg daily	$112.00 (150 mg daily)	Edema, fatigue, anxiety, rash, dry skin, bone pain, myalgia, cough	1–7 hrs	24–36 hrs	Recommend prior authorization by medical director. Generally not appropriate in hospice patients. Must be palliating a symptom and have monitoring guidelines.
Erythromycin (E-Mycin, Erytab)	Infection (Respiratory, Skin) N&V (Gastric Stasis)/Macrolide	250–500 mg QID 10–14 days (4 gms/day)	$10.00/course (250 mg QID 3 10 days)	Abdominal pain, diarrhea	4 h	1–3 h	Beneficial for gastric stasis if patient cannot tolerate metoclopramide due to EPS. No EPS. Good for Parkinson's gastroparesis.
Escitalopram (Lexapro)	Depression/Serotonin Reuptake Inhibitor	10–20 mg daily (20 mg/day)	$2.10 (10 mg daily)	Headache, nausea	5 hrs	27–32 hrs	Onset of effect in 3 weeks. All doses of tablets cost about the same; Reliability of reputed faster onset of action unclear.

Drug	Class/Use	Dose	Cost	Side Effects			Comments
Esomeprazole (Nexium)	Gastritis/Proton Pump Inhibitor	20–40 mg daily-BID	**$4.00 (20 mg daily)**	Headache, dizziness	1.5 hrs	1–1.5 hrs	Drug of choice is Prilosec OTC. Evaluate the need to continue. Can step down to H2. All PPIs have similar efficacy: 40 mg costs the same as 20 mg.
Estazolam (Prosom)	Insomnia/ Benzodiazepine	0.5–2 mg QHS	$0.85 (1 mg QHS)	Somnolence, weakness	0.5–1.6 hrs	10–24 hrs	Short duration of action. Not recommended.
Exemestane (Aromasin)	Cancer/Antineoplastic, Aromatase Inactivator	25 mg daily	**$8.40 (25 mg daily)**	Hypertension, fatigue, insomnia, hot flases	1.2 hrs	24 hrs	
Famotidine (Pepcid)	GI/2 Antagonists; Dysphagia	10–40 mg daily-BID	$1.35 (20 mg BID)	Dizziness, headache	1–3 hrs	2.5–3.5 hrs	OTC products more cost effective than prescription forms. Geriatric/Renal dose is 10 mg BID or 20 mg daily.
Fentanyl Patch (Duragesic)	Nociceptive Pain/Opioids	Various	$20.00 (100 mcg q72h)	Hypotension, confusion, diaphoresis	—	17 hrs	Use only if patient is unable to take oral medication. Difficult to titrate. Steady state levels may not be established until 6 days after dose change. May have a role in patients when the oral route is unavailable. Schedule II controlled substance. Matrix product may be cut. Variable absorption in geriatric and cachectic patients. Do not apply heat to patch. Some patients require 48 hour dosing.
Fentanyl buccal tablets (Fentora)	Nociceptive Pain/Opioid	Various		Hypotension, confusion, diaphoresis	45 min	3–12 hrs	Expensive.
Fentanyl Transmucosal (Actiq)	Nociceptive Pain/Opioid	Various	**$32. 00 (200 mcg QID)**	Hypotension, confusion, diaphoresis	90 min	7 hrs	Expensive.

*Drugs in Italics: Not generally recommended in hospice patients
**MDD = Maximun Daily Dose
***BOLD-not available as a generic

Drug Information Table

Generic (Example of Trade)*	Indication/Drug Class	Dosage Range (MDD**)	2007 Avg. Cost/Day for Therapy (Dose for Cost Comparison)***	Adverse Effects	Onset to Peak	T1/2	Comments
Filgastrim (Neupogen)	Neutrapenia/Colony Stimulating Factor	Indivdualized	$4000.00/course	Fever, petechiae, rash splenomegaly, chronic neutropenia, bone pain, epistaxis, headache, nausea	—	—	Not appropriate in hospice patients.
Fluconazole (Diflucan)	Infection/Systemic Fungal (Thrush, Vaginal)/Antifungal	200 mg po on day 1, then 100 mg daily for a total of 7–10 days of therapy; 150 mg × 1 dose vaginal	$54.60/course (100 mg daily × 7 days)	Headache, dizziness	1–3 h	6–8 h	Expensive. Can reduce dose and frequency in geriatric or renally compromised patients. Can be crushed. Considerably more expensive than nystatin.
Flunisolide (AeroBid)	Respiratory/Inhaled Corticosteroid	1–4 puffs BID (8 INH/day)	$77.00/MDI (2 puffs BID)	Headache, bad after taste	—	1.8 hrs	Oral corticosteroids provide greater symptom relief in end stage disease.
Fluocinonide (Lidex)	Pruritus/Rash Topical Corticosteroid	Apply BID-QID	$62.00/tube		—	—	More expensive than hydrocortisone cream.
Fluoxetine (Prozac)	Depression, Anxiety/Serotonin Reuptake Inhibitor	10–60 mg daily (80 mg/day)	$1.15 (20 mg daily)	Insomnia, headache, anxiety, nausea, diarrhea, weakness, somnolence	6–8 hrs	1–3 days & 4–16 days (metabolite)	Onset of effect 3–4 weeks. Long half life may add benefit to patients once they can no longer swallow. No abrupt withdraw symptoms. Cost the same for 10 & 20 mg. Least expensive Serotonin Reuptake Inhibitor.
Flurazepam (Dalmane)	Insomnia/Benzodiazepine	15–30 mg at bedtime (60 mg/day)	$0.35 (15 mg QHS)	Confusion, dizziness, drowsiness, blurred vision	3–6 hrs	2.3 hrs	Long half-life; avoid in geriatric patients.

Drug	Classification	Dose (MDD**)	Cost	Side Effects			Notes
Fluticasone (Flovent)	Respiratory/Inhaled Corticosteroid	88–400 mcg BID	$3.60 (220 mcg BID)	Headache, throat irritation, cough, bronchitis	—	—	Oral corticosteroids provide greater symptom relief in end stage disease.
Fosinopril (Monopril)	Cardovascular/ACE Inhibitors	10–80 mg daily (40 mg/day)	$1.00 (20 mg daily)	Dizziness	~3 hrs	12 hrs	2nd line based on cost. Dry cough and angioedema side effects. No significant difference between ACE Inhibitors.
Fulvestrant (Faslodex)	Breast Cancer/ Antineoplastic Estrogen Receptor Blocker	250 mg Monthly	**250 mg monthly**	Vasodialation, pain, headache, hot flushes, nausea, vomiting, abdominal pain	7–9 days	~40 days	Not generally appropriate in hospice patients.
Furosemide (Lasix)	Fluid Retention/Loop Diuretic	10–120 mg daily-BID	$0.10 (40 mg daily)	Acute hypotension, photosensitivity,	0.5–2 h	30 min	Drug of choice for pulmonary congestion and dependent edema. Last daily dose should be no later than afternoon.
Gabapentin (Neurontin)	Neuropathic Pain, Hiccups, Agitation/ Anticonvulsant.	100–1800 mg TID (3600 mg/day)	$3.70 (300 mg TID)	Fatigue, visual disturbances, tremor, weight gain, dyspepsia, sedation, dizziness	—	5–7 hrs	Doses should be titrated to at least 900 mg/day. Start low and titrate slow. Current anticonvulsant of choice in neuropathic pain; expensive; Requires at least a week for effect.
Galantamine (Reminyl)	Dementia/ Cholinesterase Inhibitors	4–12 mg BID	**$4.40 (8 mg BID)**	Nausea, vomiting, diarrhea	1–5 hrs	7 hrs	May not be beneficial for end-stage dementia. Can cause GI side effects.
Gefitinib (Iressa)	Lung Cancer/ Antineoplastic Tyrosine Kinase Inhibitor	250–500 mg daily	**$57.00 (250 mg daily)**	Rash, acne, dry skin, diarrhea, nausea, vomiting	3–7 hrs	—	Generally not appropriate in hospice patients. Must be palliating a symptom and have monitoring guidelines (PPS). Recommend discontinuing when out of current supply.

*Drugs in Italics: Not generally recommended in hospice patients
**MDD = Maximun Daily Dose
***BOLD-not available as a generic

Drug Information Table

Generic (Example of Trade)*	Indication/Drug Class	Dosage Range (MDD**)	2007 Avg. Cost/Day for Therapy (Dose for Cost Comparison)***	Adverse Effects	Onset to Peak	T1/2	Comments
Glipizide (Glucotrol)	Hyperglycemia/Oral Hyperglycemic Agents	5–20 mg daily-BID (40 mg/day)	$0.40 (10 mg daily)	Edema, hypoglycemia	1–3 hrs	2–5 hrs	Only covered by hospice if hyperglycemia due to terminal diagnosis or related treatment. Monitor for hypoglycemia.
Glyburide (Micronase, Diabeta)	Hyperglycemia/Oral Hyperglycemic Agents	2.5–10 mg BID (20 mg/day)	$0.55 (5 mg BID)	Hypoglycemia	2–4 hrs	4–10 hrs	Only covered by hospice if hyperglycemia due to terminal diagnosis or related treatment. Monitor for hypoglycemia.
Glycerin (Glycerin)	Constipation/Osmotic Laxative	1 supp daily-BID	$1.00 (1 supp daily)	—	—	—	Suppositories only. Indicated for hard dry stool in rectal vault.
Glycopyrrolate (Robinul)	Nausea & Vomiting/ Abdominal Spasm/ Cramping, Bowel Obstruction, Terminal Secretions, Visceral Pain/Anticholinergic	1–2 mg BID-TID; 0.1–0.2 mg TID-QID (Inj) (1.2 mg/day-parenteral 12 mg/day—oral)	$13.35 (2 mg TID; 0.2 mg QID (inj))	Constipation, dry mouth, mydriasis, blurred vision, urinary retention, drowsiness, tachycardia, sedating, confusion	1–45 min	20–40 min	Tablets expensive. Does not cross blood brain barrier therefore minimizes CNS side effects (eg sedation, confusion). Potent drying effect; about 5 times as potent as atropine.
Goserelin Acetate (Zoladex)	Prostate Cancer/ Antineoplastic: Gonadotropin Releasing Hormone Agonist	10.8 mg every 3 mos/ 3.6 mg monthly	**$450.00/ month**	Headache, depression, insomnia, hot flashes, diaphoresis	12–15 days (male), 8–22 days (female)	2–4 hrs	Not generally appropriate in hospice patients.
Granisetron (Kytril)	Nausea & Vomiting/ 5HT3 Antagonist	1 mg daily	**$60.00 (1 mg daily)**	Headache, constipation, weakness	—	5–9 hrs	Expensive. Recommended alternative: Metoclopramide 10–20 mg q4–6h + Haloperidol 1 mg q4hprn. Primarily beneficial for chemotherapy-induced nausea & vomiting, not as effective in other types of nausea & vomiting.

Drug	Indication	Dose (MDD**)	Cost	Side Effects	Onset	Half-life	Comments
Guaifenesin (Robitussin)	Cough, Thick Secretions/ Expectorant	5–30mL q4h; 200–400 mg PO q4h (2400 mg/day)	$2.60 (15mL q4h)		—	~1 hr	First line therapy. Must have good fluid intake for optimal effect. Need minimum daily dose of 60mL. If immediate release is effective converting to sustained release may increase adherence.
Guaifenesin/Codeine (Robitussin AC)	Cough/Expectorant/ Suppressant	5–10mL po q4h ATC or prn (600 mg/day)	$2.30 (5mL q4h)	Dizziness, drowsiness, stomach pain	1/4–8 h	8–Mar	Not as readily available as DM or hydrocodone preps. Causes more constipation and CNS side effects than hydrocodone containing preparations. If regular doses are used consider initiating a stool softener/stimulant laxative to prevent constipation.
Guaifenesin/ Dextromethorphan (Robitussin DM)	Cough/Expectorant/ Suppressant	5–10mL po q4h (120 mg/day DM)	$2.60 (5mL q4h)	Dizziness, drowsiness, stomach pain	< 1/2–6 h	Unknown	First line therapy.
Guaifenesin SR (Mucinex)	Cough/Expectorant	600 mg 1–2 tabs BID (2400 mg/day)	$0.90 (600 mg BID)		—	~1 hr	Do not crush, chew or break tablet. Take with full glass of water without regard to meals. Use of the extended release product may increase adherence if product is effective and needed around the clock.
Haloperidol (Haldol)	Nausea & Vomiting (Chemoreceptor Trigger Zone), Delirium, Agitation, Anxiety, Bowel Obstruction. Hiccups/ Neuroleptics	0.5–2 mg q4–12h (100 mg/day)	$0.20 (1 mg BID)	Extrapyramidal effect, tardive dyskinesia, insomnia, anxiety, drowsiness	3–6 h	17 h	Also used for other symptoms- N/V, agitation, delirium, hallucinations; not significantly sedating, can often dose q12h; 2 mg/mL oral solution can be given PO/SL/PR. Low doses have few side effects; Useful if anxious patient unable to tolerate benzodiazepines; May produce extrapyramidal symptoms, including akathisia (which can mimic anxiety); May produce movement disorders. Associated with prolongation of QT interval. Most commonly used and studied medication for delirium. Tablets can be used rectally.

*Drugs in Italics: Not generally recommended in hospice patients
**MDD = Maximun Daily Dose
***BOLD-not available as a generic

Drug Information Table

Generic (Example of Trade)*	Indication/Drug Class	Dosage Range (MDD**)	2007 Avg. Cost/Day for Therapy (Dose for Cost Comparison)***	Adverse Effects	Onset to Peak	T1/2	Comments
Heparin (Heparin)	Cardiac/Anticoagulants	DVT/PE prophylaxis: 5,000units sq q8–12h	$4.00 (5000 units q8h)	Fever, chills, bruising	20–30 minutes	1.5 hrs	Evaluate continued need for DVT prophylaxis.
Hydralazine (Apresoline)	Cardiac/Vasodilator	10–100 mg BID	$0.50 (50 mg BID)	Increased heart rate, flushing	20–30 minutes	2–8 hrs	Monitor for hypotension.
Hydrochlorothiazide (Oretic)	Fluid Retention/Thiazide Diuretic	12.5–100 mg daily	$0.10 (25 mg daily)	Photosensitivity, orthostatic hypotension	1–2.5 hrs	5.6–14.8 hrs	JNCVII Preferred for hypertension.
Hydrocodone/ Homatropine (Hycodan)	Cough/Suppressant	5–10mL po q4h	$7.50 (5mL q4h)	Dizziness, drowsiness, nausea, vomiting	—	—	Drying effect not always beneficial. Less constipation and less CNS effects than codeine containing preparations. If regular doses are used consider initiating a stool softener/stimulant laxative to prevent constipation.
Hydrocodone/ Chlorpheniramine (Tussionex)	Cough/Suppressant	5mL q12h	$5.00 (5mL q12h)	Dizziness, drowsiness, nausea, vomiting	—	—	Expensive. Drying effect not always beneficial.
Hydrocodone/Ibuprofen (Vicoprofen)	Nociceptive Pain/ Combination NSAID & Opioid	1 tab q4–6h (16 tablets/day)	$12.00 (2 tabs 5 mg/200 mg q4h)	Dizziness, drowsiness, nausea, vomiting	—	—	Expensive. Give low dose opioid and ibuprofen separately.

Drug	Indication/Class	Dose	Cost	Side Effects	Onset	Duration	Comments
Hydrocodone-APAP (Lortab, Vicodin)	Nociceptive Pain, Dyspnea/Combination Opioid/Non-opioid	1–2 tabs q4–6h; (APAP: 4000 mg/day;geriatrics 3000 mg/day)	$2.00 (5/500 2 tabs q6h)	Dizziness, drowsiness, nausea, vomiting	—	—	Monitor acetaminophen dose. Do not exceed 4 grams of acetaminophen per day. Avoid other medications, including OTCs that contain acetaminophen.
Hydrocortisone Cream (Cortaid)	Pruritus/Rash/Topical Corticosteroid	Apply BID/QID (4 applications/day)	$5.25/tube	Itching, dry skin, burning	—	—	May worsen skin infections (especially fungal). Liberal use can lead to significant systemic absorption. Prolonged use will cause thinning of the skin.
Hydromorphone (Dilaudid)	Dyspnea, Nociceptive Pain/Opioids	Various	$2.10 (2 mg q4h)	Sedation, anorexia, dizziness, dysphoria, nausea/vomiting, constipation	1–6 h	10–20 h	No long acting dosage form available. Alternative to morphine in renal failure patients. Approximately 4 times more potent than morphine. For opioid tolerant patients, increase the baseline opioid dose by 25%–50% and titrate. For breakthrough symptoms, 30%–50% of the amount taken over 4 hours can be given q 1 hour, as needed. Schedule II controlled substance. Hydromorphone 10 mg/ mL injuction (most potent opioid per volume) good for SQ. Less neurotoxicity than morphine.
Hydroxyzine (Atarax/ Vistaril)	Pruritus, Anxiety, Nausea & Vomiting (Vestibular)/ Antihistamine	Hydroxyzine HCL 10–25 mg po q4–6h or Hydroxyzine pamoate 25 mg po q4–6h (400 mg/day)	$1.00 (25 mg QID)	Very sedating	1/4–4 h	2–8 h	3rd line after benzodiazepines or low dose neuroleptics for anxiety. Sedating. Use cautiously in ambulatory geriatric patients. Also used for other symptoms—anxiety, insomia, itch. Antihistamine with some anxiolytic properties. IM injection is painful.

*Drugs in Italics: Not generally recommended in hospice patients
**MDD = Maximun Daily Dose
***BOLD-not available as a generic

Drug Information Table

Generic (Example of Trade)*	Indication/Drug Class	Dosage Range (MDD**)	2007 Avg. Cost/Day for Therapy (Dose for Cost Comparison)***	Adverse Effects	Onset to Peak	T1/2	Comments
Hyoscyamine (Levsin)	Secretions, Nausea & Vomiting, Abdominal Spasm, Cramping, Urinary Spasms, Bowel Obstruction, Dysphagia, Visceral Pain/Anticholinergic	0.125–0.25 mg q4–6h; 0.25–0.5 mg IV/IM/SQ q6h (1.5 mg/day)	$0.80 tabs; $4.80 liq (0.125 mg q4h)	Dry mouth, drowsiness, blurred vision, dizziness, decreased sweating, constipation, nausea, loss of taste, headache, tachycardia, difficulty sleeping, or nervousness, confusion	20–30 min	3.5 h	Liquid expensive. SL tablets leave chalky residue; Contributes to constipation. Do not exceed 12 tablets per 24 hours. Available in sublingual formulation for administration in patients who cannot swallow. Not recommended in the elderly.
Ibuprofen (Motrin)	Fever, Nociceptive, Bone Pain/Mixed COX NSAID	400–800 mg q6–8 hr (3.2 gm/day)	$0.30 (400 mg q6h)	Dyspepsia, nausea, abdominal pain, fluid retention, tinnitus, rash, GI bleed, acute renal failure, constipation, headache, dirrhea, flatulance	20 min–2 h	2–4 h	Monitor for GI distress; avoid in patients with renal insufficiency. Less GI upset than naproxen. May cause an increase in systolic blood pressure (all NSAIDs). May cause edema (all NSAIDs). PPIs may be useful for gastric protection in selected "at risk" patients (all NSAIDs). Opioid sparing. Maximum daily dose = 3200 mg. Weigh risk-benefit in patients with renal insufficiency.
Imipramine (Tofranil)	Neuropathic Pain, Depression/Tricyclic Antidepressant	25–300 mg QHS or in divided doses (300 mg/day)	$1.75 (150 mg QHS)	Orthostasis, dizziness, drowsiness, urinary rentention	—	6–18 hrs	Do not start as first line agent. Can increase dose for antidepressant effect if on for other indications. Optimal effect in 4–6 weeks. Less severe side effects compared to amitriptyline.
Indomethacin (indocin)	Fever, Nociceptive, Bone Pain/Mixed COX NSAID	25–50 mg BID-TID (200 mg/day)	$0.80 (50 mg TID)	Headache, nausea, abdominal cramps	20 min–4 h	12–15 h	Highest incidence of GI distress and CNS effects. Avoid in patients with renal insufficiency. Maximum daily dose = 200 mg/day. Weigh risk-benefit in patients with renal insufficiency.

Drug	Class	Dose	Cost	Side Effects	Onset	Half-life	Comments
Insulin Glargine (Lantus)	Hyperglycemia/Insulin	Based on patient	**$76.00/vial**	Hypoglycemia, weight gain, injection site irritation	No peak	—	Only covered by hospice if hyperglycemia due to terminal diagnosis or related treatment. Monitor for hypoglycemia.
Insulin, Human NPH/Regular (Humulin 70/30)	Hyperglycemia/Insulin	Based on patient	**$36.50/vial**	Hypoglycemia, weight gain, injection site irritation	2–12 hrs	—	Only covered by hospice if hyperglycemia due to terminal diagnosis or related treatment. Monitor for hypoglycemia.
Insulin, Human NPH (Humulin N)	Hyperglycemia/Insulin	Based on patient	$35.15/vial	Hypoglycemia, weight gain, injection site irritation	6–12 hrs	—	Only covered by hospice if hyperglycemia due to terminal diagnosis or related treatment. Monitor for hypoglycemia.
Insulin, Human Regular (Humulin R)	Hyperglycemia/Insulin	Based on patient	$35.15/vial	Hypoglycemia, weight gain, injection site irritation	2–4 hrs	—	Only covered by hospice if hyperglycemia due to terminal diagnosis or related treatment. Monitor for hypoglycemia.
Insulin, Lispro (Humalog)	Hyperglycemia/Insulin	Based on patient	$78.50/vial	Hypoglycemia, weight gain, injection site irritation	30–90 minutes	—	Only covered by hospice if hyperglycemia due to terminal diagnosis or related treatment. Monitor for hypoglycemia.
Ipraropium MDI/Neb Soln (Atrovent)	Bronchodilators/Anticholinergic Short Acting	2 puffs QID ; 500mcg q6–8h (12 INH/day)	$38.00 /MDI; $1.92 (2 puffs QID; 500 mcg q6h)	Cough, dry mouth, nervousness, dizziness, headache, bronchospasms	5 min–2 h	1.6 h	As patient declines, change inhaler to nebulizer. Minimal efficacy in lung cancer. Albuterol alone usually sufficient.
Irbesartan (Avapro)	Cardiovascular/Angiotensin Receptor Blocker	150–300 mg daily (300 mg/day)	**$1.50 (150 mg daily)**	Hyperkalemia, orthostatic hypotension, dizziness, fatigue	1–2 h	11–15 h	Second line after ACE Inhibitors. Expensive.
Isosorbide Dinitrate (Isordil)	Cardiovascular/Antianginal	5–20 mg sl q2h, Immediate release: 5–40 mg po QID, Sustained release: 40 mg po q8–12h (160 mg/day)	$2.40 (10 mg QID)	Hypotension, tachycardia, flushing, peripheral edema, headache, lightheadedness, dizziness, restlessness, nausea, blurred vison,	SL: 2–10; Oral: 45–60 m	1–4 h; metabolite 5 h	Monitor for hypotension.

*Drugs in Italics: Not generally recommended in hospice patients
**MDD = Maximun Daily Dose
***BOLD-not available as a generic

Drug Information Table

Generic (Example of Trade)*	Indication/Drug Class	Dosage Range (MDD**)	2007 Avg. Cost/Day for Therapy (Dose for Cost Comparison)***	Adverse Effects	Onset to Peak	T1/2	Comments
Isosorbide Mononitrate (Imdur)	Cardiovascular/ Antianginal	Imdur 30–120 mg po daily, Ismo 20 mg po bid (dose 7 hours apart; 8am & 3pm) (240 mg/day)	$0.50 (30 mg daily)	Headache, dizziness, nausea	30–60 m	4 h	Do not crush. Monitor for hypotension.
Itraconazole (Sporanox)	Infection (Systemic Fungal)/Antifungal	100–200 mg daily-BID (400 mg/day)	$338.55/course (100 mg BID × 3wks)	Nausea, edema, hypertension, headache, fatigue		Intial: 21 +/−5 hr	Very expensive. Not recommended.
Ketamine (Ketolar)	Neuropathic Pain/ Dissociative Anesthetic, NMDA Antagonist	0.4 mg/kg (IM: 8 mg/kg; IV: 4.5 mg/kg)	$11.35 (5 mg q8h)	Hypertension, tachycardia, hallucinations, vivid dreams, tonic-clonic movements, tremor, diplopia, nausea, anorexia	1–2 m	11–17 m	
Ketoconazole (Nizoral)	Infection (Systemic Fungal)/Antifungal	200 mg dailyx 1–10 days (400 mg/day)	$29.15/course (200 mg daily × 7 days)	Pruritus, nausea, abdominal pain	1–2 h	Initial: 2 h; terminal: 8 h	Multiple drug interactions.
Ketorolac (Toradol)	Nociceptive, Bone Pain/ Mixed COX NSAID	IV: 60 mg initially, then 30 mg q6h IM: 30 mg q6h PO: 20 mg initially then 10 mg q6h (Oral: 40 mg/day; Parenteral: 120 mg/day, not to exceed 5 days)	$0.85 (10 mg daily)	Headache, gastrointestinal pain, dyspepsia, nausea, edema, hypertension	2–3 h	2–8 h; prolonged in elderly by 30–50%	IV/IM administration should NOT exceed 5 days.

Drug	Indication/Class	Dose	Cost	Side Effects	Onset	Half-life	Comments
Lactulose (Chronulac)	Constipation/Osmotic Laxative	15–30mL daily-BID (120 mL/day)	$2.55 (30mL BID)	Flatulence, abdominal distention, belching, abdominal pain, diarrhea, anorexia, nausea, vomiting, electrolyte disorders	24–48 h	Unknown	Sorbitol 70% more cost effective than lactulose. Dependent on adequate hydration. Not sufficient without stimulant if patient is on an opioid. Drug of choice for hepatic encephalopathy. Kristalose expensive. More expensive than stimulants with no improved efficacy. Associated with increased cramping and flatulence. Onset 24–48 hours.
Lansoprazole (Prevacid)	Gastritis/Proton Pump Inhibitors	15–30 mg daily-BID (120 mg/day)	$4.00 (30 mg daily)	Diarrhea, nausea, rash, abdominal pain, headache, taste changes	0–1.7 h	< 2 h	M Prilosec OTC more cost effective. Evaluate need for therapy. Can step down to H2. All PPIs have similar efficacy: Cost of 15 & 30 mg the same.
Letrozole (Femara)	Breast Cancer/ Antineoplastic: Aromatase Inhibitor	2.5 mg daily	**$7.30 (2.5 mg daily)**	Headache, fatigue, hot flashes, nausea, bone pain, back pain, dyspnea, insomnia,	2–6 w to ss	2 d	Generally not appropriate in hospice patients. Must be palliating a symptom and have monitoring guidelines (PPS). Recommend discontinuing.
Leuprolide (Lupron)	Prostate Canxer/ Antineoplastic: Gonadotropine Releasing Hormone Agonist	0.3 mg/kg every 30 days SQ: Eligard: 7.5 mg monthly or 22.5 mg Q3months; Lupron: 1 mg/day:Viadur: 65 mg implanted Q12months IM: 7.5 mg Qmonth or 22.5 Q3months	**$625.00/month**	Angina, atrial fib, hot flashes, edema, hypertension, tachycardia, agitation, confusion, dizziness, fatigue, fever, headache, insomnia, decrease bone density, breast enlargement, hirsutism, decreased libido	2–4 w	IV:3 h	Generally not appropriate in hospice patients. Must be palliating a symptom and have monitoring guidelines (PPS). Recommend discontinuing.
Levadopa-Carbidopa (Sinemet)	Parkinson's/Dopamine Agonist	Various (200 mg carbidopa; 2000 mg levodopa/day)	$1.30 (25 mg–100 mg TID)	Hypotension, dizziness, confusion, headache, hallucinations, delusions, agitation, somnolence, on-off phenomenon, decreased mental acuity	IR: 0.5–2 h ER: 2–3 h	1.5–2 h	Do not crush SR dosage forms.

*Drugs in Italics: Not generally recommended in hospice patients
**MDD = Maximun Daily Dose
***BOLD-not available as a generic

Drug Information Table

Generic (Example of Trade)*	Indication/Drug Class	Dosage Range (MDD**)	2007 Avg. Cost/Day for Therapy (Dose for Cost Comparison)***	Adverse Effects	Onset to Peak	T1/2	Comments
Levalbuterol (Xoponex)	Bronchodilators/Short Acting Beta Agonists	1 unit q6–8h (12 INH/day)	**$8.90 (1.25 mg/3mL q8h)**	Increased serum glucose, decreased serum potassium, tremor, nervousness, anxiety, tachycardia, flu-like syndrome	5 min–2 h	5–6 h	Indicated if albuterol caused bronchospasm or excessive side effects. Should be dosed no more frequently than q6–8 hours.
Levofloxacin (Levaquin)	Infection (Respiratory)/ Quinolone	250–500 mg daily × 7–10 days (750 mg/day)	**$112.00/course (500 mg daily × 7 days)**	Headache, insomnia, dizziness, nausea, pharyngitis	1–2 h	6–8 h	
Levothyroxine (Synthroid)	Hypothyroidism/Thyroid Replacement	Based on patient (300 mcg/day)	$0.45 (0.1 mg daily)	Flushing, tachycardia, anxiety, insomnia, hyperactivity, nervousness	2–4 h	Euthyroid: 6–7 d; hypothyroid: 9–10 d; hyperthyroid: 3–4 d	Related to terminal diagnosis only for patients with thyroidectomy due to terminal diagnosis.
Lidocaine/Prilocaine (EMLA)	Pain/Local Anesthetic	Apply q4–6h	$42.00/ tube	Hyperpigmentation, itching, rash, burning	2–3 h	Lidocaine: 1.5–2 h prilocaine: 10–150 m	Expensive. Onset 1–2 hrs. Duration of action 4 hrs.
Lidocaine Nebulized (Xylocaine Without Epinephrine)	Cough/Local Anesthetic	Nebulize diluted in normal saline QID	$3.20 (1% 4mL q4h)	Bronchospasm	?	?	1–2% Lidocaine 1–4mL nebulized q4hprn. Don't eat or drink for 30 min after nebulizing lidocaine to prevent aspiration.

Drug	Indication/Class	Dose (MDD**)	Cost	Side Effects	Onset	Half-life	Comments
Lidocaine Oint (Xylocaine)	Pain, Pruritus/Local Anesthetic	Apply QID (320 mg/day)	$13.00/tube	Contact dermatitis, itching, petechia, rash	3–5 m	1.5–2 h	Alternative to expensive Lidoderm patch. Frequent use can lead to significant absorption (and possible cardiac arrhythmias).
Lidocaine Oral (Xylocaine Viscous)	Pain/Local Anesthetic	5–10mL q4h (1200 mg/day)	$4.80 (10mL q4h)	Drowsiness, confusion, headache, dizziness, slurred speech, arrhythmias, heart block		Biphasic elimination 7–30m followed by 1.5–2 h	
Lidocaine Patch (Lidoderm Patch)	Neuropathic Pain/Local Anesthetic	Apply for 12 hours off 12 hours (3 patches/application)	**$5.95 (1 patch daily)**	Contact dermatitis, itching, petechia, rash	1–2 h	36–54 h	Expensive. Not recommended. Patches may be cut before removing backing. Do not shave area; clip hair to short length before applying patch.
Lisinopril (Prinivil/Zestril)	Cardiovascular/ACE Inhibitors	5–40 mg daily (40 mg/day)	$0.60 (20 mg daily)	Hypotension, dizziness, headache, hyperkalemia, cough	6 h	11–12 h	Dry cough and angioedema side effects. No significant difference between ACE Inhibitors.
Loperamide (Immodium AD)	Diarrhea/Antidiarrheal	2 tabs now then 1 tab after each loose stool (max 8 tabs/day) (16 mg/day)	$1.40 (2 QID)	Constipation, nausea, abdominal pain	5 h	7–14 h	Available OTC. Not recommended in patients with bacterial diarrhea.
Loratadine (Claritin)	Pruritus/Antihistamines	10 mg daily (10 mg/day)	$0.15 (10 mg daily)	Headache, somnolence, fatigue, xerostomia	8–12 h	12–15 h	Expensive. Minimal sedation.

*Drugs in Italics: Not generally recommended in hospice patients
**MDD = Maximun Daily Dose
*****BOLD-not available as a generic**

Drug Information Table

Generic (Example of Trade)*	Indication/Drug Class	Dosage Range (MDD**)	2007 Avg. Cost/Day for Therapy (Dose for Cost Comparison)***	Adverse Effects	Onset to Peak	T1/2	Comments
Lorazepam (Ativan)	Anxiety, Agitation, Insomnia, Nausea & Vomiting From Anxiety, Dyspnea, Acute Seizures/Benzodiazepine	0.5 mg–1 mg q4-6h; Seizure abortive dose 2 mg q15min × 4 doses (10 mg/day)	$1.40 (0.5 mg q6h)	Sedation, dizziness, weakness, ataxia, depression, antegrade anemesia	1–6 h	10–20 h	Benzodiazepines are drugs of choice for anxiety. Lorazepam more expensive than alprazolam or diazepam. Use tablets instead of Intensol, Benzodiazepines not first line in delirium and can worsen delirium. Intensol is expensive. All drugs in class may produce paradoxical agitation in elderly, demented or brain-injured patients-start with test dose; Short-acting; No active metabolites; Most reliably absorbed drug in class when administered parenterally. Benzodiazepines can decrease anxiety associated with breathlessness, however should be reserved as second line after opioids. Begin with low doses and titrate to effect. Breakthrough doses may be necessary to settle dyspnea. Can be used together with opioids with careful titration of each agent. Best for short-term or intermittent use; Tolerance to sedating effects develops with longer use. Benzodiazepine of choice in hospice. Treats anxiety that causes or exacerbates nausea and vomiting. Indirect anti-emetic effect.

Drug	Classification	Dose	Cost	Side Effects	Onset	Duration	Notes
Losartan (Cozaar)	Cardiovascular/ Angiotensin Receptor Blocker	25–50 mg daily-BID (100 mg/day)	**$1.45 (50 mg daily)**	Chest pain, fatigue, hypoglycemia, diarrhea, weakness	1 h	1.5–2 h	Second line after ACE Inhibitors. Expensive.
Low Molecular Weight Heparin (Lovenox, Fragmin)	Cardiovascular/ Anticoagulants	1 mg/kg BID or 1.5 mg/kg daily prophylaxytic dose	**$70.00 (80 mg daily)**	Hemorrhage, fever, nausea,	3–5 h	4.5–7 h	Evaluate appropriateness. Expensive! Convert to Coumadin if possible. Need about 4 days of overlap of LMWH and Coumadin.
Magnesium Hydroxide (Milk of Magnesia)	Constipation/Osmotic Laxative	15–30mL daily-BID (60 mL/day)	$0.45 (30mL daily)	Diarrhea, nausea, vomiting, abdominal cramps, alkalosis, electrolyte disorders	1/2–3 h	Unknown	Not sufficient without stimulant if patient is on an opioid. Encourage fluid intake.
Meclizine (Antivert)	Nausea & Vomiting (Vestibular)/ Antihistamine	12.5–25 mg TID-QID (100mg/day)	$0.75 (25 mg TID)	Drowsiness, excitation, hypotension, tachycardia, blurred vision, dry mouth, confusion	1 h	6 h	Drug of choice for vertigo. Sedating.

*Drugs in Italics: Not generally recommended in hospice patients
**MDD = Maximun Daily Dose
*****BOLD**-not available as a generic

Drug Information Table

Generic (Example of Trade)*	Indication/Drug Class	Dosage Range (MDD**)	2007 Avg. Cost/Day for Therapy (Dose for Cost Comparison)***	Adverse Effects	Onset to Peak	T1/2	Comments
Megestrol Acetate (Megace)	Anorexia/Progestin	400–800 mg daily; initial dose 160 mg PO daily; Maximum dose in anorexia 800 mg PO daily (800 mg/day)	$10.75 (800 mg daily)	Thromboembolic disorder	1–5 h	1 h	Megace has less overall benefit to patient in last few weeks of life than corticosteroids. Corticosteroid efficacy equivalent to megestrol for treatment of anorexia for 6–8 weeks. Weight gain is not a goal of hospice care. Megestrol can increase risk of hypercoagulation; First line for long term therapy (3 months); Avoid use in patients with history of DVT; Risk of thromboembolism and hyperglycemia-monitor patients; Monitor for efficacy every two weeks, if no response increase dose by 160 mg po daily; Elixir is preferred due to decreased pill burden and is more cost-effective; Clinical trial have shown there is no benefit at doses above 800 mg/day.
Memantine (Namenda)	Dementia/NMDA Antagonist	5–10 mg daily-BID (20 mg/day)	$4.55 (10 mg daily)	Hypertension, dizziness, confusion, headache, hallucinations, constipation	3–7 h	60–80 h	Limited benefit in end-stage Alzheimer's dementia.
Meperidine (Demerol)	Nociceptive Pain/Opioids	Various (600 mg/day)	$4.25 (50 mg q4h)	Hypotension, fatigue, drowsiness, headache, restlessness, hallucinations, seizures	SQ: 1 h Oral: 2 h	Parent: 2.5–4 h metabolite: 15–30 h	Toxic metabolite: Never use in chronic pain management.
Metaxalone (Skelaxin)	Muscle Spasm/Muscle Relaxant	400–800 mg TID-QID (3200 mg/day)	$12.30 (800 mg QID)	Nausea, vomitting, headache, drowsiness, irritability	3 h	8–9 h	Sedative/hypnotic class.

Drug	Class	Dose	Cost	Side Effects	Onset	Half-life	Comments
Metformin (Glucophage)	Hyperglycemia/Oral Hyperglycemic Agents	1500–2000 mg daily (2500 mg/day)	$1.90 (2000 mg daily)	Nausea, vomitting, diarrhea, flatulence, weakness	ER: 4–8 h	6.2 h	Only covered by hospice if hyperglycemia due to terminal diagnosis or related treatment. Contraindicated in renal failure.
Methadone (Methadose)	Nociceptive & Neuropathic Pain/NMDA Antagonist Opioid	Various	$0.55 (20 mg TID)	Dizziness, sedation, nausea/vomiting, sweating, flushing, dry mouth, constipation, QT prolongation, arrhythmias	Onset 2 h	23 h	Extremely effective for both nociceptive and neuropathic pain. Inexpensive. **Must be dosed and titrated by experienced clinicians.** Monitor for accumulation. Absorbed sublingually. Long half/life-routine dose titrations should only be done approximately every 3-6 days. Equianalgesic doses vary widely between patients. Patient specific dose titration required. Excessive sedation may signal overdose. Schedule II controlled substance. Long and variable half-life (average ~25 hrs). Multiple drug interactions. Dosage adjustment needed only in severe renal insufficiency (GRF <10mL/min).
Methylcellulose (Citrucel)	Diarrhea/Bulking Agent	2–4 caplets 1–3 times daily, or 1 TBSP 1–3 times daily	$0.65 (19g BID)	None reported	Unknown	Unknown	Not useful in dehydrated patients; must take with plenty of fluid.
Methylphenidate (Ritalin)	Depression, Excessive Sedation/ Psychostimulants	2.5–10 mg qAM—BID (last dose before 2pm (60 mg/day)	$1.00 (5 mg BID)	Insomnia, nervousness, tachycardia, anorexia, headache, dyskinesia, abdominal pain, angina	1–3 h	3–4 h	Drug of choice for depression if patient has less than 2–3 weeks to live. Onset of action immediately. Can use in combination with Serotonin Reuptake Inhibitor for first 2 weeks of therapy. Frequently requires twice daily dosing.

*Drugs in Italics: Not generally recommended in hospice patients
**MDD = Maximun Daily Dose
***BOLD-not available as a generic

Drug Information Table

Generic (Example of Trade)*	Indication/Drug Class	Dosage Range (MDD**)	2007 Avg. Cost/Day for Therapy (Dose for Cost Comparison)***	Adverse Effects	Onset to Peak	T1/2	Comments
Metoclopramide (Reglan)	Nausea & Vomiting (Gastric Stasis) Hiccups, Partial Bowel Obstruction/Gastric Stimulant Antiemetic	5–20 mg q4–6h (120 mg/day)	$4.85 (10 mg QID)	Extrapyramidal symptoms, drowsiness, confusion, seizures, dizziness	1/2–1 h	4–6 h	Drug of choice for gastric stasis or squashed stomach. Monitor for confusion and EPS. Can cause confusion in elderly. Doses up to 120 mg/day have been reported to be of benefit. Useful for gastric distension mediated hiccups. Promotes gastric emptying; also has anti-emetic properties. Has 5-HT4 agonist action in the gut. Starting dose for elderly=5 mg TID-QID. D2 antagonist.
Metolazone (Zaroxolyn)	Fluid Retention/Thiazide Diuretic	2.5–20 mg daily (20 mg/day)	$1.25 (5 mg daily)	Orthostatic hypotension, dizziness, drowsiness, purpura rash, abdominal pain, nausea	60 m	20 h	Use only if furosemide ineffective alone. Give 1/2 hour before loop diuretics for optimal effect. Very potent. Watch for dehydration and hypokalemia.
Metoprolol (Lopressor)	Cardiovascular/Beta Blocker	12.5–100 mg po daily-TID (450 mg/day)	$0.40 (50 mg BID)	Bradycardia, hypotension, dizziness, fatigue, pruritus, rash	1.5–4 h	3–8 h	Toprol XL cannot be crushed. Abrupt discontinuation can cause rebound hypertension.
Metronidazole (Flagyl)	Infections (C. Diff., Skin, Vaginal)/Antibiotic	250–500 mg QID for 10–14 days (4 gm/day)	$10.00/course (500 mg TID × 10 days)	Ataxia, dizziness, headache, rash, disulfriam-like reaction, nausea	1–3 h	6–8 h	Do not take with alcohol. May be used topically. Drug of choice for C.difficile & Giardia infection. May be used empirically if diarrhea follow course of antibiotics.
Mexiletine (Mexitil)	Cardiac/Antiarrhythmic	200–300 mg q8h (1200 mg/day)	$ 1.90 (100 mg TID)	Dyspepsia, dizziness, tremor, palpitations, tinnitus	1–3 h	6–8 h	Expensive. Questionable efficacy. Multiple side effects.

Drug	Indication/Class	Dose	Cost	Side Effects	Onset	Half-life	Comments
Miconazole (Monistat)	Topical/Vaginal Infection/ Antifungal	Tinea: use for no longer than 4 weeks, vaginal candiasis treatment for up to 7 days	$17.00/course; $6.80/tube (200 mg daily × 3 days)	Contact dermatitis, burning, maceration, itching	1–3 h	6–8 h	
Midazolam (Versed)	Delirium, Agitation/ Benzodiazepine	10–15 mg IV loading dose, then 40–120 mg/24hr SQ infusion	$7.50 (5 mg/ mL vial)	Nausea, vomiting, sedation, headache, confusion, ataxia, metallic taste	1/2–1 h (IM)	1.2–12.3 h	Benzodiazepines not first line in delirium and can worsen delirium. Use only for palliative sedation.
Mineral Oil/Enema only (Fleets Mineral Oil Enema)	Constipation/Lubricant	PRN 118 mL as single dose	$2.80 (1 PR daily prn)	Abd cramping, diarrhea, nausea, lipid pneumonitis with aspiration, hemorrhoids	2–15 m	Unknown	Avoid using mineral oil orally. Try frozen pea size Vaseline balls rolled in sugar. 1–4 PO daily prn for high, hard impactions.
Mirtazapine (Remeron)	Anorexia, Insomnia, Depression/Atypical Antidepressant	7.5–45 mg HS (45 mg/day)	$1.45 (15 mg QHS)	Somnolence, constipation, xerostomia, increased appetite, weight gain	2 h	20–40 h	Second line to Serotonin Reuptake Inhibitor . Also used for other symptoms-anorexia, insomnia (doses <15 mg). 45 mg tabs and disintegrating tabs not generic; cost for all tablet sizes very similar; Consider in patients with concurrent insomnia or depression combined with appetite/weight loss; Lower doses are more sedating (7.5 mg–15 mg) while higher doses are more effective for depression. Enhances central 5HT and NE. Histamine (H1) antagonist. 5HT3 antagonist-antiemetic. Alpha-2 antagonist antidepressant. Histamine H1 antagonist, 5HT2 antagonist.

*Drugs in Italics: Not generally recommended in hospice patients
**MDD = Maximun Daily Dose
***BOLD-not available as a generic

Drug Information Table

Generic (Example of Trade)*	Indication/Drug Class	Dosage Range (MDD**)	2007 Avg. Cost/Day for Therapy (Dose for Cost Comparison)***	Adverse Effects	Onset to Peak	T1/2	Comments
Montelukast (Singulair)	Respiratory/Leukotriene Receptor Antagonist	10 mg daily	$3.00 (10 mg daily)	Dizziness, fatigue, abdominal pain, cough, flu-like symptoms	10 mg: 3–4 h; 5 mg: 2–2.5 h; 4 mg: 2 h	2.7–5.5 h	Indicated for asthma. Evaluate efficacy and discontinue as patient declines.
Morphine 24 hr SR (Avinza)	Nociceptive Pain/Opioid	Various	$13.25 (180 mg daily)	Somnolence, constipation, nausea, hypotension, vomiting, dry mouth, urinary retention, pruitus, miosis	0.5–1 h	2.5–3 h	Use only if patient needs a 24 hour product, if a sprinkle dose is needed, or if they need it via G-tube. Kadian has less predictable 24hr duration. Avinza and Kadian capsules may be opened and the pellets may be sprinkled on food or put down feeding tube.
Morphine 8–12 hr SR (MS Contin)	Nociceptive Pain/Opioids	Various	$9.40 (100 mg BID)	Somnolence, constipation, nausea, hypotension, vomiting, dry mouth, urinary retention, pruitus, miosis	1/2–1 h	2.5–3 h	Endo brand most cost effective. Can give tablets rectally. Dose requirements should be established using immediate release formulations. Sustained release preparations should not be used for dose findings. Schedule II controlled substance. Glucuronide metabolites accumulate in renal insufficiency and with high doses causing neurotoxicity. Do not crush.

Drug	Indication/Class	Dose (MDD**)	Cost	Side Effects	Onset	Half-life	Comments
Morphine IR (Roxanol)	Nociceptive Pain, Dyspnea/Opioid	Various	$18.15/30mL (5 mg q4h)	Somnolence, constipation, nausea, hypotension, vomiting, dry mouth, urinary retention, pruitus, miosis	45 min	2.6 h	Sustained release may be appropriate if patient requiring frequent PRN doses. For opioid tolerant patients, increase the baseline opioid dose by 25%–50% and titrate. For breakthrough symptoms, 30%–50% of the amount taken over 4 hours can be given q 1 hour, as needed. Consideration of inpatient hospice/palliative care setting may be helpful for patients with severe dyspnea, due to the necessity of close monitoring. Addition of benzodiazepines may also be necessary if anxiety is a significant contributor to breathlessness. Studies have been inconsistent regarding the efficacy of nebulized morphine. An interdisciplinary team should be involved in any interventions for severe dyspnea which may include palliative sedation. Schedule II controlled substance. Glucuronide metabolities accumulate in renal insufficiency and with high doses causing neurotoxicity.
Moxifloxacin (Avelox)	Infection (Respiratory)/Quinolone	400 mg daily × 7–14 days (400 mg/day)	$104.00/course (400 mg daily × 10 days)	Nausea, diarrhea	1–3 h	12 h	Expensive.
Mupirocin (Bactroban)	Topical Infection/Topical Antibiotic	Apply TID for 10 days	$44.00/tube	Dizziness, headache, dry skin, burning, edema	Unknown	Unknown	Expensive. Use Neosporin unless positive for MRSA.
Nabumatone (Relafen)	Nociceptive, Bone Pain/Mixed COX NSAID	50 mg BID-TID (2000 mg/day)	$1.35 (500 mg BID)	Abdominal pain, diarrhea, dyspepsia, edema, dizziness, headache	Serum: 2.5–4 h synovial: 4–12 h	24 h	Alternative to COX II NSAID. Once a day dosing beneficial. Onset of action takes several days. Expensive.

*Drugs in Italics: Not generally recommended in hospice patients
**MDD = Maximun Daily Dose
***BOLD-not available as a generic

Drug Information Table

Generic (Example of Trade)*	Indication/Drug Class	Dosage Range (MDD**)	2007 Avg. Cost/Day for Therapy (Dose for Cost Comparison)***	Adverse Effects	Onset to Peak	T1/2	Comments
Naproxen (Naprosyn)	Nociceptive, Bone Pain, Fever/Mixed COX NSAID	250–500 mg BID-TID (1250 mg/day)	$0.60 (500 mg BID)	Dyspepsia, nausea, abdominal pain, fluid retention, tinnitus, rash, GI bleed, acute renal failure, constipation, headache, diarrhea, flatulance	20 min–2 h	2–4 h	Can dose BID for better compliance. Opioid sparing. Maximum daily dose = 1250 mg/day (expressed as naproxen base, not naproxen sodium). Aleve® (naproxen sodium) 220 mg=naproxen base 200 mg + 20 mg sodium. Weigh risk-benefit in patients with renal insufficiency. Preferred agent for tumor fever.
Nebulized Furosemide	Dyspnea/Diuretic	20–40 mg BID-QID	$9.00 (20 mg QID)	Transient nausea, cough, risk of bronchospasm, potential diuresis	30 min–2 h	Unknown	
Nebulized Opioids (fentanyl preferred)	Dyspnea/Opioids	q1–4h	$14.75 (50mcg Q4)	Transient nausea, cough, risk of bronchospasm	10–60 min	2–4 h	May give with albuterol. Clinical efficacy of nebulized opioids not established. Use systemic opioids and anxiolytics instead.
Nebulized Saline (Saline Dey Vials)	Dyspnea, Thick Secretions/Normal Saline	1 vial q4h prn	$0.40. vial (1 vial q4h prn)	Cough, risk of bronchospasm	30 min–2 h	N/A	Dyspnea. Use in between bronchodilator doses to prevent overutilization of active drug. Loosens secretions to make cough more productive. Suspected phrenic or vagal stimulation induced hiccups.
Neomycin/Polymyxin/ Bacitracin (Neosporin)	Topical Infection/Topical Antibiotic	Apply 1–5 times a day	$6.00/tube	Contact dermatitis, itching, swelling	2 h	6 h	
Nitrofurantion (Macrodantin)	Infection (Urinary Tract)/Antibiotic	100 mg BID × 10 days (200 mg/day)	$37.00/course (100 mg BID × 10 days)	Chest pain, confusion, dizziness, drowsiness, headache, angioedema, abd pain	30 m	20–60 m	

Drug	Indication/Class	Dosing	Cost	Side Effects		Onset	Notes
Nitroglycerin tablets, patch, paste (Nitrostat)	Cardiovascular/ Antianginal	0.4 mg SL every 5 minutes for up to 3 doses prn; 0.1–0.8 mg/hr patch (oral: 26 mg qid; SL: 0.6 mg Q5m X3; paste: 2" every 6 h; patch: 0.8 mg/hr)	$1.25 (0.4 mg/hr patch daily)	Hypotension, tachycardia, flushing, peripheral edema, headache, lightheadedness, dizziness, restlessness, nausea, blurred vison	SL:4–8 m; SR: 45–120 m; Spray: 4–10 m; paste: 30–120; patch: 60–180	1–4 m	Monitor for hypotension. Treat side effect of headache with acetaminophen.
Nizatidine (Axid)	Gastritis/H2 Antagonists	75–300 mg daily–BID (300 mg/day)	$1.80 (150 mg BID)	Headache, anxiety, dizziness, insomnia, abd pain	0.5–3 h	1–2 h	OTC products more cost effective than prescription forms. Geriatric/Renal dose is 75 mg BID or 150 mg daily.
Nortriptyline (Pamelor)	Neuropathic Pain, Depression/Tricyclic Antidepressant	25–150 mg QHS or in divided doses; 10–25 mg; Usual therapeutic range: 75–150 mg (150 mg/day)	$0.45 (75 mg QHS)	Dry mouth, drowsiness, constipation, urinary retention, tachycardia	2–6 h	14–62 h	Neuropathic pain: Onset of analgesia in about 7 days. Less severe side effects compared to amitriptyline. Not first line for depression. Can increase dose for antidepressant effect if on for other indications. Optimal effect in 4–6 weeks. Fewer drug interactions than other tricyclic antidepressants. Start low & titrate slowly. Tricyclic antidepressant. Least likely tricyclic to cause orthostasis. Alternative to desipramine; preferred by some clinicians due to good studies for neuropathic pain use.
Nystatin (Mycostatin)	Fungal Infection, Thrush/ Antifungal	Swish and swallow/spit 1 teaspoonful po QID × 7–10 days ; Apply 2–4 times a day oral cadidiasis: 400,000–600,000 QID intestinal infection: 500,000–1,000,000 q8h	$22.00/Oral course: $3.50/tube (5mL PO QID × 10 days; apply qid)	Nausea, vomitting, diarrhea, abdominal pain	1–4 h	8 h	First line therapy.

*Drugs in Italics: Not generally recommended in hospice patients
**MDD = Maximun Daily Dose
***BOLD-not available as a generic

Drug Information Table

Generic (Example of Trade)*	Indication/Drug Class	Dosage Range (MDD**)	2007 Avg. Cost/Day for Therapy (Dose for Cost Comparison)***	Adverse Effects	Onset to Peak	T1/2	Comments
Nystatin/Triamcinolone (Mycolog)	Rash, Fungal Infection/Topical Antifungal/Corticosteroid Combination	Apply 2–4 times a day apply sparingly 2–4 times daily	$8.00/tube	Dryness, foliculitis, acne, skin atrophy, burning, irritation	Unknown	Unknown	
Octreotide (Sandostatin)	GI Hypersecretion, Bowel Obstruction, Diarrhea, Visceral Pain/ Somatostatin Analog	50–600mcg/day divided BID-QID; 50–100 mcg IV/SQ q8h or continuous IV/SQ infusion initiated at 10–20 mcg/hr (1500 mcg/day)	$37.00 (50mcg TID)	Nausea, diarrhea, abdominal pain, vomiting, arthralgias	0–0.4 h	1.7 h	Try glycopyrrolate 0.2 mg SC q4h ATC, decadron 8 mg daily, and haloperidol 1 mg q4hprn first. Very expensive. For severe intractable diarrhea from carcinoid tumors. Expensive. Selectively inhibits secretion of fluids and electrolytes into the gut lumen. May be beneficial in patients with complete obstruction.
Olanzapine (Zyprexa)	Delirium, Agitation, Anxiety/Atypical Antipsychotic	2.5–20 mg daily (20 mg/day)	$7.80 (5 mg daily)	Somnolence, agitation, insomnia, headache, nervousness, hostility, dizziness	6 h	20 h	VERY expensive and sedating. Generally, no benefit over haloperidol or chlorpromazine. Can increase blood glucose levels. Useful if anxious patient unable to tolerate benzodiazepines AND "typical antipsychotics"; May produce extrapyramidal symptoms including akathisia.
Omeprazole (Prilosec OTC, Prilosec)	Gastritis/Proton Pump Inhibitors	20–40 mg daily/BID (40 mg/day)	$0.80 (OTC) : $3.10 (RX) (20 mg daily)	Headache, dizziness, diarrhea, abdominal pain, nausea	2 h	0.5–1 h	OTC form ONLY is PPI of choice. Can be given via g-tube or NG tube as simplified omeprazole solution-consult pharmacist.

Drug	Indication/Class	Dose	Cost	Side Effects	Onset	Peak	Comments
Ondansetron (Zofran)	Nausea & Vomiting/ 5HT3 Receptor Antagonist	4–8 mg TID (32 mg)	$120.00 (8 mg TID)	Headache, fatigue, constipation, diarrhea, dizziness, abdominal pain	1.7 h	3–3.5 h	Expensive. Recommended alternative: Metoclopramide 10-20 mg q4–6h + Haloperidol 1 mg q4hprn. Primarily beneficial for chemotherapy induced nausea & vomiting, not as effective in other types of nausea & vomiting.
Ophthalmic Lubricant (Lacrilube)	Dry Eyes/Lubricant	Apply PRN every 2 hours	$6.00/tube	None reported	Unknown	Unknown	Leaves film on eyes.
Oxybutynin IR (Ditropan)	Urinary Spasms & Frequency/ Anticholinergic	5–10 mg TID (30 mg/day)	$3.00 (5 mg q8h)	Dry mouth, drowsiness, blurred vision, dizziness, decreased sweating, constipation, nausea, loss of taste, headache, difficulty sleeping, or nervousness	3–6 h	2–3 h	Can't crush SR tabs.
Oxycodone (Roxicodone)	Nociceptive Pain, Dyspnea/Opioids	Various	$1.95 (5 mg q4h)	Somnolence, dizziness, pruritus, nausea, constipation, vomitting, respiratory depression	0.5–1 h	2–3 h	More expensive than morphine. Preferred over morphine in patients with significant renal insufficiency who are not candidates for hydromorphone or methadone. For opioid tolerant patients, increase the baseline opioid dose by 25%–50% and titrate. For breakthrough symptoms, 30%–50% of the amount taken over 4 hours can be given q 1 hour, as needed. May be helpful for patient with dyspnea. Addition of benzodiazepines may also be necessary if anxiety is a significant contributor to breathlessness.

*Drugs in Italics: Not generally recommended in hospice patients
**MDD = Maximun Daily Dose
***BOLD-not available as a generic

Drug Information Table

Generic (Example of Trade)*	Indication/Drug Class	Dosage Range (MDD**)	2007 Avg. Cost/Day for Therapy (Dose for Cost Comparison)***	Adverse Effects	Onset to Peak	T1/2	Comments
Oxycodone + APAP (Perocet)	Dyspnea, Nociceptive Pain/Opioid/Non-opioid Combination	1–2 tabs q4h (Acetaminophen 4000 mg/day; geriatrics 3000 mg/day)	$2.80 (2 tabs q4h)	Somnolence, dizziness, pruritus, nausea, constipation, vomitting, respiratory depression	0.5–1 h	2–3 h	Do not exceed 4 grams of acetaminophen per day. Avoid other medications, including OTCs that contain acetaminophen. Schedule II controlled substance. Elderly dosing of oxycodone is 1/2 adult starting dose.
Oxycodone SR (OxyContin)	Nociceptive Pain, Dyspnea/Opioids	Various q8-12h	**$16.45 (80 mg BID)**	Somnolence, dizziness, pruritus, nausea, constipation, vomitting, respiratory depression	10 min–1 h	5 h	Most expensive long action opioid. Little advantage over morphine SR. Approximatly 1.5 times more potent than morphine. Dose requirements should be established using immediate release forumulations. Sustained release preparations should not be used for dose finding. Schedule II controlled substance. Safer than morphine in severe renal insufficiency. Do not crush. May give rectally (unapproved route).
Oxymetazoline (Afrin)	Respiratory/ Decongestants	1–2 sprays in nose q12h (6 sprays each nostril/day)	$5.50/btl	Hypertension, dry nasal mucosa, rebound congestion	5–10 m	5–8 h	Can cause rebound congestion if used > 3 days in a row.
Pancrelipase (Multiple brands)	GI Malabsorption, Visceral Pain/Pancreatic Enzyme	30,000 IU pancreatic lipase with each meal 2500 units of lipase/kg/meal (10,000 units lipase/kg/day)	$9.00 (2 caps QID)	Nausea, abdominal cramps, constipation, diarrhea, greasy stools	Unknown	Unknown	Fatty stool from pancreatic insufficiency; +/− H2 Blocker or PPI. Use non-enteric coated products for colicky pancreatic pain.

Drug	Indication/Class	Dose (MDD**)	Cost	Side Effects	Onset	Half-life	Comments
Pantoprazole (Protonix)	Gastritis/Proton Pump Inhibitors	40 mg po daily (80 mg/day)	**$4.00 (40 mg daily)**	Headache, dizziness, diarrhea, abdominal pain, nausea	2.5 h	1 h	PPI of choice is Prilosec OTC. Protonix is the most cost effective prescription form. Evaluate the need to continue. Can step down to H2. All PPIs have similar efficacy. Do not crush.
Paregoric (Camphorated Opium)	Diarrhea/Opioid	1–2 tsp daily-QID	$5.70 (1 tsp QID)	CNS depression, drowsiness, dizziness, hypotension, respiratory depression, constipation, pruritus	—	—	Hard to find. Tastes bad. Not recommended for patients with bacterial diarrhea.
Paroxetine (Paxil)	Depression, Anxiety/ Serotonin Reuptake Inhibitor	10–60 mg daily (60 mg/day)	$1.05 (20 mg daily)	Headache, dry mouth, constipation, sexual dysfunction, appetite changes	2–8 h	21 h	Severe withdrawal if abruptly discontinued. Onset of effect in 3–4 weeks. 10, 20, 30 mg tablets cost about the same. Serotonin Reuptake Inhibitor. Highest incidence of anticholinergic side effects. Shortest half-life, withdrawl symptoms can occur with missed doses.
Pentazocine (Talwin)	Nociceptive Pain/ Agonist/Antagonist Opioid	IM, SubQ: 30-60 mg q3-4h PO: 50mg q4-6h	$6.00 (50 mg tab q4h)	Nausea; circulatory, CNS, respiratory depression	IM, SQ onset 15–30 mins; IV onset 2–3 mins	2–3 h	Agonist—Antagonist opioid: Not appropriate in chronic pain.
Pentobarbital (Nembutal)	Delirium, Agitation/ Barbiturates	50–200 mg q4–8h (3 mg/kg/hr)	$54.00 (100 mg q6h)	CNS, respiratory depression, nausea	1 min IV Onset 10–15min IM Onset	15–50 h	Expensive: Useful for palliative sedation if parenteral access available.

*Drugs in Italics: Not generally recommended in hospice patients
**MDD = Maximun Daily Dose
***BOLD-not available as a generic

Drug Information Table

Generic (Example of Trade)*	Indication/Drug Class	Dosage Range (MDD**)	2007 Avg. Cost/Day for Therapy (Dose for Cost Comparison)***	Adverse Effects	Onset to Peak	T1/2	Comments
Phenazopyridine (Pyridium)	Urinary Pain/Urinary Analgesic	100–200 mg TID × 2–3 days	$0.90 (100 mg TID)	HA, dizziness, GI upset	—	—	Good for urinary pain control when no infection present. Take with food. Turns urine red-orange.
Phenobarbital (Luminal)	Seizures/Maintenance, Delirium, Agitation/ Barbiturate	30–600 mg daily-TID (400 mg/day)	$0.25 (60 mg TID)	Somnolence, CNS excitation or depression	PO: 1–6 h; IV: ~30 mins	Children: 37–73 h; adults: 53–140 h	Sedating. Can be dosed q12h. Can be given SC or PR. Also used for other symptoms: delirium & seizures. Barbiturate. Long half-life allows maintenance dose to be taken once daily (ideally at bedtime). Signs of toxicity are drowsiness, nystagmus, ataxia.
Phenytoin (Dilantin)	Seizures/Maintenance, Hiccups/Anticonvulsants	300 mg/day or 5–6 mg/kg/day. Adjust per levels (600 mg/day)	$0.60 (100 mg TID)	IV effects: hypotension, bradycardia; Gingival hypertrophy, hypertrichosis. Toxicity effects: nystagmus, blurred vision, ataxia, osteomalacia	PO: IR: 2–3 h; XR: 4–12 h	22h (range 7–42 h)	Do not use rectally-absorption erratic and incomplete. Monitor levels for optimal effect. Miantenance anticonvulsant of choice in hospice. Long half-life allows maintenance dose to be taken once daily (ideally at bedtime). Signs of toxicity are drowsiness, diplopia, ataxia.
Pilocarpine (Salagen, Pilocarpine 1%)	Xerostomia/Cholinergic	5–10 mg TID (30 mg/day)	$0.80 (5 mg (1.5mL) TID)	Hypertension, tachcardia, diarrhea, N&V, flushing, diaphoresis	20min–1 h	3–5 h	Only effective if patient has functioning salivary glands. Try sour hard candy as first line intervention. Tablets expensive. Unpleasant side effects. Avoid taking with dairy products. May take up to 2 months for maximal effect.

Drug	Indication/Class	Dosage	Cost	Side Effects	Onset	Duration	Notes
Polyethylene Glycol/ Electrolytes (Miralax)	Constipation/Osmotic Laxative	17 gm in water daily	$1.35 (17gms daily)	N&V, bloating, GI cramps	—	—	Dependent on adequate hydration. Not sufficient without stimulant if patient is on an opioid.
Potassium Chloride (KlorCon)	Hypokalemia/Potassium Suppliment	Dosage based on patient-specific factors (IV: 40 mEq/hour; 400 mEq/day)	$0.25 (20mEq daily)	N&V, diarrhea, GI pain, flatulence	3 h	Unknown	Can dissolve K-Dur in water for tasteless oral suspension.
Pramipexole (Mirapex)	Parkinson's/Dopamine Agonist	0.5–1.5 mg TID	**$5.90 (1 mg TID)**	Postural hypotension, dizziness, HA, insomnia or somnolence, hallucinations, dyskinesia, nausea, constipation	2 h	8 h (elderly 12–14)	
Prazosin (Minipress)	Cardiovascular/Alpha Blocker	1–5 mg po bid-TID (20 mg/day)	$0.60 (2 mg BID)	Dizziness, orthostatic hypotension, palpitations, HA, drowsiness	2–4 h	2–4 h (prolonged w/ CHF)	Monitor for hypotension.
Prednisone (Deltasone)	Anorexia, Bone Pain, Nerve Compression Pain, Respiratory Inflammation, Pruritus, Excessive Sedation. Visceral Pain/ Corticosteroid	10–20 mg daily-appetite; 20–40 mg daily-BID (80 mg/day)	$0.10 (10 mg daily)	GI upset, adrenal insufficiency, steroid psychosis, hyperglycemia	1–2 h	18–36 h	Drug of choice. Least expensive corticosteroid. Use with caution in diabetics. Also used for other symptoms-inflammation, pain, mood, breathing, brain metastases, N/V, anorexia; Indicated when short term therapy may be beneficial; Also used in the conditions of bone pain, asthenia or bronchospams; More cost effective than dexamethasone; Start with low dose (10 mg po daily) and monitor for efficacy weekly, can increase dose and reassess weekly. Long term effects must be considered but the initiation of therapy should not be delayed because of undue concerns about adverse effects of prolonged use. More mineralocorticoid activity than dexamethasone.

*Drugs in Italics: Not generally recommended in hospice patients
**MDD = Maximun Daily Dose
***BOLD-not available as a generic

Drug Information Table

Generic (Example of Trade)*	Indication/Drug Class	Dosage Range (MDD**)	2007 Avg. Cost/Day for Therapy (Dose for Cost Comparison)***	Adverse Effects	Onset to Peak	T1/2	Comments
Pregabalin (Lyrica)	Neuropathic Pain/ Anticonvulsant	50 mg –100 BID-TID (600 mg/day)	$4.30 (100 mg BID)	Peripheral edema, dizziness, somnolence, ataxia, weight gain, xerostomia, tremor, blurred vision, diplopia	1.5 h (3 h w/food)	6.3 h	Onset of action in 3–5 days.
Procainamide (Pronestyl/ Procan SR)	Cardiovascular/ Antiarrhythmic	500–1000 mg q6h PO: (5 grams/day)	$3.20 (500 mg q6h)	Hypotension, rash, diarrhea, N&V; (has Black Box warnings)	Capsule: 45 mins—2.5 h; IM: 15—60 mins	2.5—4.7 h (11 h anephric)	
Prochlorperazine (Compazine)	Nausea & Vomiting (Chemoreceptor Trigger Zone)/Phenothiazine Antiemetic	5–10 mg q4–8h; (5–25 mg q4–8h PR) (40 mg/day)	$1.75 (10 mg q6h; 25 mg q6h PR)	Drowsiness, dizziness, blurred vision, extrapyramidal symptoms, rash, dry mouth, jaundice	10–40 min	10–12 h	Less versatile than haloperidol. Multiple dosage forms necessary. May cause sedation and EPS.
Promethazine (Phenergan)	Nausea & Vomiting (Chemoreceptor Trigger Zone)/Antihistamine-Phenothiazine Derivative Antiemetic	12.5–50 mg q4–8h (200 mg/day)	$1.55 PO/ $18.33 supp (25 mg q6h)	Dizziness, drowsiness, dry mouth, N&V, hypertension or hypotension	4.4 h (syrup); 6.7—8.6 h (suppository)	9–16 h	Sedating. Suppositories expensive. Less effective than haloperidol, prochlorperzine or chlorpromazine. Very sedating. May cause EPS.
Propofol (Diprovan)	Delirium, Agitation/ Anesthetic	Various	$14.05/20mL vial	Hypotension (hypertension in children), apnea, injection site burning/pain, movement hypotonia	Onset is 9–51 secs; duration is 3–10 mins	Biphasic: Initial 40 mins; Terminal 4–7 h up to 1–3 days	Other alternatives such as chlorpromazine and phenobarbital usually sufficient.

Drug	Category	Dose	Cost	Side Effects	Onset	Half-life	Comments
Propoxyphene-APAP (Darvocet N)	Nociceptive Pain/Opioid/ Non-opioid Combination	1–2 tabs q6h (Max 6 tabs/day) (Acetaminophen = 4000 mg/ day, geriatrics 3000 mg/day; Propoxyphene = 600 mg/day)	$2.80 (1 tab q4h)	Hypotension, sedation, dizziness, incoordination, disorientation, N&V, constipation, urinary retention, dyspnea	—	Parent drug: 6–12 h; Active metabolite: 30–36 h	Analgesic effect poor. Monitor acetaminophen dose. Not recommended in the elderly. Schedule IV controlled substance. Weak, ineffective opioid. Cardiotoxic metabolites.
Propranolol (Inderal)	Cardiovascular/Beta Blocker	20–80 mg BID (640 mg/day)	$0.55 (40 mg BID)	Dizziness, lethargy, depression	60–90 mins	4–6 h	Avoid in patients with COPD. Also useful for tremors. Abrupt discontinuation can cause rebound hypertension.
Pseudoephedrine (Sudafed)	Respiratory/ Decongestants	30–60 mg q4–6h (240 mg/day)	$0.50 (30 mg Q6h)	Dizziness, nervousness, restlessness, insomnia, HA, difficulty urinating	30–60 mins	9–16 h	Can exacerbate hypertension, cause restlessness, agitation and insomnia.
Psyllium (Metamucil)	Diarrhea/Bulking agent	1–2 Rounded Tbsp daily-BID 1 dose up to 3 times daily	$0.30 (1 Tbsp BID)	Abdominal cramps, bloating	2–3 days	—	For use as a bulking agent, give with minimal amount of fluid. Separate drug administration times with other medicaiton due to decreased absorption.
Quetiapine (Seroquel)	Delirium/ Agitationanxiety/Atypical Antipsychotic	25–200 mg BID-TID (800 mg/day)	**$3.20 (25 mg BID)**	Dizziness, HA, somnolence, agitation, weight gain, xerostomia	1.5 h	Mean, terminal: ~ 6 h	Expensive. Antipsychotic of choice in Parkinson's Disease for delirium/agitation due to low incidence of extrapyramidal symptoms. Otherwise, no benefit over haloperidol or chlorpromazine. Can increase blood glucose levels. Especially useful if more sedating agent is desired. Most sedating of the atypical antipsychotics.
Quinipril (Accupril)	Cardiovascular/ACE Inhibitors	10–40 mg daily (80 mg/day)	$1.15 (20 mg daily)	Dizziness, HA, cough	2–4 h	Parent drug: 0.8 h; Active metabolite: 3 h	2nd line based on cost. Dry cough and angioedema side effects. No significant difference between ACE Inhibitors.

*Drugs in Italics: Not generally recommended in hospice patients
**MDD = Maximun Daily Dose
*****BOLD-not available as a generic**

Drug Information Table

Generic (Example of Trade)*	Indication/Drug Class	Dosage Range (MDD**)	2007 Avg. Cost/Day for Therapy (Dose for Cost Comparison)***	Adverse Effects	Onset to Peak	T1/2	Comments
Rabeprazole (Aciphex)	Gastritis/ Proton Pump Inhibitor	20–40 mg daily-BID	$4.70 (20 mg daily)	HA	2–5 h	0.85–2 h	Drug of choice is Prilosec OTC. Evaluate the need to continue. Can step down to H2. All PPIs have similar efficacy.
Ramelteon (Rozerem)	Insomnia/Non-Benzodiazepine Hypnotic	8 mg HS (8 mg/day)	$3.10 (8 mg QHS)	Dizziness, fatigue, diarrhea, nausea	0.5–1.5 h	Parent: 1–2.6 h; active metabolite: 2–5 h	Expensive.
Ramipril (Altace)	Cardiovascular/ACE Inhibitor	2.5–20 mg daily (20 mg/day)	$2.95 (10 mg daily)	Cough, hypotension, hyperkalemia	~ 1 h	Effective: 13–17 h; terminal: >50 h	Expensive. Dry cough and angioedema side effects. No significant difference between ACE Inhibitors.
Ranitidine (Zantac)	Gastritis/H2 Antagonists	75–300 mg daily-BID (600 mg/day)	$0.70 (150 mg BID)	Headache, diarrhea, constipation, muscle aches, vertigo	1–3 h	4–8 h	OTC products more cost effective than prescription forms. Geriatric/Renal dose is 75 mg BID or 150 mg daily.
Riluzole (Rilutek)	ALS/Glutamate Inhibitor	50 mg q12h	$27.20 (50 mg BID)	Nausea, weakness, decrease in lung function	—	12 h	Recommend discontinuing once patient is bed bound. May be beneficial in ambulatory patients to slow progression of disease.
Risperidone (Risperdal)	Anxiety, Delirium, Agitation/Atypical Antipsychotic	0.25–3 mg daily-BID (6 mg/day)	$7.00 (0.5 mg BID)	Extrapyramidal symptoms, somnolence, insomnia, agitation, anxiety, HA, dizziness, weight gain, constipation	1–17 h	Oral: mean = 20 h; IM = 3–6 days	Generally, no benefit over haloperidol or chlorpromazine. More expensive. Can increase blood glucose levels. Orally disintegrating tablets more expensive than coventional tablets.

Drug	Category	Dose (MDD**)	Cost	Side Effects	Onset	Half-life	Comments
Rivastigmine (Exelon)	Dementia/Cholinesterase Inhibitors	1.5–6 mg BID (12 mg/day)	**$5.95 (6 mg BID)**	Dizziness, HA, N&V, diarrhea, abdominal pain, anorexia	1 h	1.5 h	Generally not indicated for end-stage dementia. Can cause GI side effects.
Salmeterol (Serevent)	Bronchodilators/Long Acting Beta Agonists	1 puff q12h 1 INH twice daily	**$120/inhaler**	Headache, pain, hypertension, URI, pharyngitis	2 h	5.5 h	Assess patient's ability to use inhaler correctly.
Salmeterol/Fluticasone (Advair)	Respiratory/Combination Long Acting Beta Agonist/Corticosteroid	1–2 puffs q12h (1 INH BID diskus; 2 INH BID HFA)	**$13.50(2 puffs BID)**	Headache, URI, pharyngitis, oral candidiasis, GI upset	See individual agents	See individual agents	Assess patient's ability to use inhaler correctly. As patient declines, change to oral corticosteroid nebulized albuterol q4–6h: usually more effective in end stage disease.
Salsalate (Disalcid)	Bone Pain/Salicylate	1gm BID/TID (3 gms/day)	$0.30 (750 mg BID)	GI upset, rash, weakness, dyspnea	3–4 days	7–8 h	Generally not used PRN. Less GI upset than other NSAIDS. Can use with coumadin. Monitor for tinnitus.
Scopolamine Patch (Transderm-Scop)	Nausea & Vomiting (Vestibular), Secretion, Bowel Obstruction, Secretions, Visceral Pain/Anticholinergic	1–3 patches q 3 days (3 patches)	**$7.90/patch (1 patch q 3 days)**	Sedating and constipating. May cause confusion and visual distrubances.	2–7 h	10–25 h	2nd line to meclizine. Scopolamine can cause CNS side effects and contributes to constipation; Atropine SL drug of choice. Onset of action of patches can take up to 4 hours. Not easily titratable. Questionable need for 3 day dosing unit. Approximately 12 hours to peak effect. Patients sometimes need multiple patches (1–3) to be effective.
Senna (Senokot)	Constipation/Stimulant	1–2 tabs daily-QID; 2–4 tabs PO daily to BID (100 mg/day)	$0.45 (2 tabs BID)	Diarrhea, nausea, vomiting, abdominal cramps, alkalosis, electrolyte disorders	6–12 h	Unknown	Available in liquid. May be used with stool softener. Comes in combination product with docusate.
Senna (+Docusate)—(Senokot S)	Constipation/Combination Stool Softener/Stimulant	1–2 tabs po QHS—TID (8 tablets/day)	$0.45 (2 tabs BID)	GI upset, urine discoloration	—	—	Drug of choice for prophylaxis and treatment of opioid induced constipation.

*Drugs in Italics: Not generally recommended in hospice patients
**MDD = Maximun Daily Dose
***BOLD-not available as a generic

Drug Information Table

Generic (Example of Trade)*	Indication/Drug Class	Dosage Range (MDD**)	2007 Avg. Cost/Day for Therapy (Dose for Cost Comparison)***	Adverse Effects	Onset to Peak	T1/2	Comments
Sertraline (Zoloft)	Depression, Anxiety/Serotonin Reuptake Inhibitor	25–200 mg daily (200 mg/day)	$2.30 (100 mg daily)	Insomnia, nausea, erectile dysfunction, weight gain or loss, agitation	4 1/2–8 1/2 h	26–65 h	Optimal effect in 3–4 weeks; Serotonin Reuptake Inhibitor.
Silver Sulfadiazine (Silvadene)	Burns/Topical Antibiotic		$10.99/jar	Pain, burning, rash, skin necrosis, skin discoloration	3–11 days	10 h	
Simethicone (Mylicon)	Gas, Hiccups/Antiflatulent	40–125 mg QID (480 mg/day)	$0.25 (80 mg QID)	Diarrhea, nausea	3 h	Unknown	Drug of choice for gas. Gastric distension mediated hiccups.
Sodium Phosphate-Biphosphate Enema (Fleets Phospho soda)	Constipation/Osmotic Laxative	one enema prn	$1.05 (1 daily)	Abdominal cramps, electrolyte imbalance	0.25–1 h	—	Use as a supplement to oral bowel regimen.
Sorbitol 70% (Sorbitol)	Constipation/Osmotic Laxative	15–30mL daily-BID	$1.40 (30mL BID)	Edema, GI upset, hyperglycemia	0.25–1 h	—	Dependent on adequate hydration. Not sufficient without stimulant if patient is on an opioid.
Spironolactone (Aldactone)	Fluid Retention/K+ Sparing Diuretic	25–200 mg daily-BID	$0.50 (25 mg BID)	CNS disorders, gynecomastia, GI upset, hyperkalemia	1-3 h	1-1.5 h	Drug of choice for ascites. Optimum treatment for ascites requires a ratio of spironolactone to furosemide 100 mg:40 mg.
Sucralfate (Carafate)	Gastritis/GI Protectant	1gm po QID	$1.42 (1gm QID)	Constipation	1–2 h	—	Give 1 hour after or 2 hours before other medication.
Sulfamethoxazole/Trimethaprim (Bactrim DS)	Infection (Respiratory, UTI)/Sulfonamide Antibiotic	800/160 mg BID 10–14 days-respiratory; BID × 7–10 days-UTI	$5.80/course (1 tab BID × 10 days)	GI upset, rash	1 h	0.75–1.5 h	Encourage fluids.

Drug	Category/Class	Dose	Cost (MDD)	Side Effects	Tmax	Half-life	Notes
Sunitinib (Sutent)	Cancer/Tyrosine Kinase Inhibitor	50 mg daily for 4 weeks then off 2 weeks	**50 mg daily**	Hypertension, LVEF decreased, edema, fatigue, dermatologic disorders, endocrine disorders, GI upset, hematologic disorders, LFTs increased, creatinine increased, dyspnea	6–12 h	40–60 h	Not generally appropriate in hospice patients.
Tamoxifen (Nolvadex)	Breast Cancer/ Antineoplastic Estrogen Receptor Antagonist	10–20 mg daily	$1.30 (20 mg daily)	Flushing, hypertension, rash, nausea, weight loss, pain, edema, depression, vaginal bleeding, weakness, amenorrhea	5 h	5–7 days	Usually not appropriate in hospice patients. Must be palliating a symptom and have monitoring guidelines (PPS). Recommend discontinuing when out of current supply.
Tamsulosin (Flomax)	Urinary Hesitancy/Alpha 1 Blocker	0.4–0.8 mg daily (0.8 mg/day)	$2.50 (0.4 mg daily)	Hypotension, headache, dizziness, rhinitis, infection, sexual dysfunction, weakness	4–7 h	14–15 h	Only covered in patients with prostate cancer who are not catheterized.
Temazepam (Restoril)	Insomnia/ Benzodiazepine	7.5–30 mg po HS (60 mg/day)	$0.40 (30 mg QHS)	Fatigue, dizziness, depression, nausea, blurred vision	1–2 h	8–10 h	Less effective if patient also on benzodiazepines for anxiety.
Temozolomide (Temodar)	Cancer/Antineoplastic: Alkalating Agent	150 mg/m2 × 5 days every 28 days	**$1910.00/course (250 mg daily × 5 days)**	Fatigue, seizure, headache, edema, GI upset, hematoligic disorders	1 h	2 h	Usually not appropriate in hospice patients. Must be palliating a symptom and have monitoring guidelines (PPS). Recommend discontinuing when out of current supply.
Terazosin (Hytrin)	Cardiovascular/Alpha Blocker	1 mg daily (20 mg/day)	$0.45 (2 mg daily)	Dizziness, headache, muscle weakness, hypotension	1–2 h	9–12 h	Monitor for hypotension.
Thalidomide (Thalomid)	Cancer/Antineoplastic	100–300 mg/day (400 mg/day)	**$29.45 (50 mg daily)**	Drowsiness, dizziness, orthostatic hypotension, rash, fever	3–6 h	5–7 h	Usually not appropriate in hospice patients. Must be palliating a symptom and have monitoring guidelines (PPS). Recommend discontinuing when out of current supply.

*Drugs in Italics: Not generally recommended in hospice patients
**MDD = Maximun Daily Dose
*****BOLD-not available as a generic**

Drug Information Table

Generic (Example of Trade)*	Indication/Drug Class	Dosage Range (MDD**)	2007 Avg. Cost/Day for Therapy (Dose for Cost Comparison)***	Adverse Effects	Onset to Peak	T1/2	Comments
Theophylline (Theodur)	Respiratory/ Methylxanthine Bronchodilator	100–300 mg BID; 300–600 mg q24h (900 mg/day)	$0.70 (300 mg BID)	Nausea, headache, vomiting, insomnia, rash, nervousness	Liquid: 1 h; tablet ec: 5 h; tablet uncoated: 2 h	Highly variable	Do not initiate as new therapy. Consider discontinuing. Monitor for theophylline toxicity as patient declines. Do not crush sustained release forms.
Thymol/Menthol/ Glycerin/Calamine (Calmoseptine®)	Excorated Skin/Topical Protectant		$5.90 /Tube	Irritation	—	—	Good barrier for peri-area.
Tiotropium (Spiriva)	Bronchodilator/ Anticholinergic Long Acting	1 cap inhaled daily (1 cap INH/day)	**$4.50 (1 cap inhaled daily)**	Xerostomia, Upper respiratory infection	5 min–2 h	1.6 h	Only appropriate if once a day dosing is necessary and patient is able to use inhaler correctly. Not usually beneficial as patient declines.
Tizanidine (Zanaflex)	Muscle Spasm/Alpha2 Adrenergic Agent	2–4 mg TID (36 mg/day)	$2.70 (4 mg TID)	Hypotension, dry mouth, weakness, somnolence, dizziness	1–1.5 h	2 h	Antispastic class; prominent sedation a potential side effect or benefit.
Tolterodine (Detrol)	Urinary Frequency/ Anticholinergic	1–2 mg BID; 2–4 mg LA daily (4 mg/day)	**$4.00 (2 mg BID)**	Dry mouth, headache, fatigue, dizziness, GI upset, dysuria	IR: 1–2 h ER: 2–6 h	IR: 2 h ER: 7 h	
Topiramate (Topamax)	Siezures, Neuropathic Pain/Anticonvulsant	200–1600 mg daily (3600 mg/day)	**$7.50 (400 mg daily)**	CNS abnormalities, GI upset, weight loss, parasthesia, nystagmus, URI	2–3 h	5–7 h	Expensive. Not recommended.
Torsemide (Demedex)	Fluid Retention/Loop Diuretic	10–100 mg daily-BID (200 mg/day)	$1.50 (40 mg daily)	Headache, GI upset, ECG abnormality, dizziness, weakness	1–4 h	2–4 h	Use only if tolerance to the effects of furosemide occurs.

Drug	Class/Use	Dose (MDD**)	Cost	Side Effects	Onset	Duration	Comments
Tramadol (Ultram)	Pain/Non-opioid Analgesic	50–100 mg q4-6h (400 mg/day;elderly 300 mg/day;renal 200 mg/day)	$8.20 (100 mg q6h)	Dizziness, constipation, nausea/vomiting, dysphoria, seizures	IR: 2 h; ER: 12 h	6-8 h	Titrate slowly to full dose to minimize side effects. Lowers seizure threshold; use with caution in patient with sezure potential. No antiinflammatory activity. Major mechanism of action is inhibition of serotonin and norepineprhine reuptake. VERY weak opioid activity. Is not a controlled substance.
Trazodone (Desyrel)	Insomnia/Antidepressant	25-200 mg HS (600 mg/day)	$0.30 (50 mg QHS)	Drowsiness, nausea/vomiting, bitter taste, priapism, temor, hypotension	1–2 h	5–9 h	Drug of choice for patients also taking benzodiazepines for anxiety. Unlikely to have significant antidepressant effect at doses used for sleep. Daytime sedation common at higher doses. Orthostasis at higher doses.
Triamcinolone (Kenalog)	Pruritus, Rash/Topical Corticosteroid	Apply 2–4 times a day	$19.00/tube	GI upset, Cushing's-like syndrome, hypertension, appetite increased	8–10 h	18–36 h	
Triamcinolone (Azmacort)	Respiratory/Inhaled Corticosteroid	200-400mcg 3-4 times a day (1600 mcg/day)	**$131.00/inhaler (2 puffs TID)**	Burning, irritation, skin atrophy	—	—	Oral corticosteroids provide greater symptom relief in end stage disease.
Triamterene/Hydrochlorothiazide (Dyazide)	Fluid Retention/K+ Sparing Diuretic	1 tab/cap daily 50 mg HCTZ/75 mg triamterene	$0.30 (1 daily)	Hypotension, GI upset, rash, electrolyte disorder, muscle cramps	See individual drugs	See individual drugs	For mild hypertension or edema.
Trimethobenzamide (Tigan)	Nausea & Vomiting/(Chemoreceptor Trigger Zone)/Anticholinergic Antiemetic	300 mg TID-QID	$4.00 (300 mg PO QID)	Blurred vision, headache, drowsiness, jaundice, dizziness	45 min	7–9 h	Antihistamine. Less effective than haloperidol and phenothiazines in other patients.

*Drugs in Italics: Not generally recommended in hospice patients
**MDD = Maximun Daily Dose
***BOLD-not available as a generic

Drug Information Table

Generic (Example of Trade)*	Indication/Drug Class	Dosage Range (MDD**)	2007 Avg. Cost/Day for Therapy (Dose for Cost Comparison)***	Adverse Effects	Onset to Peak	T1/2	Comments
Urea (Carmol)	Dry Skin/Topical Emollient	Apply 1—3 times a day	$12.00/tube	Transient stinging, irritation	—	—	
Ursodiol (Actigall)	Pruritus, Jaundice/ Gallstone Dissolver	300 mg BID	$4.80 (300 mg BID)	Headache, dizziness, constipation, rash, GI upset, leukopenia	—	100 h	Expensive. Monitor efficacy.
Valproic Acid, Divalproex Sodium (Depakene, Depakote, Depakote Sprinkles)	Seizures, Hiccups, Behavior/Anticonvulsant	1000-2500 mg dialy in 1–3 divided doses, 15 mg/kg/day, increased by 250 mg every 2 weeks (60 mg/kg/day)	$10.40 (250 mg QID)	Somnolence, dizziness, insomnia, nervousness, alopecia, GI upset, thrombocytopenia, tremor	4 h	9–16 h	Regular release and delayed release formulations are usually given in 2-4 divided doses/day, extended release formulation (Depakote ER) is usually given once daily. Conversion to Depakote ER from a stable dose may require an increase in the total daily dose between 8% and 20% to maintain similar serum concentrations.
Valsartan (Diovan)	Cardiovascular/ Angiotensin Receptor Blocker	40-160 mg BID (320 mg/day)	$2.10 (80 mg daily)	Dizziness, BUN increased, hypotension, hyperkalemia	2–4 h	6 h	Second line after ACE Inhibitors. Expensive.
Vancomycin (Vancocin)	Diarrhea/Antibiotic	125 mg QID for 10 days	$300.00/course (125 mg QID)	Bitter taste, N/V, chills, drug fever, eosinophilia	—	5–11 h	PO only for C.diff diarrhea, IV ineffective. Very expensive-2nd line if metronidazole ineffective. Resistance occurs quickly to enterococcus.
Venlafaxine (Effexor, Effexor SR)	Depression/Serotonin/ Norepinephrine Reuptake Inhibitor	37.5–75 mg BID-TID; SR 75–225 mg daily (375 mg/day;SR 225 mg/day)	$3.50 (150 mg SR daily)	Hypertension, tachcardia, diarrhea, N&V, flushing, diaphoresis	2 h	3–7 h	Second line to Serotonin Reuptake Inhibitors. All non-SR dosages cost about the same. Do not crush SR forms. Mixed serotonin and norepinephrine reuptake inhibitor. Requires divided dosing. Some evidence that it reduces neuropathic pain at higher doses.

Drug	Class	Dose	Cost	Side Effects	Onset	Duration	Notes
Verapamil (Calan)	Cardiac/Calcium Channel Blocker	80–120 mg TID (360 mg/day)	$2.40 (80 mg TID)	gingival hyperplasia, constipation, hypotension, edema	PO: 1–2 h I.V. 1–5 min	2–12 h	Do not crush sustained release form. Constipating.
Vitamin A & D	Excoriated Skin, Burns/ Topical Emollient	Apply PRN	$9.00/tube	irritation	—	—	
Warfarin Sodium (Coumadin)	Cardiac/Anticoagulants	titrate dose to INR = 2–3	$0.80 (5 mg daily)	bleeding, bruising, rash, GI upset, edema, asthenia, malaise	5-7 days	20–60 h	Monitor PT/INR and discontinue if risk outweighs benefit.
Zafirlukast (Accolate)	Respiratory/Leukotriene Receptor Antagonist	10-20 mg BID (40 mg/day)	**$2.87 (20 mg BID)**	headache, GI upset, myalgia	3 h	10 h	Indicated for asthma. Evaluate efficacy and discontinue as patient declines.
Zaleplon (Sonata)	Insomnia/ Benzodiazepine/like Hypnotic	5–20 mg HS (20 mg/day)	**$3.45 (10 mg QHS)**	headache, dizziness, nausea, asthenia, somnolence, abdominal pain, tremor, eye pain	1 h	1 h	Expensive. Short duration of action. Not recommended.
Zinc Oxide (Desitin)	Excoriated Skin, Burns/ Topical Protectant		$4.42/tube	skin sensitivity, irritation	—	—	
Ziprasidone (Geodon)	Delirium, Agitation/ Atypical Antipsychotic	20–80 mg BID (160 mg/day)	**$10.50 (20 mg BID)**	EPS, somnolence, headache, dizziness, nausea, chest pain, weight gain	PO: 6-8 h I.M.: < 60 min	PO: 7 h I.M.: 2-5 h	Generally, no benefit over haloperidol or chlorpromazine. More expensive. Can increase blood glucose levels.
Zolpidem (Ambien)	Insomnia/ Benzodiazepine/Like Hypnotic	5–10 mg HS (10 mg/day;12.5 mg CR/day)	$4.05 (10 mg QHS)	headache, drowsiness, myalgias, nausea, dizziness	2 h	2 h	Expensive. Short duration of action. Not recommended. Little to no anxiolytic effect. No clear advantage over benzodiazepines.

www.Lexi.com Accessed 12-20-07

*Drugs in Italics: Not generally recommended in hospice patients
**MDD = Maximun Daily Dose
***BOLD-not available as a generic